VISUAL ARTHROSCOPY SERIES

Arthroscopic Techniques of the Knee

A VISUAL GUIDE

Visual Arthroscopy Series

Series Editors, James R. Andrews and Tal S. David

VISUAL ARTHROSCOPY SERIES

Arthroscopic Techniques of the Knee

A VISUAL GUIDE

THOMAS J. GILL, MD

MASSACHUSETTS GENERAL HOSPITAL

BOSTON, MASSACHUSETTS

SLACK
INCORPORATED

www.slackbooks.com

ISBN: 978-1-55642-858-6

Copyright © 2009 by SLACK Incorporated

Cover illustration © 2008 iStock International Inc. Sebastian Kaulitzki

All rights reserved. No part of this book may be reproduced, stored in a retrieval system or transmitted in any form or by any means, electronic, mechanical, photocopying, recording or otherwise, without written permission from the publisher, except for brief quotations embodied in critical articles and reviews.

The procedures and practices described in this book should be implemented in a manner consistent with the professional standards set for the circumstances that apply in each specific situation. Every effort has been made to confirm the accuracy of the information presented and to correctly relate generally accepted practices. The authors, editor, and publisher cannot accept responsibility for errors or exclusions or for the outcome of the material presented herein. There is no expressed or implied warranty of this book or information imparted by it. Care has been taken to ensure that drug selection and dosages are in accordance with currently accepted/recommended practice. Due to continuing research, changes in government policy and regulations, and various effects of drug reactions and interactions, it is recommended that the reader carefully review all materials and literature provided for each drug, especially those that are new or not frequently used. Any review or mention of specific companies or products is not intended as an endorsement by the author or publisher.

SLACK Incorporated uses a review process to evaluate submitted material. Prior to publication, educators or clinicians provide important feedback on the content that we publish. We welcome feedback on this work.

Published by: SLACK Incorporated
                6900 Grove Road
                Thorofare, NJ 08086 USA
                Telephone: 856-848-1000
                Fax: 856-853-5991
                www.slackbooks.com

Contact SLACK Incorporated for more information about other books in this field or about the availability of our books from distributors outside the United States.

Library of Congress Cataloging-in-Publication Data

Arthroscopic techniques of the knee : a visual guide / editor, Thomas J. Gill.
   p. ; cm. -- (Visual arthroscopy series)
 Includes bibliographical references and index.
 ISBN 978-1-55642-858-6 (alk. paper)
 1. Knee--Endoscopic surgery--Atlases. I. Gill, Thomas J., 1964- II. Series: Visual arthroscopy series.
  [DNLM: 1. Arthroscopy--methods--Atlases. 2. Knee Joint--surgery--Atlases. 3. Anterior Cruciate Ligament--surgery--Atlases. 4. Posterior Cruciate Ligament--surgery--Atlases. WE 17 A7875 2009]
 RD561.A76 2009
 617.5'82059--dc22
                                    2009002880

For permission to reprint material in another publication, contact SLACK Incorporated. Authorization to photocopy items for internal, personal, or academic use is granted by SLACK Incorporated provided that the appropriate fee is paid directly to Copyright Clearance Center. Prior to photocopying items, please contact the Copyright Clearance Center at 222 Rosewood Drive, Danvers, MA 01923 USA; phone: 978-750-8400; web site: www.copyright.com; email: info@copyright.com

Last digit is print number: 10 9 8 7 6 5 4 3 2 1

DEDICATION

Arthroscopic Techniques of the Knee: A Visual Guide is dedicated to the orthopedic surgical residents, sports medicine fellows, and practicing orthopedic surgeons who have taught me so much throughout my own career, and to those who continually pursue education and better clinical outcomes in the field of minimally invasive knee surgery.

Many of us have been influenced by technically gifted and compassionate surgical educators. I have had the distinct honor to have pursued my fellowship training in reconstructive surgery under several such teachers. Today, there is scarcely a "simple" knee arthroscopy or complex arthroscopic-assisted surgical reconstruction of a dislocated knee where I do not think back to the principles of 2 of my own teachers—Dr. Richard Steadman (who has graciously contributed to this text) and Professor Reinhold Ganz. My approach to knee surgery today incorporates many of the tenets taught to me during my training with them. Dr. Steadman was a model for how to interact with patients in the office. His compassionate and sincere approach to everyone whom he treated was a paradigm. He constantly tried to develop minimally invasive techniques such as microfracture to preserve knee joints, avoid the need for total joint arthroplasty, and keep people of all ages physically active for as long as possible. From Professor Ganz, I learned something that is a lifelong gift, both for my sports medicine practice and for life in general. Rather than simply trying to teach me the technical details of *how* he performed specific procedures, he stressed how to actually *think* about problems when confronted by new challenges. He taught me to always question why I believed what I believed to be true. Professor Ganz stressed the need to go back always to the original scientific data on a subject and to study it for myself rather than relying on the interpretations of others. He stressed the need to challenge the status quo, not accept "conventional wisdom" as gospel, and seek new and better treatments for our patients.

This book is also dedicated to my wife, Kathleen, and children, Ty, Olivia, and Rebecca. Their smiles and support have continuously taught me new ways to laugh, live, and learn.

Contents

Dedication .... *v*
Acknowledgments .... *ix*
About the Editor .... *xi*
Contributing Authors .... *xiii*

Chapter 1   Positioning and Set-Up 1
Matthew H. Griffith, MD and Peter D. Asnis, MD

Chapter 2   Anesthesia for Knee Surgery 15
Lisa Wollman, MD

Chapter 3   Diagnostic Arthroscopy of the Knee—The 10-Point Exam 27
Matthew J. Matava, MD and Evan D. Ellis, MD

Chapter 4   Techniques of Meniscal Repair 45
Asheesh Bedi, MD and Russell F. Warren, MD

Chapter 5   Microfracture 63
Luke S. Oh, MD and Thomas J. Gill, MD

Chapter 6   Osteochondral Transplantation 73
Michael J. DeFranco, MD; Allison G. McNickle, MS; and Brian J. Cole, MD, MBA

Chapter 7   Autologous Chondrocyte Implantation 83
Andreas H. Gomoll, MD and Tom Minas, MD, MS

Chapter 8   Pediatric Osteochondral Injuries 93
Dennis E. Kramer, MD and Mininder S. Kocher, MD, MPH

Chapter 9   Single-Bundle ACL Reconstruction Using Patellar Tendon Grafts:
Transtibial Endoscopic Hybrid Technique 105
Jerome J. Da Silva, MD; Champ L. Baker III, MD; and Bernard R. Bach Jr, MD

Chapter 10   Anatomic Double-Bundle ACL Reconstruction 123
Susan S. Jordan, MD; Wei Shen, MD, PhD; and Freddie H. Fu, MD, DSc

Chapter 11   ACL—Arthroscopically Assisted Internal Fixation of Tibial Spine Avulsion
Fractures 135
Bojan Zoric, MD and William Sterett, MD

Chapter 12   Single-Bundle Posterior Cruciate Ligament Reconstruction:
Arthroscopic Transtibial Technique 147
Luke S. Oh, MD and Thomas J. Gill, MD

Chapter 13	Posterior Cruciate Ligament Reconstruction: Single-Bundle Tibial Inlay Technique 171
	Lutul D. Farrow, MD and John A. Bergfeld, MD
Chapter 14	Transtibial Double-Bundle PCL Reconstruction... 189
	Mathew W. Pombo, MD; Brian Forsythe, MD; Randy Mascarenhas, MD; and Christopher D. Harner, MD
Chapter 15	Arthroscopic Treatment of Arthrofibrosis of the Knee 209
	J. Richard Steadman, MD

Index 221

Acknowledgments

The contributing authors in this book have served as educators and mentors to many of us. This textbook is meant to serve as an "ongoing mentorship" in which nationally reknowned leaders in the field of arthroscopic knee surgery present their own advice on how to optimally treat difficult knee problems in a minimally invasive fashion while avoiding complications and technical errors. Specifically, they were asked to present and illustrate their current, detailed step-by-step technique for a given topic in arthroscopic knee surgery as if they were teaching their own fellows in the operating room. They were asked to draw on their years of experience to offer special "pearls and pitfalls" as if the reader were alongside them in the operating room. By doing so, it is hoped that we can all provide better arthroscopic surgical outcomes for all of our patients.

About the Editor

Thomas J. Gill, MD received his medical degree from Harvard Medical School after graduating Phi Beta Kappa and Magna Cum Laude in Biology from Harvard College, He interned in general surgery at the Massachusetts General Hospital and completed his orthopedic surgery training in the Harvard Combined Orthopaedic Residency Program. Upon finishing his training, Dr. Gill was awarded the Maurice E. Muller Scholarship to study reconstructive surgery in Bern, Switzerland and in other European academic centers. He then completed his fellowship training in sports medicine and shoulder surgery at the Steadman Hawkins Clinic in Vail, Colorado.

Dr. Gill is Chief of the Sports Medicine Service at the Massachusetts General Hospital and an Associate Professor of Orthopaedic Surgery at Harvard Medical School. He has a strong commitment to education as course director or faculty member with many CME courses and as the Director of the Harvard/MGH Sports Medicine Fellowship Program. The research program that he established is extensive, and it spans the range of clinical and basic research and has a multi-institutional base.

Dr. Gill is a national leader in the field of sports medicine. He serves as medical director for the Boston Red Sox, head team physician for the New England Patriots, and team physician for the Boston Bruins. He is a fellow of the American Association of Orthopedic Surgeons and a member of the American Orthopedic Society for Sports Medicine; the American Orthopedic Association; and the Team Physician Societies of Major League Baseball, the National Football League, and the National Hockey League. He has been elected to the Herodicus Society.

Dr. Gill's primary clinical and research interests focus on knee and shoulder injuries. He has a particular interest in the biomechanics of the knee and shoulder and in tissue engineering techniques for joint preservation and cartilage repair in the knee. His studies have appeared in many articles and chapters on basic science and clinical issues involving the knee and in his book *Complications of Shoulder Surgery*.

Contributing Authors

Peter D. Asnis, MD (Chapter 1)
Department of Sports Medicine
Massachusetts General Hospital
Harvard University Medical School
Boston, MA

Bernard R. Bach Jr, MD (Chapter 9)
Division of Sports Medicine
Department of Orthopaedic Surgery
RUSH University Medical Center
Chicago, IL

Champ L. Baker III, MD (Chapter 9)
Division of Sports Medicine
Department of Orthopaedic Surgery
RUSH University Medical Center
Chicago, IL

Asheesh Bedi, MD (Chapter 4)
Hospital for Special Surgery
New York, NY

John A. Bergfeld, MD (Chapter 13)
Cleveland Clinic
Cleveland, OH

Brian J. Cole, MD, MBA (Chapter 6)
Department of Orthopaedic Surgery
RUSH University Medical Center
Chicago, IL

Jerome J. Da Silva, MD (Chapter 9)
Division of Sports Medicine
Department of Orthopaedic Surgery
RUSH University Medical Center
Chicago, IL

Michael J. DeFranco, MD (Chapter 6)
Department of Orthopaedic Surgery
RUSH University Medical Center
Chicago, IL

Evan D. Ellis, MD (Chapter 3)
Department of Orthopedic Surgery
Washington University School of Medicine
St. Louis, MO

Lutul D. Farrow, MD (Chapter 13)
University of Arizona College of Medicine
Department of Orthopaedic Surgery
Arizona Institute for Sports Medicine
Tucson, AZ

Brian Forsythe, MD (Chapter 14)
OAK Orthopaedics
Frankfort, IL

Freddie H. Fu, MD, DSc (Chapter 10)
Department of Orthopaedics
University of Pittsburgh Medical Center
Pittsburgh, PA

Andreas H. Gomoll, MD (Chapter 7)
Department of Orthopaedic Surgery
Harvard Medical School
Brigham and Women's Hospital
Boston, MA

Matthew H. Griffith, MD (Chapter 1)
Department of Sports Medicine
Massachusetts General Hospital
Harvard University Medical School
Boston, MA

Christopher D. Harner, MD (Chapter 14)
Blue Cross of Western Pennsylvania
University of Pittsburgh School of Medicine
UPMC Center for Sports Medicine
Pittsburgh, PA

Susan S. Jordan, MD (Chapter 10)
Department of Orthopaedics
University of Pittsburgh Medical Center
Pittsburgh, PA

Mininder S. Kocher, MD, MPH (Chapter 8)
Division of Sports Medicine
Department of Orthopaedic Surgery
Childrens Hospital Boston
Harvard Medical School
Boston, MA

Contributing Authors

Dennis E. Kramer, MD (Chapter 8)
Division of Sports Medicine
Department of Orthopaedic Surgery
Childrens Hospital Boston
Harvard Medical School
Boston, MA

Randy Mascarenhas, MD (Chapter 14)
Department of Orthopaedic Surgery
University of Pittsburgh School of Medicine
Pittsburgh, PA

Matthew J. Matava, MD (Chapter 3)
Department of Orthopedic Surgery
Washington University School of Medicine
St. Louis, MO

Allison G. McNickle, MS (Chapter 6)
Department of Orthopaedic Surgery
RUSH University Medical Center
Chicago, IL

Tom Minas, MD, MS (Chapter 7)
Department of Orthopedic Surgery
Harvard Medical School
Brigham and Women's Hospital
Boston, MA

Luke S. Oh, MD (Chapters 5 and 12)
Massachusetts General Hospital
Boston, MA

Mathew W. Pombo, MD (Chapter 14)
The Sports Medicine & Orthopaedic Institute of Gwinnett
Duluth, GA

Wei Shen, MD, PhD (Chapter 10)
Department of Orthopaedics
University of Pittsburgh Medical School
Pittsburgh, PA

J. Richard Steadman, MD (Chapter 15)
Steadman Hawkins Clinic
Steadman Hawkins Research Foundation
Vail, CO

William Sterett, MD (Chapter 11)
Steadman Hawkins Clinic
Vail, CO

Russell F. Warren, MD (Chapter 4)
Hospital for Special Surgery
New York, NY

Lisa Wollman, MD (Chapter 2)
Harvard Medical School
Massachusetts General Hospital
Boston, MA

Bojan Zoric, MD (Chapter 11)
Stetson Powell Orthopaedics & Sports Medicine
Burbank, CA

Positioning and Set-Up

Matthew H. Griffith, MD and Peter D. Asnis, MD

Preoperative planning and preparation are essential to successful arthroscopic surgery of the knee. The surgeon must have a thorough understanding of the arthroscopic equipment commonly used and must know what additional instruments are available if needed. Care must be taken to accurately identify the pathology to be treated and to develop a well thought-out treatment plan. It is also important to consider potential problems that could arise during surgery and to be prepared to deal with them. Lack of preparation can leave the surgeon waiting on required instruments. This wastes time and money as well as increases the patient's anesthesia time.

PATIENT POSITIONING

The patient is placed supine on the operating table. If additional open procedures are planned on the lateral aspect of the knee, a bump is placed under the ipsilateral buttock to improve visualization. For most arthroscopic procedures, the patient should be placed low enough on the table so that the popliteal fossa is at or below the break in the table (Figure 1-1). This allows flexion of the knee to 90 degrees if the surgeon wishes to drop the foot of the table. A pad or folded blanket placed under the distal thighs will prevent hip hyperextension and will facilitate flexion of the knee to 90 degrees, which is desired during arthroscopic ligament reconstructions. This padding may have the additional benefit of preventing soft tissue injury or venous compression on the break of the table in procedures where prolonged knee flexion is used.

A tourniquet may be applied high on the thigh over a layer of cotton padding. The use of a tourniquet is surgeon-specific, but it may prove valuable in improving visualization during cruciate ligament reconstruction or in cases where bleeding is encountered. A thorough understanding of proper tourniquet use and potential complications (including neurovascular injury) is critical to ensure patient safety. Ideally, tourniquet time should be kept under 2 hours. Tourniquet pressure seldom needs to be placed above 280 mm, except in cases of very large diameter thighs.

After the patient is positioned satisfactorily, an examination under anesthesia is performed and recorded. This includes range of motion and a thorough ligament examination. The contralateral knee is used for comparison.

A lateral post or a leg holder may be used to stabilize the leg. The lateral post allows valgus stress to be placed across the joint to open the medial compartment for visualization and safe instrumentation (Figure 1-2). The post should be positioned so that when the lower extremity is abducted, it should contact the mid-thigh and allow valgus stress to be applied. The benefits

Figure 1-1. The patient is positioned supine on the operating table with the popliteal fossa at the break of the table.

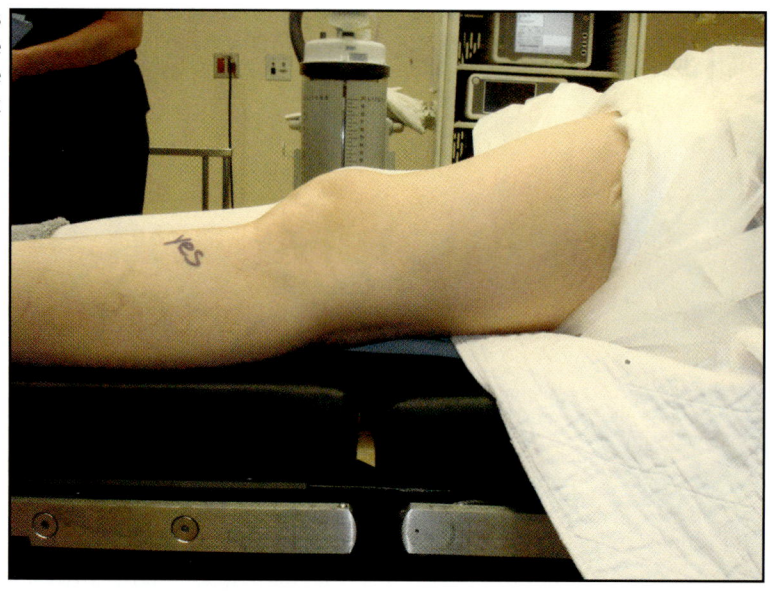

Figure 1-2. The lateral post is placed at the level of the mid-thigh.

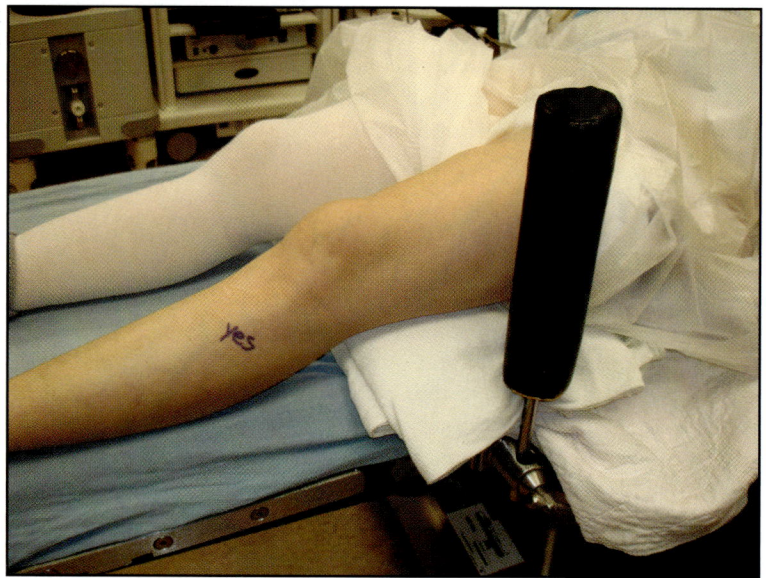

of a lateral post are that it leaves the leg free during the procedure and it can be used with most patients without difficulty. However, an assistant may be required to apply sufficient valgus force with the knee extended to visualize the posterior aspect of the medial meniscus in tight knees. Risks involved with using a lateral post include direct soft tissue injury, rupture of the medial collateral ligament (MCL), or fracture if excessive force is applied.

A leg holder may be applied high on the thigh at the level of the tourniquet. The leg holder is a clamp that encircles the thigh, stabilizing it to the table. When using a leg holder, it is important to position the patient with the knee distal to the break in the table so that 90 degrees of knee flexion is possible. The leg holder may be advantageous because it securely stabilizes the thigh and allows higher valgus and varus forces to be applied without requiring an assistant. Disadvantages include that the limb is not free for full motion during the surgery and the leg holder may be impossible

Positioning and Set-Up **3**

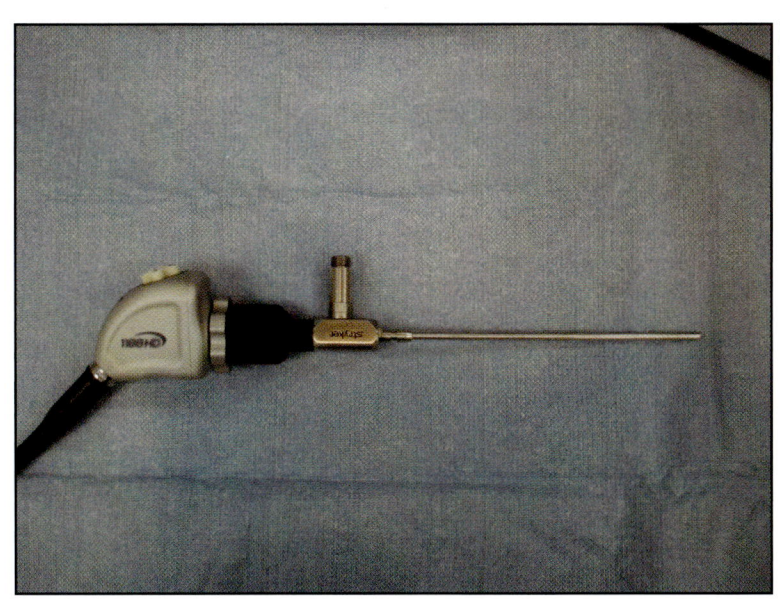

Figure 1-3. An arthroscope with camera attachment.

to use in obese patients. Risks of using a leg holder are similar to those noted previously for the lateral post.

After setup is complete, the leg is prepped to the level of the tourniquet, and drapes are applied using sterile technique. Antibiotics are given intravenously, and a correct surgical site "time-out" is performed with the operating room staff before beginning the procedure.

ARTHROSCOPES

Arthroscopy cannot be performed without adequate visualization (Figure 1-3). To introduce the arthroscope into the joint, the cannula is first introduced through the skin incision over a blunt obturator. Most scope cannulas have attachments for inflow and suction to aid in fluid management (Figure 1-4). The obturator is removed from the cannula, and the arthroscope is inserted and locked into place.

Arthroscopes with various viewing angles are available. The most common scope used in knee arthroscopy is a 30-degree prism, and this viewing angle is adequate for most arthroscopic procedures. A 70-degree scope is useful in posterior cruciate ligament (PCL) reconstruction. It also may be helpful when addressing a displaced meniscal tear or a loose body in the posterior aspect of the joint. Cameras should allow recording of arthroscopic pictures and videos. The fiber-optic light source attaches to the camera to illuminate the joint for visualization. The light source and video unit are usually positioned on an arthroscopic tower (Figure 1-5). The equipment tower should be located on the contralateral side of the table to allow easy viewing of the monitor and convenient organization of cables and tubing (Figure 1-6).

SHAVERS AND BURRS

An arthroscopic shaver has many uses in knee arthroscopy, including débridement of meniscal or chondral injuries and resecting loose bodies, fat pads, synovium, or remnants of torn ligaments. The shaver tip is cylindrical and has a hole to expose the cutting blades. There are a variety

Figure 1-4. Cannula for the arthroscope with obturator in place.

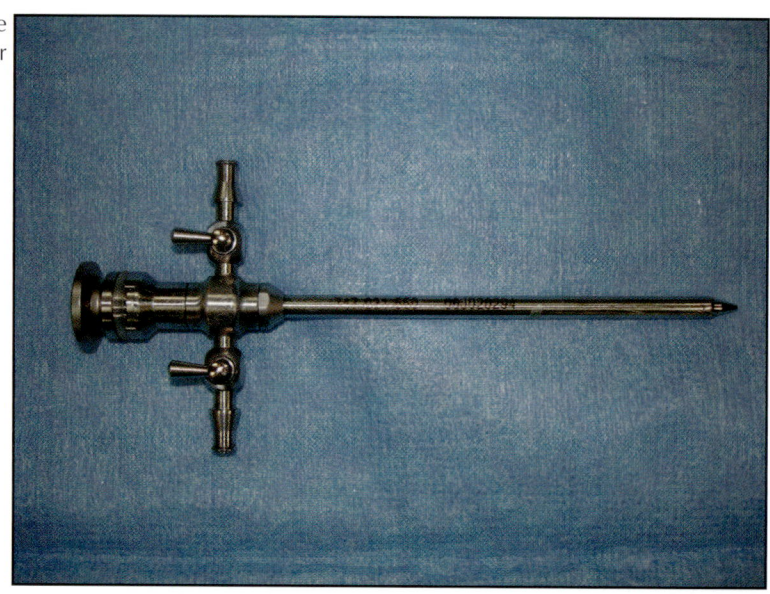

Figure 1-5. An arthroscopic tower allows equipment to be organized.

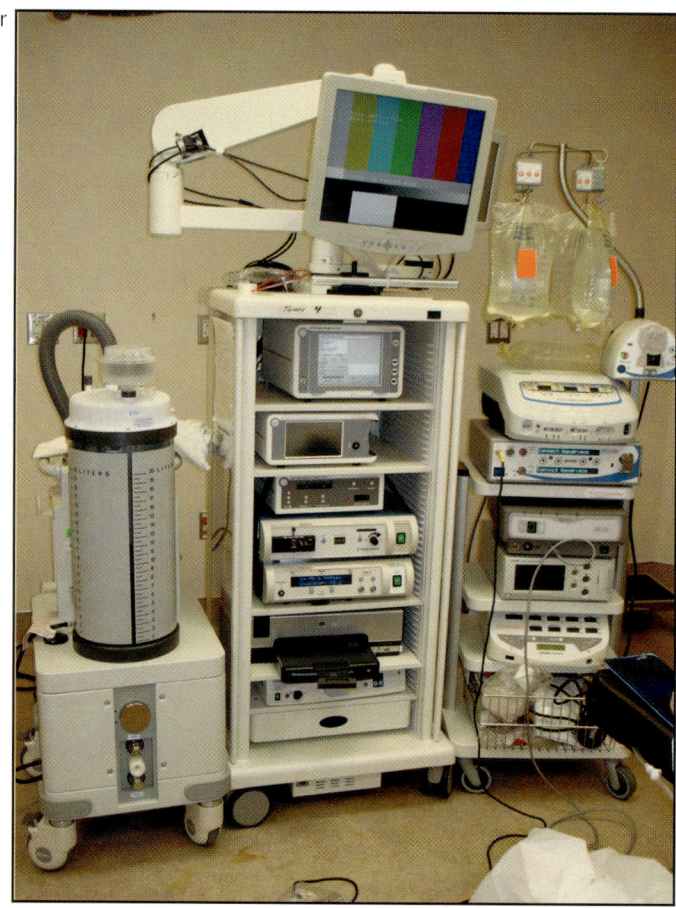

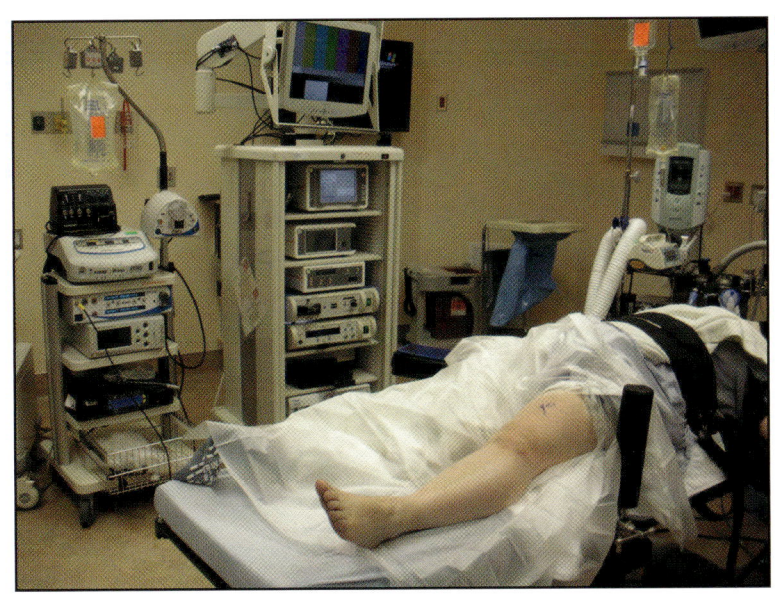

Figure 1-6. Standard operating room set-up with the arthroscopic tower opposite the operative side.

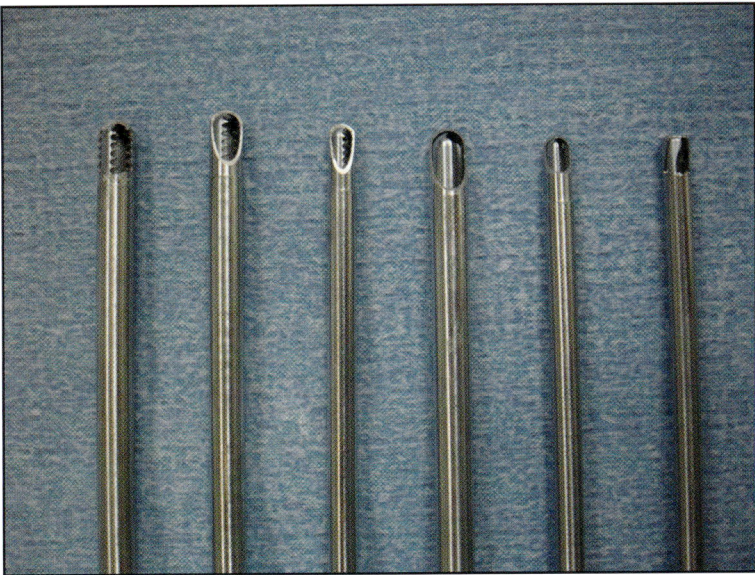

Figure 1-7. Arthroscopic shavers.

of hole configurations (full-radius, slotted, end-cutting) and blade types (smooth, serrated). It is important to understand the different types of shavers so that the proper instrument is selected. This will allow efficient and safe treatment of the pathology. A slotted shaver with a smooth blade is less aggressive and would be more appropriate for performing a chondroplasty. A full-radius shaver with a serrated blade is more aggressive and would be useful in resection of a torn anterior cruciate ligament (ACL) stump or torn meniscus. Shavers are also available in a variety of diameters (Figure 1-7). Larger shavers allow more aggressive tissue resection. A suction attachment allows loose tissue to be pulled into the blades of the shaver, facilitating resection and minimizing the risk of leaving loose fragments within the joint.

Arthroscopic burrs are available in various shapes and sizes (Figure 1-8). A burr allows a very aggressive resection and is usually reserved for bony work. Burr usage may produce significant

Figure 1-8. Arthroscopic burrs.

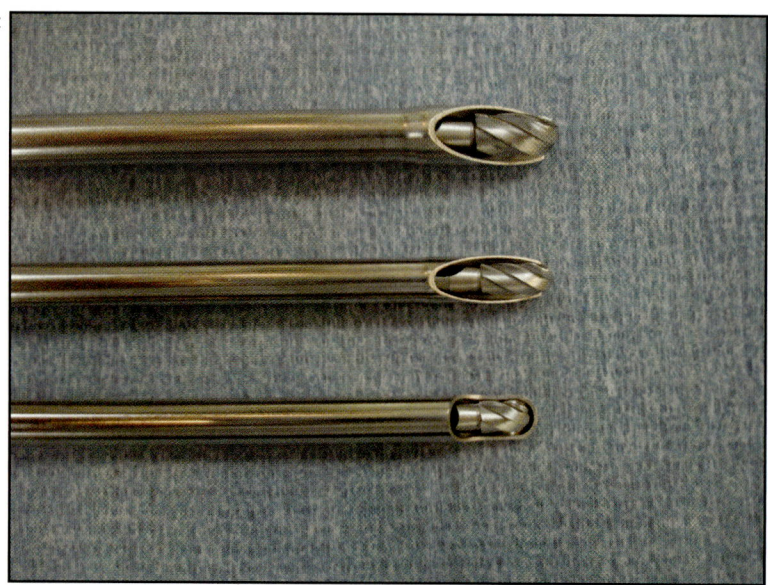

debris within the joint, and it is important to maintain suction through the burr tip and have adequate fluid flow from the arthroscopic pump inflow. Larger diameter shavers and burrs have the potential to rapidly suction fluid from the joint during usage. Without adequate pump inflow, the arthroscopic fluid can be quickly evacuated from the joint, obscuring visualization and decreasing the effectiveness of the instrument. It is important to have a pump that can provide enough flow to keep up with the shaver or burr that is being used.

ELECTROCAUTERY

Arthroscopic cautery devices are either monopolar or bipolar.[1-3] Monopolar radiofrequency devices produce tissue heating by alternating current that passes from the probe tip through the tissue to the grounding pad on the patient. The path that the energy takes (through capsule, cartilage, fluid, etc) is dependent in part on the characteristics of the tissue. In bipolar radiofrequency devices, both the energy source and ground are on the probe tip. Therefore, the energy passes through the fluid or tissue located between the poles of the probe following the path of least resistance. Bipolar electrocautery devices are more frequently used in knee arthroscopy (Figure 1-9).

There are several electrocautery systems available. Electrocautery can be very useful in controlling bleeding and débriding soft tissue. Some authors advocate contouring of cartilage irregularities using a radiofrequency probe.[4] However, several studies have demonstrated the possibility of significant surrounding chondrocyte death using this technique,[1,5,6] and we do not use it for this indication. In addition, fluid temperatures within the joint may reach levels potentially damaging to cartilage.[2,7] Studies have shown the benefit of maintaining fluid flow within the joint during electrocautery usage to prevent chondral injury.[2,7]

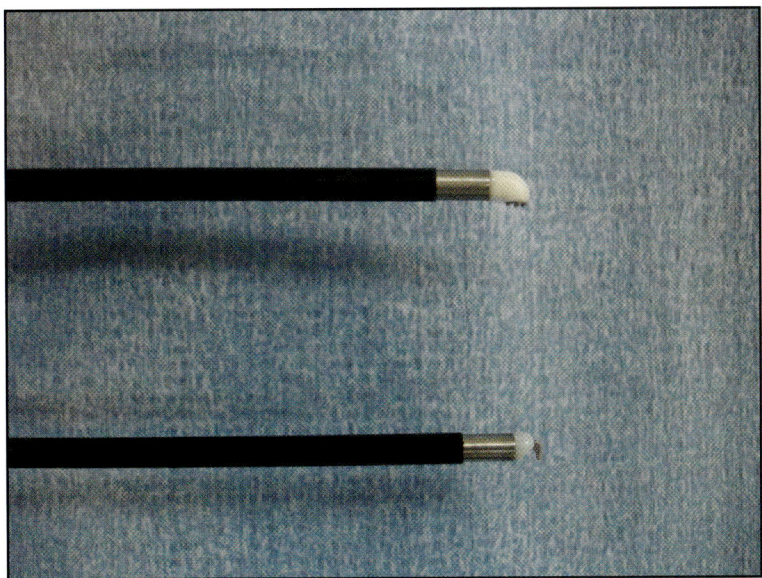

Figure 1-9. Electrocautery devices.

FLUID MANAGEMENT

Distention of the joint with saline allows improved visualization during arthroscopy. Some surgeons use gravity inflow, which has the benefit of minimizing risks related to a pressurized pump but provides less joint distension and is less effective in controlling bleeding. There are many arthroscopic fluid infusion systems available, and these vary in design and features. Fluid pumps have the benefit of more reliable fluid delivery, improved visualization, and minimized bleeding within the joint. Fluid is usually driven by either a diaphragm or roller pump and is regulated by either a pressure setting or a combination of pressure and flow settings. Fluid pumps that have separate control of pressure and flow have been shown to provide improved visualization during arthroscopic procedures.[8] Separate control of flow, especially when outflow and suction are also regulated, provides consistent fluid flow and joint distension. It is also beneficial for the pump to have a feature that provides on-demand short duration bursts of increased flow when bleeding is encountered.

For most arthroscopic procedures, inflow can be connected to the sheath of the arthroscope. The primary determinant of the maximum flow rate that can be achieved is the diameter of the inflow cannula. Therefore, if higher flow is required, a separate inflow portal may be beneficial. Caution must be taken when using a fluid infusion system because most pumps allow pressure settings that are well above values that are considered safe during knee arthroscopy. However, one study found a poor correlation between the pressure setting on the fluid pump and the actual intra-articular pressures during pump usage.[9]

Intra-articular pressures greater than 120 mm Hg have been shown to increase the risk of capsular rupture and fluid extravasation.[9,10] There have been several reports of complications related to the use of an arthroscopic fluid pump, including compartment syndrome, nerve injury, and capsular rupture.[11-15] In general, we use a pressure setting of 60 mm Hg during knee arthroscopy.

Figure 1-10. Anatomic landmarks are drawn out with a surgical marker. Portals are marked out. A = inferolateral, B = inferomedial, C = superolateral, D = superomedial.

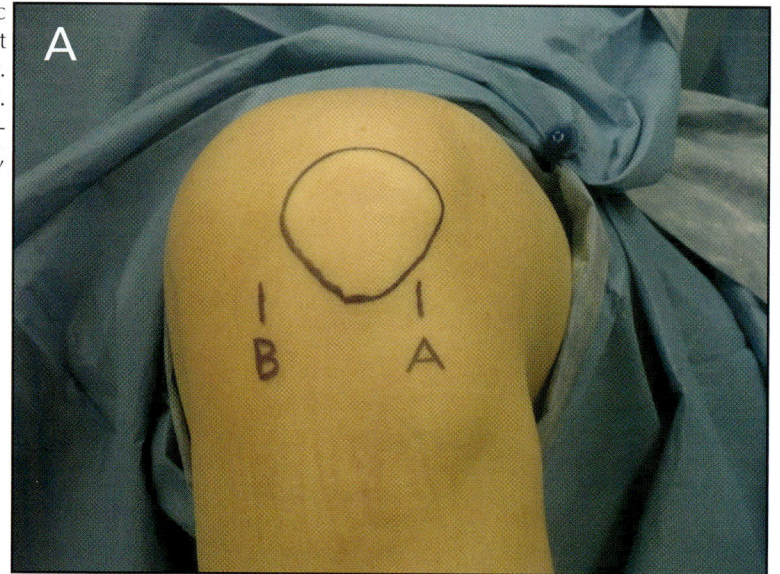

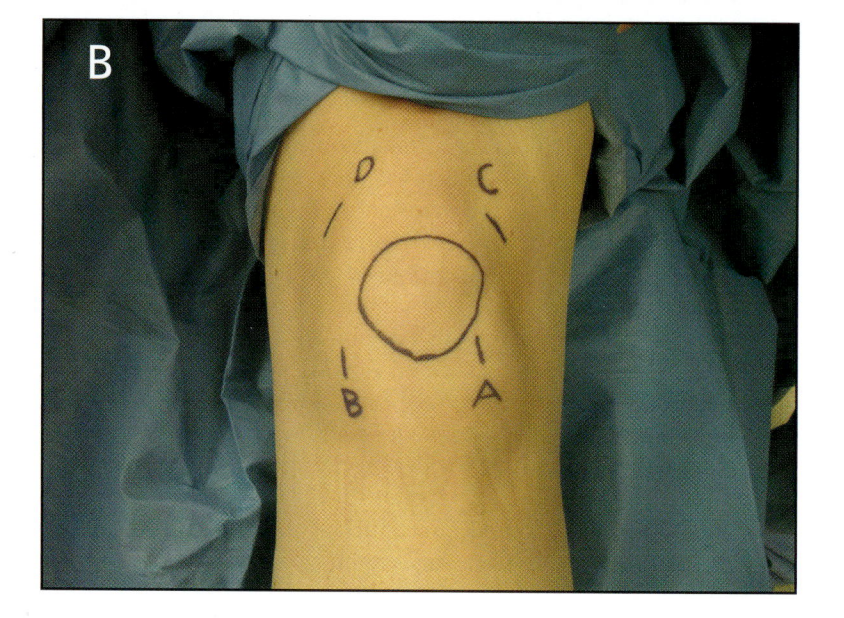

PORTALS

LANDMARKS

Palpating bony and soft tissue landmarks is helpful in determining the proper location to place portals. Important landmarks include the patella, patellar tendon, medial and lateral femoral condyles, and the proximal tibial joint line. It may be helpful to draw out the landmarks with a surgical marker before beginning the operation (Figure 1-10).

INFEROLATERAL

The inferolateral portal is the standard viewing portal in knee arthroscopy. It is the first portal established during arthroscopy, and it allows visualization of the entire joint (with the exception of the posterolateral joint and anterior horn of the lateral meniscus). This portal is located lateral to the patellar tendon in the soft spot between the patella, lateral femoral condyle, and proximal-lateral tibia. It may be helpful to flex the knee to 90 degrees to better define the landmarks. The portal should be several millimeters below the level of the inferior pole of the patella. If the portal is too low, it may contact the tibial eminence and prevent proper visualization of the medial joint, or it may damage the meniscus upon instrument insertion. It may also make it difficult to introduce the cannula into the patellofemoral joint.

The portal is established using a #11 scalpel. A skin incision measuring about 5 mm is made, and the blade is passed through the capsule. Depending on surgeon preference, the skin incision can be made vertical, horizontal, or oblique with Langer's lines. We prefer vertical incisions because they pull the portal edges together with knee flexion. It is advised to make the capsulotomy with the blade directed cephalad to avoid injury to the anterior horn of the lateral meniscus. The scope cannula with obturator is then inserted through the portal, aiming toward the intercondylar notch to avoid cartilage injury. With the knee in extension, the cannula is then advanced under the patella and into the suprapatellar pouch. The inflow system is attached to the cannula, and the joint is distended with fluid. The camera is then inserted and arthroscopy begun.

INFEROMEDIAL

The inferomedial portal is the most common portal used for instrumentation during knee arthroscopy. It is located in the soft spot medial to the patellar tendon between the medial femoral condyle, patella, and proximal-medial tibia. A spinal needle may be used to determine the desired portal location while visualizing the anteromedial joint from the inferolateral portal. It is important not to make this portal too low or instruments may contact the anterior tibia, preventing access to the posterior aspect of the joint.

SUPEROMEDIAL AND SUPEROLATERAL

The superomedial portal is located 4 cm proximal to the medial pole of the patella.[16] The superolateral portal is in a similar location above the superolateral patella between the quadriceps tendon and iliotibial band. These portals are most commonly used if an additional inflow is desired. The superolateral portal is usually preferred because less muscle must be penetrated during portal placement, and this may result in less postoperative pain. However, superomedial portals are less likely to be complicated by fistula formation due to the thick muscle layer under the skin incision. One or both of these portals may also be useful when performing more extensive procedures within the patellofemoral joint, such as removal of loose bodies, synovectomy, and lateral release.

These portals are established by making a 5-mm skin incision in Langer's lines. A cannula is inserted using a blunt obturator, aiming deep to the quadriceps tendon and patella to enter the suprapatellar pouch.

POSTEROMEDIAL

The posteromedial portal is useful in PCL reconstruction and débridement or repair of tears of the posterior aspect of the medial meniscus.[8,17-19] This portal is established with the knee in 90 degrees of flexion. This aids in palpation of landmarks and moves the sartorial branch of the saphenous nerve more posteriorly. The portal is located about 2 cm posterior to the medial femoral epicondyle and about 1 to 2 cm above the joint line. This places it behind the MCL and

Figure 1-11. Posteromedial portal location 2 cm posterior to the medial femoral epicondyle and about 1 to 2 cm above the joint line. This places it posterior to the MCL and proximal to the semimembranosus insertion.

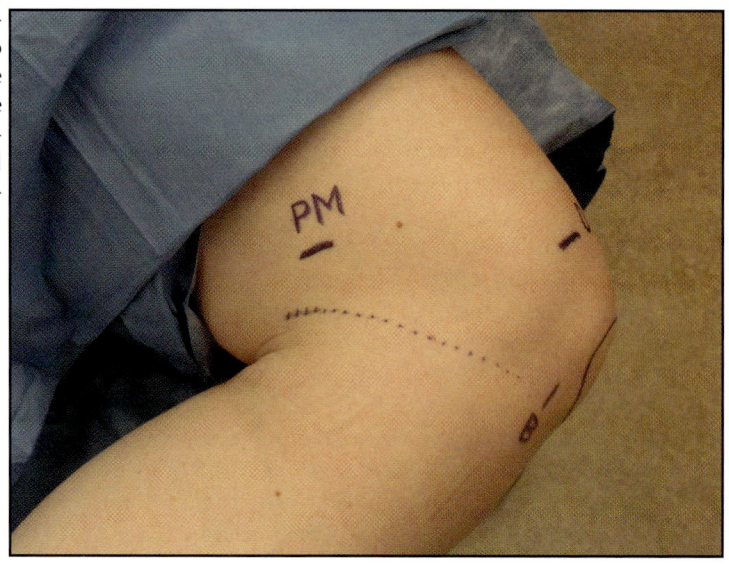

above the semimembranosus tendon in a palpable soft spot (Figure 1-11). The arthroscope is driven into the intercondylar notch and below the femoral insertion of the PCL to enter the posteromedial compartment. Distending the joint with fluid aids in visualization and identification of landmarks. Trans-illumination may reveal the saphenous vein and nerve (sartorial branch) posteriorly. A spinal needle is placed through the soft spot into the posteromedial joint under direct visualization, aiming slightly distal and anterior (Figure 1-12A). The skin is then incised with a #11 blade scalpel, and a blunt trochar or hemostat is used to spread down to capsule (Figure 1-12B). A plastic cannula can then be inserted over a switching stick or blunt obturator.

SUMMARY

Preparation is essential to a successful knee arthroscopy. There are many arthroscopic instruments available. The surgeon should select his or her preferred instruments and become comfortable with them. It is also important to understand how the video, pump, and shaver systems work because a knowledgeable representative or staff member may not be available to troubleshoot problems.

The surgeon should be familiar with the standard arthroscopic portals and accessory portals. A thorough understanding of knee anatomy is critical. Superficial landmarks are used to determine proper portal location, and spinal needle localization may be used when needed. Proper setup and portal placement will help to enable safe, efficient, and effective knee arthroscopy.

TIPS AND PEARLS

- ✔ Make a preoperative plan for each case which includes patient positioning, equipment needed, and possible alternative procedures or bailouts.
- ✔ Develop a thorough understanding of all equipment being used.
- ✔ Position the patient carefully with the popliteal fossa at or below the break in the table.

Positioning and Set-Up 11

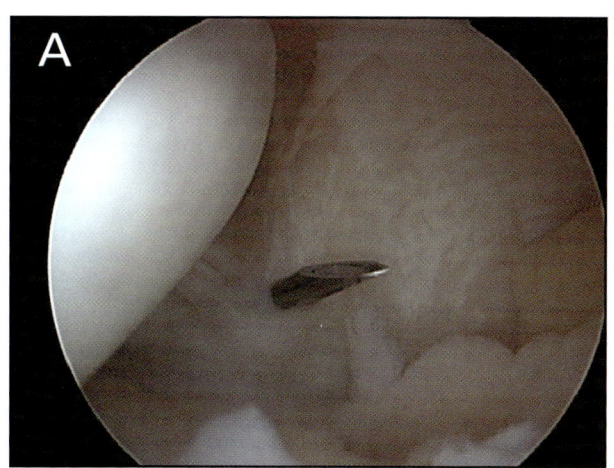

Figure 1-12. Viewing the posteromedial joint with a 30-degree arthroscope, a spinal needle is introduced under direct visualization (A). The skin is incised, and a blunt trochar (B) or hemostat is used to dilate the capsule to allow for cannula insertion.

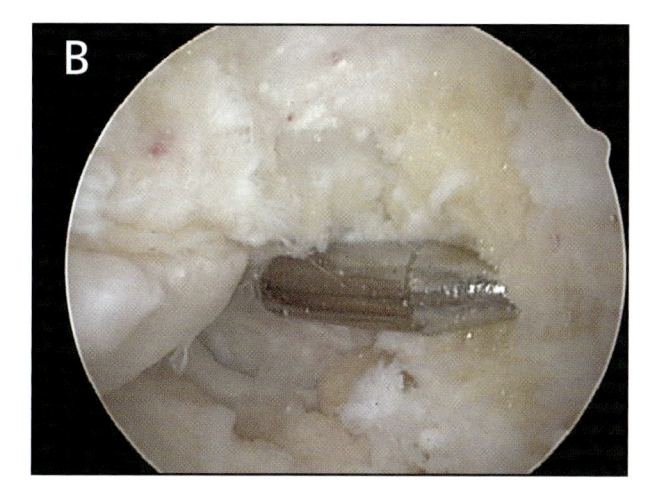

- ✔ Apply a tourniquet for use in ligament reconstructions or when bleeding is encountered.
- ✔ A lateral post is helpful for applying the valgus force required to fully access the medial compartment.
- ✔ Use a fluid pump that can distend the joint and maintain flow during shaver, burr, and electrocautery usage.
- ✔ Use local landmarks to identify proper portal locations. Once the viewing portal is established, a spinal needle can be used to confirm other portal locations before the skin is incised.

PITFALLS

- ✘ Poor preparation may leave the surgeon lacking instruments critical to the procedure or may require staff to search for equipment causing a delay during the case.
- ✘ Inadequate understanding of the equipment may lead to patient injury, equipment breakage, or the inability to troubleshoot a problem.

✘ Improper portal placement may make the procedure difficult or impossible and may require additional skin incisions.

REFERENCES

1. Edwards RB 3rd, Lu Y, Nho S, Cole BJ, Markel MD. Thermal chondroplasty of chondromalacic human cartilage. An ex vivo comparison of bipolar and monopolar radiofrequency devices. *Am J Sports Med.* 2002;30(1):90-97.
2. Lu Y, Bogdanske J, Lopez M, Cole BJ, Markel MD. Effect of simulated shoulder thermal capsulorrhaphy using radiofrequency energy on glenohumeral fluid temperature. *Arthroscopy.* 2005;21(5):592-596.
3. Lu Y, Edwards RB 3rd, Cole BJ, Markel MD. Thermal chondroplasty with radiofrequency energy: an in vitro comparison of bipolar and monopolar radiofrequency devices. *Am J Sports Med.* 2001;29(1):42-49.
4. Kaplan L, Uribe JW. The acute effects of radiofrequency energy in articular cartilage: an in vitro study. *Arthroscopy.* 2000;16(1):2-5.
5. Lu Y, Edwards RB 3rd, Nho S, Cole BJ, Markel MD. Lavage solution temperature influences depth of chondrocyte death and surface contouring during thermal chondroplasty with temperature-controlled monopolar radiofrequency energy. *Am J Sports Med.* 2002;30(5):667-673.
6. Lu Y, Edwards RB 3rd, Nho S, Heiner JP, Cole BJ, Markel MD. Thermal chondroplasty with bipolar and monopolar radiofrequency energy: effect of treatment time on chondrocyte death and surface contouring. *Arthroscopy.* 2002;18(7):779-788.
7. Griffith MH, Good CR, Shindle MK, Wanich T, Warren RF. The effect of radiofrequency energy on glenohumeral fluid temperature during shoulder arthroscopy. Presented at the American Academy of Orthopaedic Surgeons Annual Meeting; March 2008; San Francisco, CA.
8. Ogilvie-Harris DJ, Biggs DJ, Mackay M, Weisleder L. Posterior portals for arthroscopic surgery of the knee. *Arthroscopy.* 1994;10(6):608-613.
9. Muellner T, Menth-Chiari WA, Reihsner R, Eberhardsteiner J, Engebretsen L. Accuracy of pressure and flow capacities of four arthroscopic fluid management systems. *Arthroscopy.* 2001;17(7):760-764.
10. Sperber A, Wredmark T. Tensile properties of the knee-joint capsule at an elevated intraarticular pressure. *Acta Orthop Scand.* 1998;69(5):484-488.
11. Abbushi W, Egbert R, Pichelmeier R, Kovacs J. Compartment syndrome of the forearm due to infusion and transfusion using a pressure pump. *Anasthesiol Intensivmed Notfallmed Schmerzther.* 1991;26(6):348-351.
12. Belanger M, Fadale P. Compartment syndrome of the leg after arthroscopic examination of a tibial plateau fracture: case report and review of the literature. *Arthroscopy.* 1997;13(5):646-651.
13. Bomberg BC, Hurley PE, Clark CA, McLaughlin CS. Complications associated with the use of an infusion pump during knee arthroscopy. *Arthroscopy.* 1992;8(2):224-228.
14. DiStefano VJ, Kalman VR, O'Malley JS. Femoral nerve palsy after arthroscopic surgery with an infusion pump irrigation system: a report of three cases. *Am J Orthop.* 1996;25(2):145-148.
15. Sorrentino F, Eggli S, Stricker U, Ballmer FT, Hertel R. Missed compartment syndrome after anterior cruciate ligament-plasty following continuous peridural anesthesia. *Unfallchirurg.* 1998;101(6):491-494.
16. Schreiber SN. Proximal superomedial portal in arthroscopy of the knee. *Arthroscopy.* 1991;7(2):246-251.
17. Boytim MJ, Smith JP, Fischer DA, Quick DC. Arthroscopic posteromedial visualization of the knee. *Clin Orthop Relat Res.* 1995;310:82-86.
18. Gold DL, Schaner PJ, Sapega AA. The posteromedial portal in knee arthroscopy: an analysis of diagnostic and surgical utility. *Arthroscopy.* 1995;11(2):139-145.
19. Kramer DE, Bahk MS, Cascio BM, Cosgarea AJ. Posterior knee arthroscopy: anatomy, technique, application. *J Bone Joint Surg Am.* 2006;88(Suppl 4):110-121.

Anesthesia for Knee Surgery

Lisa Wollman, MD

Anesthesia for surgeries of the knee has changed dramatically in recent years, as procedures are done increasingly on an outpatient basis requiring shorter-acting drugs and alternatives for pain management. As almost all of these cases are elective and performed on relatively healthy individuals, basic anesthetic principles apply. Patient care is optimal when the anesthesiologist is knowledgeable of the surgical anatomy and specific details of the planned procedure and when medical issues relevant to the case are communicated preoperatively. Clinicians with an expertise in regional techniques and the use of ultrasound can dramatically affect the perioperative course for patients undergoing these surgeries.

AMBULATORY VERSUS INPATIENT ANESTHESIA

The national shift of formerly inpatient procedures to outpatient surgicenters is expected to continue into the foreseeable future. Outpatient surgeries are appropriate to consider on American Society of Anesthesiologists (ASA) Class 1 and 2 patients as well as selected groups of Class 3 and 4 patients, specifically those who are medically stable on current regimens. However, recent studies suggest that admissions and complications are more a function of the type of procedure and length of surgery as well as patient age rather than the actual ASA classification.

American Society of Anesthesiologists Classifications:
* ASA 1—Healthy patient
* ASA 2—Mild systemic disease without limitations
* ASA 3—Severe disease limiting activity
* ASA 4—Incapacitating disease with threat to life
* ASA 5—Not expected to survive 24 hours

Patients in Class 3 and 4 that should be operated on in a hospital setting include those who:
* Require complex extended monitoring for cardiac disease
* Are morbidly obese
* Have significant respiratory disease such as sleep apnea and chronic obstructive pulmonary disease (COPD)
* Have had postoperative complications in the past
* Present challenging pain issues if regional anesthesia is not an option

Preoperative Issues

Laboratory Studies

In healthy patients undergoing knee surgery, the need for preoperative testing is minimal; in fact, routine laboratory screening tests are rarely useful. According to current guidelines, hematologic studies are indicated if there are concerns about preoperative or intraoperative blood loss, anemia, or coagulopathy. Generally, a hematocrit of 30% or higher is safe for elective procedures; lower values should be evaluated for an etiology and possible comorbidities. Healthy patients do not need a hematocrit. Platelet function workup is only indicated in patients with easy bruising, excessive bleeding, or a positive family history. Coagulation studies should be ordered only if the patient has a history of bleeding, recent anticoagulation use, liver disease, or persistent systemic illness.

Chemistry studies are necessary if the history or physical exam suggest possible abnormalities, such as in the case of patients with renal or hepatic disease, patients with diabetes, patients on diuretics, or patients on chronic aminoglycoside antibiotics.

Electrocardiogram (ECG) is indicated in patients with risk factors for coronary artery disease or patients who are 50 years and older.

Chest x-ray is clinically indicated only in patients with acute respiratory symptoms or known malignancies.

The following are the current ASA fasting guidelines for patients:
* Intake of clear liquids until 2 hours preoperatively
* Solid foods until 8 hours preoperatively
* Medications should be continued with sips of water on the day of surgery except for anticoagulants, diuretics, and regular insulin. Long-acting insulin should be taken in half of the usual dose. (Diabetics should be scheduled as early in the day as the schedule permits.)

Preoperative Consultation

Such a meeting can expedite the evaluation and preinduction time on the day of surgery but is not necessary in most healthy, ambulatory patients. Most information can be obtained from the medical record and from the patient in a phone conversation. In patients with a significant level of apprehension and anxiety, anxiolytics may need to be prescribed at this time. A brief physical exam and review of any significant changes in medical status can be done just prior to surgery at the time of confirmation of the last oral intake and consent is obtained.

Informed Consent

This discussion should be a conversation about general anesthesia, regional anesthesia, and the various combinations thereof as well as a list of the possible complications from the most frequent to many remote, possible risks. For general anesthesia, these include sore throat, airway trauma, dental injury, allergic reactions, nausea and vomiting, intraoperative awareness, stroke, bleeding, postoperative intensive care unit (ICU) admission, and death. When regional anesthesia is planned, the conversation needs to be a more detailed review of the risks of specific to the procedure. Namely, the complications of peripheral nerve blocks include the following:
* Nerve injury
* Failure of regional anesthesia requiring general anesthesia
* Systemic toxicity of local anesthetics including seizures and cardiovascular collapse from inadvertent intravascular injection

* Infection
* Local hematoma/tissue trauma
* Catheter migration
* Difficulty with catheter removal

ANESTHETIC MANAGEMENT

Monitoring

In addition to the continual presence of an anesthetist, there is necessary standard monitoring, which must be applied to ensure safety and quality care for all patients. Standard monitors include the following:

* Oxygen analyzer
* Pulse oximetry (oxygenation)
* Capnography (ventilation)
* ECG
* Blood pressure (cuff or arterial line)

Additional monitors may be indicated for temperature, central nervous system level of consciousness (Bispectral Index Digital Electroencephalogram [BIS Aspect Medical Systems, Newton, MA]), and neuromuscular blockade.

Premedication

Anxiolytics

Benzodiazepines enhance the inhibitory tone of GABA (γ-aminobutyric acid) receptors, thereby facilitating the sedation and amnesia with general and regional anesthesia. These medications are quite effective in the treatment of anxiety; the selection of drug is based on the length of desired effect.

Diazepam (Valium, Hoffman-LaRoche Inc, Nutley, NJ) or lorazepam (Ativan, Biovail Corp, Mississauga, Canada) is often given orally for anxiety as needed prior to the day of surgery. The effect of these drugs lasts many hours, with half-lives of 10 and 20 hours, respectively.

Midazolam is usually given intravenously 10 to 50 µg/kg with an onset of 2 to 3 minutes and a half-life of less than 2 hours.

All of these drugs have beneficial anticonvulsant and muscle relaxant effects, which increase in a dose-dependent manner. They do not produce any appreciable analgesia.

Opioids

There are many choices of opioids, all of which provide analgesia but differ in potency, length of action, and side effects. The most commonly used drugs for block placement include fentanyl given intravenously in 1 to 2 µg/kg doses with effects lasting 30 to 60 minutes and remifentanil given intravenously in 0.3 to 0.5 µg/kg doses with effects lasting 5 to 10 minutes.

Longer-acting narcotics, such as morphine, meperidine (Demerol, Hospira, Inc, Lake Forest, IL), and hydromorphone (Dilaudid, Purdue Pharma L. P., Cranberry, NJ), are used intravenously for immediate postoperative pain management.

All of these agents produce analgesia, sedation, decreased need for other anesthetics, and respiratory depression.

All narcotics can cause nausea, vomiting, and urinary retention. Naloxone is a pure opioid antagonist used to reverse undesired effects of central nervous system depression. Administration can cause sudden hypertension, tachycardia, and the abrupt onset of pain.

Aspiration Prophylaxis

Treatment is often indicated in patients with extreme anxiety, morbid obesity, hiatal hernia, or severe gastroesophageal reflux. Pharmacologic options include the following:

* Ranitidine (Zantac, GlaxoSmithKline, Middlesex, United Kingdom) 150 mg orally or 50 mg intravenously blocks histamine H_2 receptors
* Bicitra 30 mL orally is a nonparticulate antacid
* Metoclopramide (Reglan, Alaven Pharmaceutical LLC, Marietta, GA) 10 mg orally or intravenously promotes gastric emptying

GENERAL ANESTHESIA

Propofol (2,6 diisopropylphenol) is the most commonly used induction and continuous sedation agent in adults; it has the desirable effects of short duration, rapid unconsciousness, good depression of pharyngeal reflexes, and reducing the incidence of postoperative nausea and vomiting.

Maintenance of anesthesia involves a variety of volatile and intravenous agents; muscle relaxation is not necessary for most of the surgeries discussed in this text.

NEUROAXIAL ANESTHESIA

Spinal anesthesia is a fast, reliable technique for orthopedic procedures of the knee and lower extremity in cases where general anesthesia is less desirable; duration is titratable by drug and concentration choice. In the ambulatory setting, however, 1% to 10% of patients may complain of post dural puncture headaches (PDPH). Healthy women younger than 40 years are at the greatest risk. Other complications that are not uncommon include urinary retention and transient neurologic symptoms/radicular irritation.

Epidural anesthesia can be used to decrease the likelihood of PDPH; a continuous catheter can be used to redose local anesthetics if needed for longer procedures. Urinary retention can also be a problem in these patients.

For these reasons, general anesthesia, in conjunction with peripheral nerve blocks, is often the more desirable technique.

REGIONAL ANESTHESIA

The most commonly used local anesthetics for peripheral nerve blocks for orthopedic surgeries include mepivacaine, lidocaine, bupivacaine, and ropivacaine. Mepivacaine has a concentration of 1% to 2%, a fast onset, and lasts for 3 to 5 hours. Lidocaine has a concentration of 1% to 2%, a fast onset, and a duration of 1 to 3 hours. Bupivacaine has a concentration of 0.25% to 0.5%, a slow onset, and a duration of 6 to 20 hours. Ropivacaine has a concentration of 0.5%, a slow onset, and a duration of 6 to 8 hours.

In a 70-kg patient, it is safe to use 20 to 40 cc of each of these drugs individually; they are often used in combination in lesser volumes to maximize the desired effect and minimize toxicities. Epinephrine should be added to all local anesthetics in concentrations of 1:200,000 to 1:400,000. The addition of epinephrine facilitates the detection of intravascular injection (tachycardia and hypertension), causes local vasoconstriction to decrease bleeding, increases the intensity of the block by direct neuronal alpha agonism, may prolong the duration of the block, decreases systemic toxicity by slowing the rate of absorption into the circulation, and may decrease the time to onset of the block.

Clinically, patients undergoing knee surgery are most often going to have general anesthesia, and the block is primarily for postoperative analgesia. Therefore, rapid onset is less important than maximizing the length of the block; bupivacaine is the most desirable drug for this reason.

Anti-Emetics

Nausea and vomiting continue to be an issue in ambulatory surgery and anesthesia. Predisposing factors include female gender, history of motion sickness, narcotic administration, pain, and, perhaps, anterior cruciate ligament (ACL) and posterior cruciate ligament (PCL) repair procedures. There are, however, many pharmacologic choices to treat this common complaint.

Ondansetron (Zofran, GlaxoSmithKline) 2 to 4 mg intravenously every 8 hours is probably the safest choice with the fewest possible side effects. When using scopolamine 1.5-mg transdermal patch, care is needed in handling because eye contact may cause long-lasting dilated pupils and blurred vision. Haloperidol (Haldol, Ortho-McNeil-Janssen Pharmaceuticals, Inc, Raritan, NJ) 1 mg intravenously is contraindicated in patients with Parkinson's disease due to rare dystonic reactions. Dexamethasone 4 mg intravenously can be repeated if needed. Patients can experience a rare Addisonian crisis and extremely rare osteonecrosis.

Postoperative Pain

Pain management is the most common problem interfering with the time to discharging ambulatory patients. Upon arrival to the post-anesthesia care unit (PACU), if a patient has pain, supplemental intravenous opioids, such as fentanyl, meperidine, morphine, or dilaudid, are indicated. In the case of most surgeries of the knee, intravenous ketorolac (Toradol, Roche Palo Alto, LLC, Palo Alto, CA), a nonsteroidal anti-inflammatory analgesic, can be given safely as an adjunct to narcotics. Recent data may, in fact, show that the use of this class of drug in the perioperative period may lead to better long-term results as far as increased range of motion and decreased long-term pain. The dose is 15 to 30 mg intravenously every 6 hours as needed. This class of drugs needs to be used cautiously in patients with a history of peptic ulcer disease, renal disease, or a history of bleeding problems. Once the patient is able to take oral medications, ibuprofen and acetaminophen can be added to any opioid regimen.

Regional Anesthesia

Although peripheral nerve blockade can be an excellent alternative to general anesthesia for many orthopedic procedures of the lower extremity, it is often used in addition to general anesthesia for postoperative pain management in quadriceps and ACL and PCL repair surgeries. This is primarily because a femoral nerve block is almost never adequate as the sole anesthetic; this requires blockade of both the lumbar and sacral plexuses, requiring multiple injections, thereby making this technique less desirable for both clinicians and patients. However, it is possible to block both the femoral and sciatic nerves in cases where regional anesthesia is preferable but central neuraxial blocks are contraindicated.

Femoral Nerve Block/3-in-1 Block

Indications for femoral nerve blockade include operations of the anterior portion of the thigh (both superficial and deep) and as an adjunct to general anesthesia for joint surgery of the knee. The femoral nerve arises from L2-L4 and is the largest branch of the lumbar plexus. The nerve

Figure 2-1. Femoral nerve anatomy.

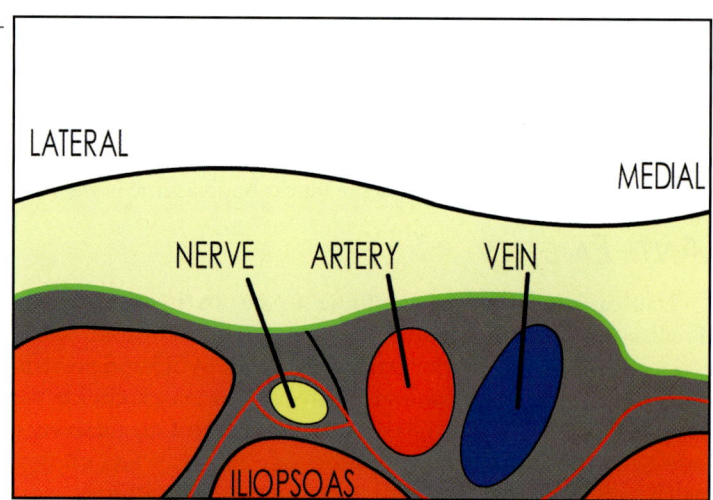

Figure 2-2. Ultrasound anatomy for the femoral nerve.

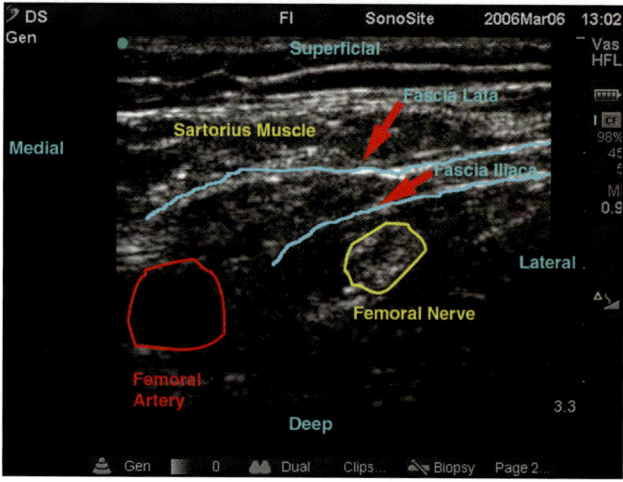

exits the psoas muscle, passes anteriorly to the iliopsoas and under the inguinal ligament, becoming superficial in the anterior thigh. The nerve is found deep to the fascia lata and fascia iliacus, which separate the nerve from the femoral artery and vein. At the inguinal ligament and distal to it, the nerve is slightly deeper and lateral to the artery; the vein is medial to the artery (Figures 2-1 and 2-2).

A number of techniques exist for locating the nerve, and block success rates are often highly operator dependent. Although practices vary among clinicians, it is safest to perform blocks on patients with the least amount of sedation possible and not under general anesthesia. In patients where pain is a challenge to manage in the PACU, a postoperative block can be performed safely following emergence.

Nerve Stimulator

The use of a nerve stimulator for block placement has been the most widely used approach—most often in an awake but sedated patient. A current of 0.1 to 1.0 mA at a frequency of 1 to 2 pulses/second is an appropriate setting. The groin is prepped in sterile fashion, and the point for needle insertion is anesthetized. The positive lead is grounded on the patient; the negative lead is attached to the needle. A roughly 2-inch, 22-gauge, short beveled, insulated needle is inserted

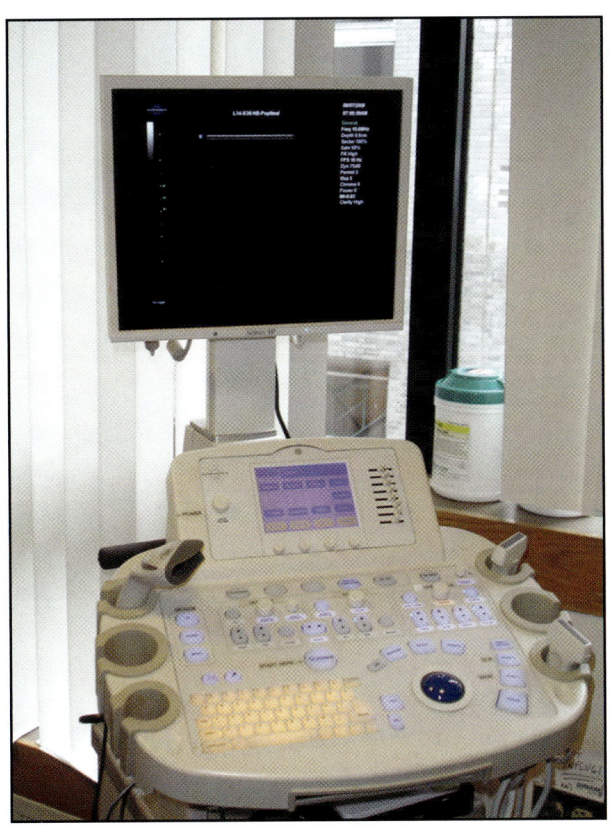

Figure 2-3. Portable ultrasound machine for block placement.

perpendicular to the skin and advanced until a patellar twitch is elicited. Some knee extension and thigh adduction may also indicate femoral nerve stimulation. Once stimulation is achieved, the electrical amplitude is dialed down to less than 0.3 to 0.5 mA. If the stimulation extinguishes in this range, it suggests that the needle is in close proximity to the nerve and not intraneural. At this point, with no pain reported by the patient and a negative aspiration, local anesthetic is injected. A volume of 20 mL is probably sufficient to block the femoral nerve; often up to 40 mL is used for greater spread to additionally block the lateral femoral cutaneous and obturator nerves.

Ultrasound Guidance

One of the most exciting advances in regional anesthesia has been the introduction of ultrasound technology (Figure 2-3). Ultrasound for peripheral nerve blocks use frequencies from 1 to 15 MHz; high frequency increases the resolution at the expense of penetration and low frequency increases the depth of penetration at the expense of resolution. Most nerve blocks require intermediate depth and frequency. Successful imaging requires the insertion of the needle, the advancement direction, and the endpoint of the tip to all be properly aligned in the center of the probe and, therefore, the ultrasound beam. This allows for full visualization of the shaft of the needle. The probe is most commonly placed at the site of where the needle insertion would be using traditional block technique. The needle appears as a hyperechoic white line and should be continually visualized throughout injection. In cases where the nerve is challenging to identify, the use of color Doppler can be useful to identify the blood vessels.

Figure 2-4. Femoral nerve block placement.

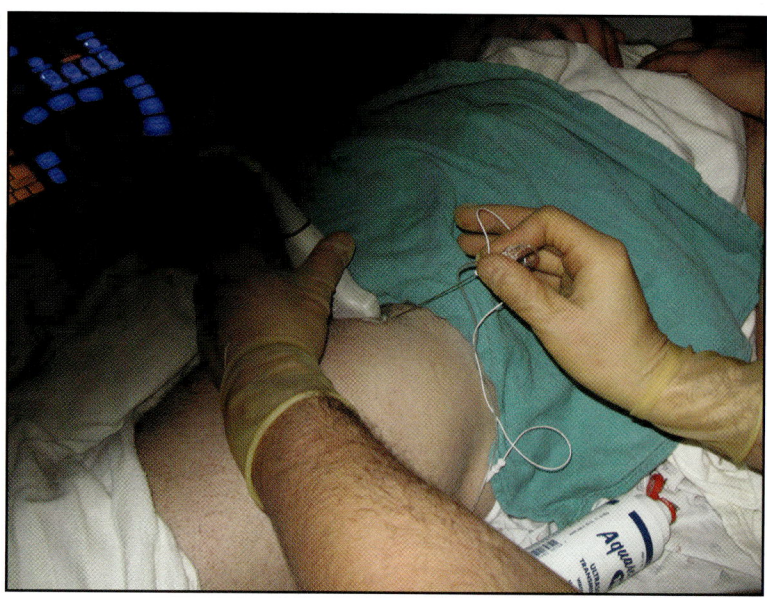

Fascia Iliaca/Femoral Nerve Block

The block (Figure 2-4) is performed with the patient in the supine position, and the probe is placed under the femoral artery at the level of the femoral crease. Moving the probe laterally brings the nerve into view and the artery to the lateral view of the image. Two fascial layers (the superficial fascia lata and the deeper fascia iliaca) can be visualized lying over the iliopsoas muscle.

Needle entry is roughly 2 cm lateral to the probe. The needle length needs to be at least 50 mm and is advanced at a 45- to 60-degree angle to the skin. Often, 2 distinct "pops" can be appreciated, which indicates loss of resistance as the fascial layers are penetrated. The needle should be deep to these layers; local anesthetic can be injected after a negative aspiration.

The block can take considerable time to set up (20 to 40 minutes) when bupivacaine is used, so planning for early placement of the block is desirable for the onset of surgical anesthesia. If the block is used in conjunction with general anesthesia for surgeries of the knee joint, timing is less of an issue. The extra case preparation time when a block is planned mandates an earlier start for the anesthesia team for the first case of the day and often requires a second anesthesia team for "to follow" cases to help avoid delays in operating room turnover times.

Complications

Blocks should only be performed on patients in a fully monitored setting, with oxygen delivery available, emergency airway equipment accessible, and with benzodiazepines and intralipid infusion ready to be administered in the case of an intravascular injection. Test doses and intermittent aspiration during injection should be mandatory regardless of technique used to minimize this risk. Rare but possible complications of lower extremity blocks include the following:
* Over sedation requiring airway support
* Seizures secondary to neurotoxicity of local anesthetics
* Cardiovascular collapse secondary to intravascular injection
* Allergic reactions

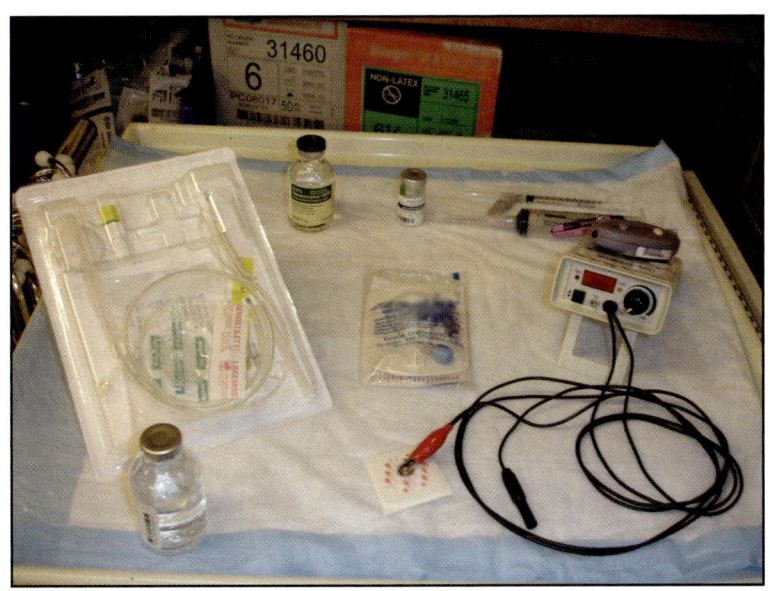

Figure 2-5. Equipment for femoral catheter placement.

* Nerve damage either by needle trauma by excessive trauma or intraneural injection
* Small hematoma especially if the artery is inadvertently punctured
* Failure of block—a patient may still complain of marked knee pain in the setting of a successful femoral nerve block as the posterior obturator nerve often has an articular branch supplying the posterior aspect of the knee. Posterior knee surgery, PCL reconstruction, and total knee replacement require sciatic nerve block as well.

CONTRAINDICATIONS

Not all patients are candidates for regional anesthesia. Absolute contraindications include lack of consent and nerve blockade interfering with the planned procedure.

Relative contraindications include coagulopathy, infection at site, the inability to communicate with the patient, anatomic abnormalities, and neurologic conditions, such as multiple sclerosis, polio, diabetic neuropathy, trauma, and muscular dystrophy.

INDWELLING PERIPHERAL NERVE CATHETERS

In appropriately selected patients, postoperative analgesia can be continued over a period of days with an infusion of local anesthesia through a catheter placed in a sheath surrounding the femoral nerve (Figure 2-5). This can significantly reduce the systemic narcotic requirement and has minimal risk of complications. Most studies seem to report better pain control with continuous catheters when compared to single shot blocks and epidural anesthesia. Contraindications include the presence of a femoral artery graft, possible lower extremity compartment syndrome, trauma, and previously mentioned contraindications for regional technique.

The success rate and ease of placement of such catheters has been greatly improved by the introduction of stimulating catheters and needles and ultrasound. There are several commercial varieties of these stimulation catheters; most have a Touhey tipped, insulated needle and a catheter with a stylet and female adaptor to accept a cable for the nerve stimulator. The catheter is placed in the same fashion as a single shot block; the catheter is gradually advanced beyond the tip of the needle for 3 to 10 cm. Patella stimulation should continue without paresthesia as the catheter is advanced; the catheter must always be withdrawn back into the needle prior to repositioning. Location of the catheter should be confirmed by ultrasound prior to drug injection; the needle can then be removed. The key to a successful continuous block is the prevention of catheter dislodgement; they are best secured by tunneling under the skin for several centimeters in the lateral direction and using skin glue for an adhesive dressing.

The drug of choice for infusion is variable among institutions; most anesthesiologists use some formulation of low concentrations of bupivacaine (0.1% to 0.25%) or ropivacaine (0.2% to 0.5%). Sterile care of these catheters and dressings is necessary; the entry site should be watched for signs of infection. Catheter follow-up requires a team of anesthesiologists trained in regional techniques and may be done on an inpatient or outpatient basis with the proper support staff.

BIBLIOGRAPHY

Dunn P, Alston T, Baker K, Davison JK, Kwo J, Rosow C. *Clinical Anesthesia Procedures of the Massachusetts General Hospital*. 7th ed. Philadelphia, PA: Lippincott Williams & Wilkins; 2007.

Tsui BCH, Bhargava R, Dillane D. *Atlas of Ultrasound and Nerve Stimulation-Guided Regional Anesthesia*. New York, NY: Springer Science+Business Media, LLC; 2007.

Diagnostic Arthroscopy of the Knee—The 10-Point Exam

Matthew J. Matava, MD and Evan D. Ellis, MD

Surgical Goals

Performing a thorough diagnostic arthroscopy is a crucial step to the beginning of any arthroscopic procedure of the knee. When performed correctly, it is a quick, efficient technique that can help document and confirm either suspected or unsuspected conditions of the knee. Therefore, it is extremely important that the surgeon develop a routine sequence in which to perform the procedure so as not to miss any relevant pathology.

In this chapter, we will describe the sequence in which we evaluate the knee arthroscopically with a method that ensures the proper evaluation of each compartment in a systematic fashion. The surgeon should be well-versed in the design and function of the components of the arthroscope and camera. All modern arthroscopes allow free rotation within their cannula, which provides the surgeon with the opportunity to increase the breadth of view so as to navigate around corners of obstruction. The experienced arthroscopist takes maximal advantage of which combination of camera and arthroscope manipulations allows for the optimal field of view. It is recommended that the intended view of interest be such that the joint surface is kept horizontal during most situations. This is much easier to do in the knee than in other joints, such as the shoulder, where patient position (ie, lateral decubitus) dictates the plane of orientation.

If the camera is rotated by the surgeon's hand and the arthroscope is held still, there will be a "laundromat" effect with rotation of the field of view around the axis of the arthroscope. If the arthroscope is rotated while the camera position is maintained, a "roller coaster" effect will result whereby the image appears to move up and down as the field of view remains horizontal. It should be kept in mind that some regions of the knee (ie, posterior compartments) are best viewed with a 70-degree arthroscope.

It is imperative that the surgeon become familiar with the different types of arthroscopes (ie, 30 degree, 70 degree) and have more than one of each type available in the event that damage occurs (typically the optics at the tip) to one of the lenses. A poorly functioning arthroscope can severely compromise the ability to view the joint in a panoramic fashion irrespective of surgeon expertise. Satisfactory joint distention is also mandatory to maintain proper hemostasis so as to optimize the surgeon's view. This may be regulated by either an increase in intra-articular fluid pressure, use of epinephrine in the fluid, or through the inflation of a tourniquet.

The surgeon may prefer to either complete the entire diagnostic arthroscopy before focusing on the area(s) of pathology or address each condition as it is encountered. It is our preference to treat each pathologic process as it is viewed in order to most efficiently complete the operative

Figure 3-1. Outflow cannula correctly positioned in the suprapatellar pouch.

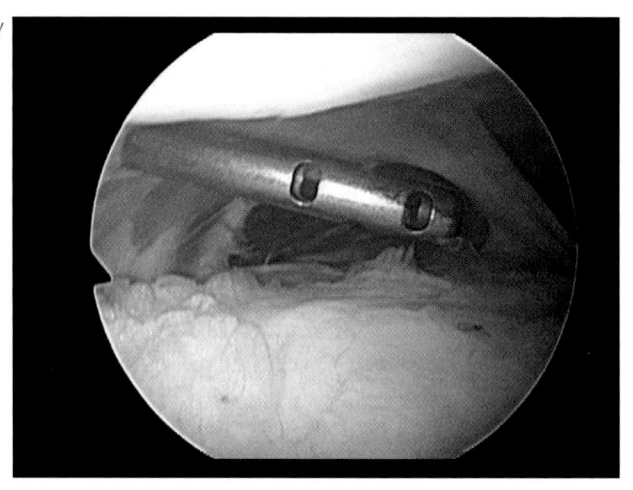

procedure without making redundant passes through the knee. Therefore, all 3 standard knee portals are made at the beginning of the procedure so that instrumentation (ie, probe, shaver, biters) can be inserted into the joint as needed. The focus of this chapter will be limited to the complete diagnostic knee examination without discussion of pathologic processes or structural defects.

SUPRAPATELLAR POUCH

The patient is positioned supine with the end of the operating table bent 90 degrees and the thigh held stationary in a leg holder, thus suspending the extremity with the knee at the level of the surgeon's umbilicus. Placement of the operating table in a slight Trendelenburg position can fine-tune the location of the knee for ease of maneuvering instruments through the joint with optimal varus or valgus stress to the knee, as needed. The contralateral limb should be supported with the hip flexed and abducted and the knee allowed to rest flexed. This position reduces strain on the anterior hip joint as well as the femoral nerve that may occur if the well limb is supported only under the thigh and the knee is unsupported in a flexed position over the end of the operating table.

A superomedial or superolateral portal is created in the manner described in Chapter 1. The outflow cannula with a blunt trocar is first placed into the suprapatellar pouch from the superomedial or superolateral portal with the knee extended (Figure 3-1). We prefer a blunt trocar to penetrate the joint in most situations to prevent articular damage. The cannula is swept proximally and distally to free it from the synovium. As the trocar is removed, the surgeon may note the expression of joint fluid from the cannula, confirming an intra-articular position. Absence of expressed fluid in a knee with an effusion is an indication of intra-synovial placement of the cannula necessitating re-positioning. However, a "dry" joint without an effusion typically is devoid of any synovial fluid expression even with correct intra-articular placement of the cannula. The surgeon may inject fluid into the joint prior to the placement of any cannulas to distend the joint space. We prefer gravity drainage once the outflow portal is established.

The knee is passively placed at 90 degrees of flexion, and the anterolateral and anteromedial portals are created with a #11 scalpel. The portal incisions are made with the blade facing superiorly and aimed at a 45-degree angle from midline through the fat pad toward the intercondylar notch. In general, the anteromedial portal is best naturally positioned approximately 5 to 10 mm more proximal than the anterolateral portal. The arthroscopic cannula and blunt trocar with the inflow tubing attached is introduced via the anterolateral portal into the notch with gentle pressure in line with the direction of the portal incision. The cannula and trocar should move freely in

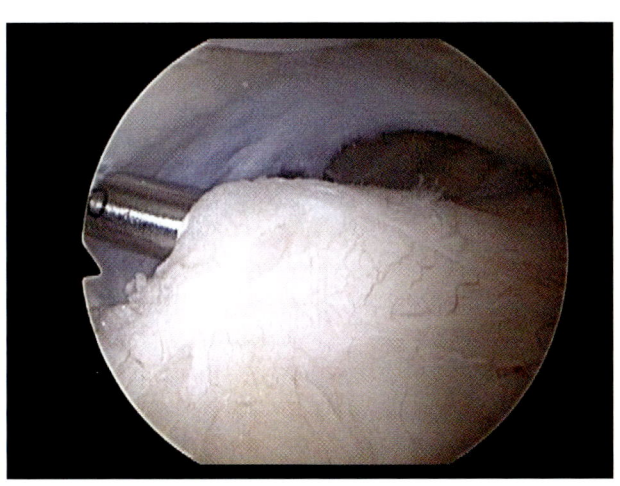

Figure 3-2. Outflow cannula incorrectly positioned within the synovium of the suprapatellar pouch.

and out of the portal to ensure ease of cannula movement throughout the joint. The knee is then slowly moved into full extension, and the cannula with the trocar still in place is driven superiorly into the midline of the suprapatellar pouch with an alternating clockwise, counter-clockwise motion. This rotating motion prevents inadvertent articular damage from the edge of the cannula as it is being advanced. The trocar is removed, and the 30-degree arthroscope with the camera attached is inserted into the cannula and locked into place.

Once the viewing arthroscope is in the joint, it is important to first assess whether the outflow cannula is truly in the joint. This cannula is most commonly misplaced in the synovium of the suprapatellar pouch (Figure 3-2). Several clues exist to this problem and are listed in the pearls on p. 40. If the cannula is not immediately visualized, it must be replaced with the trocar before continuing with the diagnostic examination.

The camera should be focused at this point on either a small blood vessel in the synovium or an object at a maximal viewing distance. Focusing on an object in the foreground often results in an absence of focus of objects in the distance.

The articular surface of the quadriceps tendon is often seen superiorly proximal to the patella, as is the muscle belly of the articularis genu. A suprapatellar plica is occasionally present that obscures these structures as a synovial veil partitioning off a portion of the suprapatellar pouch.[1] Loose bodies may hide within the pouch enclosed by this plica. The surgeon should also assess this area of the knee for synovial hypertrophy indicative of an inflammatory disorder (ie, rheumatoid arthritis) or soft-tissue masses (ie, hemangioma, lipoma arborescens, pigmented villonodular synovitis), which are frequently found in this area.[2]

PATELLOFEMORAL JOINT

The arthroscope should be withdrawn slightly and oriented superiorly to evaluate the undersurface of the patella. It is important to visualize the entire surface of the patellar cartilage (Figure 3-3). This can be performed simply by sweeping the arthroscope from medial to lateral. Alternatively, if the knee is particularly "tight," the surgeon may choose to manually translate the patella from side to side with his or her free hand while holding the arthroscope stationary in the trochlear groove. A 70-degree arthroscope can be used to better evaluate the articular surface for a more direct view, if necessary.

The arthroscope should next be directed posteriorly and withdrawn slightly to evaluate the relationship of the patella to the trochlear groove (Figure 3-4). The knee should be slowly taken from extension to flexion while the surgeon is evaluating the groove for any signs of trochlear

Figure 3-3. Appearance of the articular surface of the patella from the anterolateral portal using a 30-degree arthroscope.

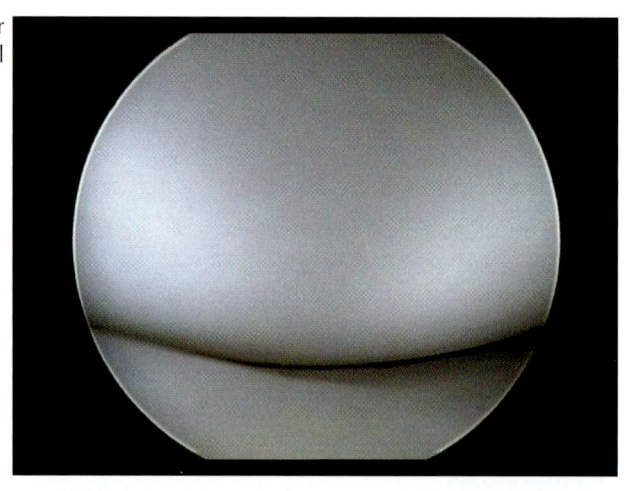

Figure 3-4. The trochlea is best viewed by retracting the arthroscope slightly and taking the knee from full extension to 90 degrees of flexion.

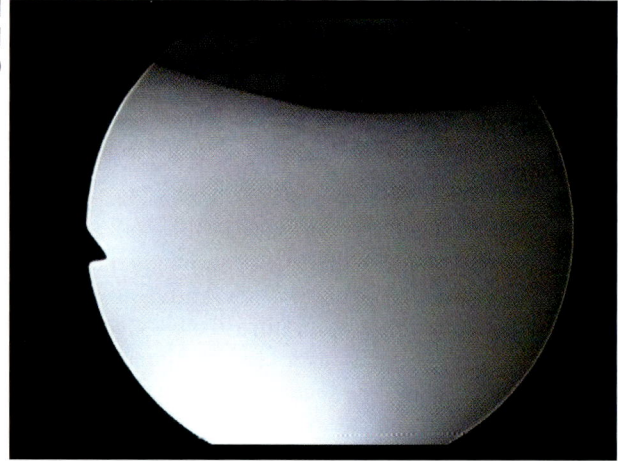

wear. At this point, the surgeon should also be able to view the superior-most aspects of both femoral condyles.

The presence of a medial synovial plica, which is variably present, lies in the coronal plane between the patella and trochlea (Figure 3-5). It may be very narrow and appear as a redundant fold of the synovial membrane, or it may be thick and broad, causing it to rub over the medial femoral condyle with knee flexion. In the latter instance, it may be the cause of frictional wear resulting in chondrosis of the condyle.[1]

LATERAL GUTTER

The knee is then brought back into extension, and the arthroscope is driven proximally past the patella. The arthroscope is then directed laterally while the camera is aimed inferiorly to navigate into the lateral gutter. The surgeon must simultaneously raise his or her hand while slightly withdrawing the arthroscope from the knee to get into the lateral gutter and avoid becoming entrapped within the patellofemoral ligament present midway down the lateral gutter (Figure 3-6). Osteophytes along the lateral femoral condyle or tightness of the lateral retinaculum may make this maneuver more difficult. Care should be taken to avoid scuffing the cartilage of the lateral femoral condyle while maneuvering into and out of the lateral gutter.

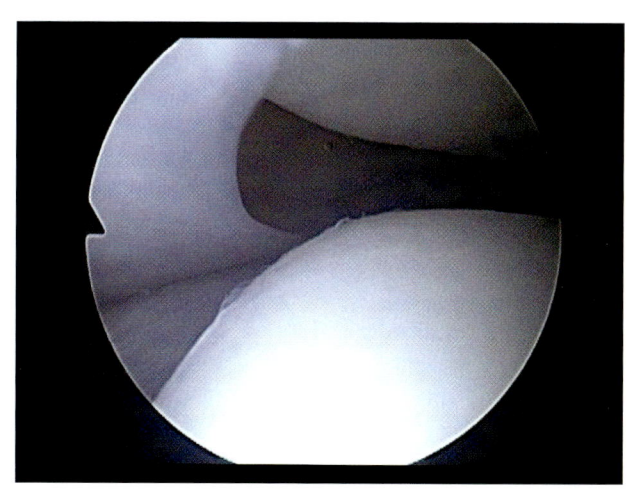

Diagnostic Arthroscopy of the Knee—The 10-Point Exam

Figure 3-5. The variably present medial synovial plica is seen in the coronal plane between the patella and trochlea in the medial aspect of the anterior compartment of the knee.

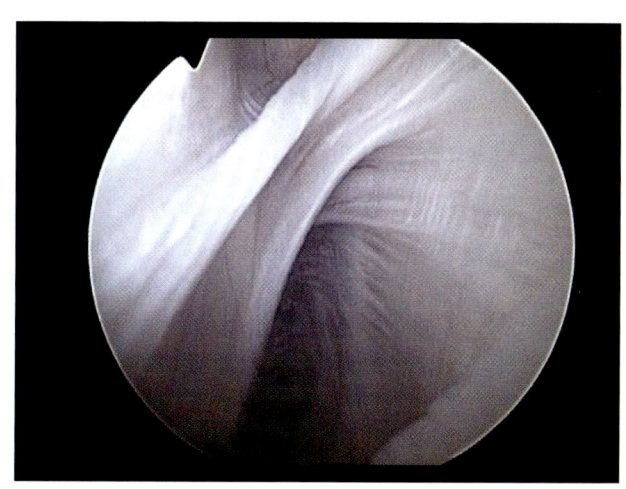

Figure 3-6. Lateral patellofemoral ligament seen midway down the lateral gutter.

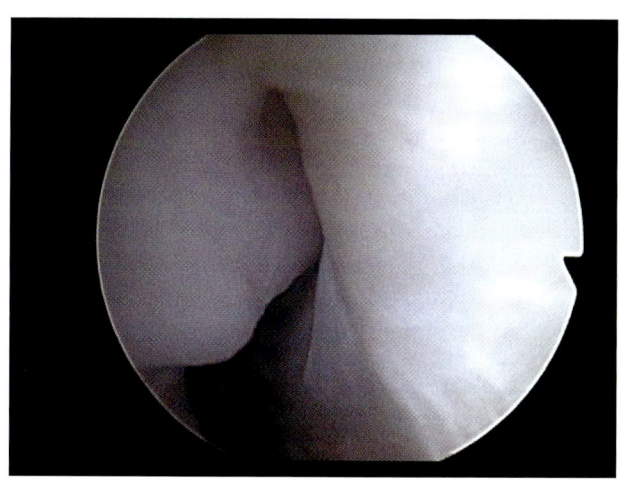

Figure 3-7. The popliteus tendon descends through the popliteus hiatus as seen with the 30-degree arthroscope from the anterolateral portal.

Figure 3-8. Medial gutter viewed from the anterolateral portal.

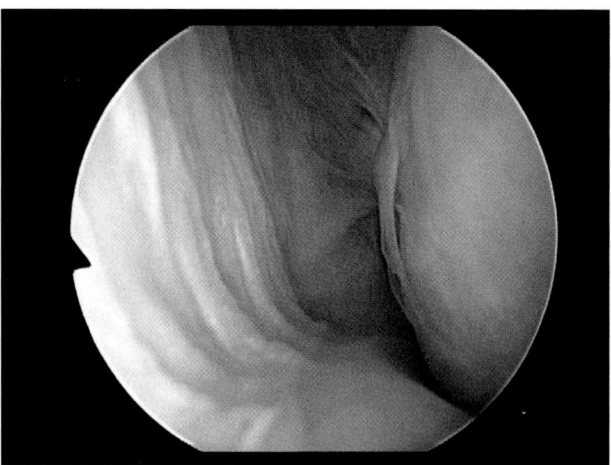

At the inferior-most portion of this gutter is the popliteus tendon, which can be seen descending through the popliteus hiatus (Figure 3-7). This tendon should be evaluated for any sign of tearing, fraying, or attenuation. This is also a common location for small loose bodies to reside. These may be brought into view by gently pressing on the posterolateral aspect of the knee to "flush" out any loose bodies from this hiatus.

MEDIAL GUTTER

To view the medial gutter, the arthroscope is brought into the suprapatellar pouch while the knee is extended. The arthroscope is then directed medially toward the gutter with the camera aimed inferiorly. The surgeon should be sure to keep the arthroscope proximal to the medial femoral condyle while moving into the medial gutter to avoid iatrogenic cartilage damage. The arthroscope is then moved distally while simultaneously backing out slightly from the knee. This helps the surgeon avoid any synovial bands and can be helpful in viewing under a prominent medial plica when one is present.[3] The knee should be slightly flexed and in varus at this time to ease maneuvering through the medial gutter (Figure 3-8).

MEDIAL COMPARTMENT

The arthroscope is slightly withdrawn from the knee and moved laterally while the knee is placed into approximately 20 degrees of flexion and 10 degrees of external rotation, as a valgus force is applied to the leg with the patient's foot locked onto the surgeon's hip or anterior pelvis.

The camera is aimed posteriorly to allow visualization of the medial compartment. The meniscus should be evaluated systematically starting with the posterior horn and working around to the anterior horn (Figure 3-9). At this point, a probe should be placed into the knee through the anteromedial portal. The probe is aimed straight toward the floor to reach the posterior horn of the medial meniscus. The meniscus should be probed from both the superior and inferior surfaces to assess its stability and evaluate for any partial-thickness tears (Figure 3-10). Moving the knee into near-full extension can enhance visualization of the posterior horn and root in a tight knee.[4] External pressure on the posteromedial aspect of the knee can help deliver the posterior horn into view. To evaluate the mid-body of the meniscus, the camera should be held in place and the arthroscope rotated approximately 180 degrees (Figure 3-11). The anterior horn of the medial meniscus is much smaller than in the lateral meniscus and can be visualized as it descends over the anterior tibial plateau. The medial tibial plateau should also be inspected with care taken to evaluate the areas covered by the medial meniscus.

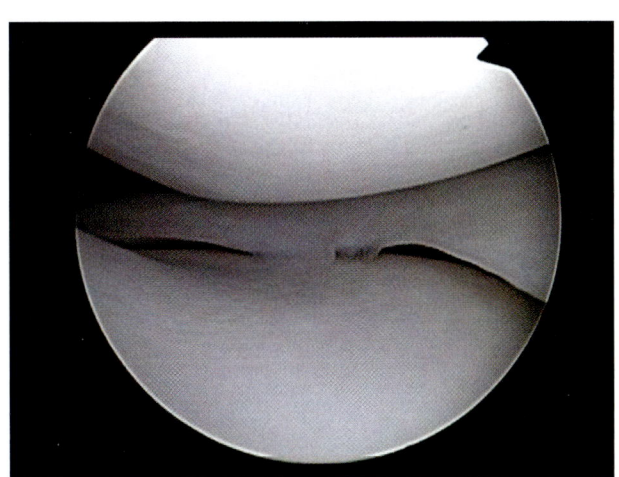

Diagnostic Arthroscopy of the Knee—The 10-Point Exam **33**

Figure 3-9. Posterior horn of the medial meniscus.

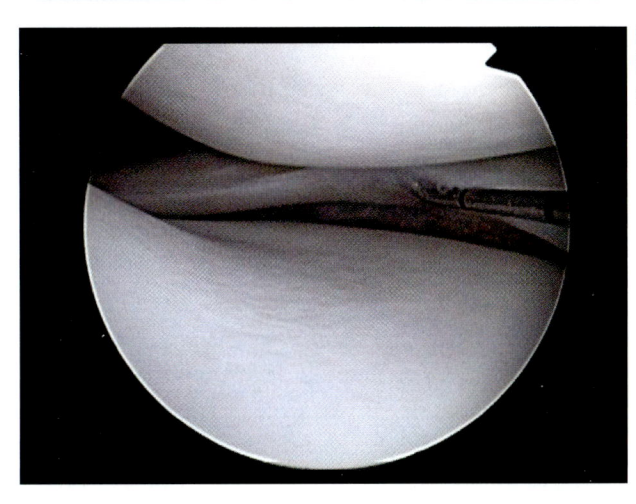

Figure 3-10. Undersurface of the posterior horn of the medial meniscus. This is occasionally the site of a partial-thickness tear.

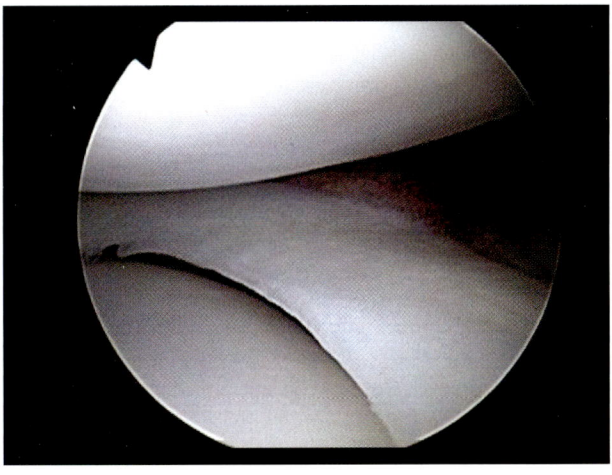

Figure 3-11. Mid-body of the medial meniscus.

Figure 3-12. Medial femoral condyle viewed by progressively flexing the knee to 90 degrees while aiming the 30-degree arthroscope superiorly.

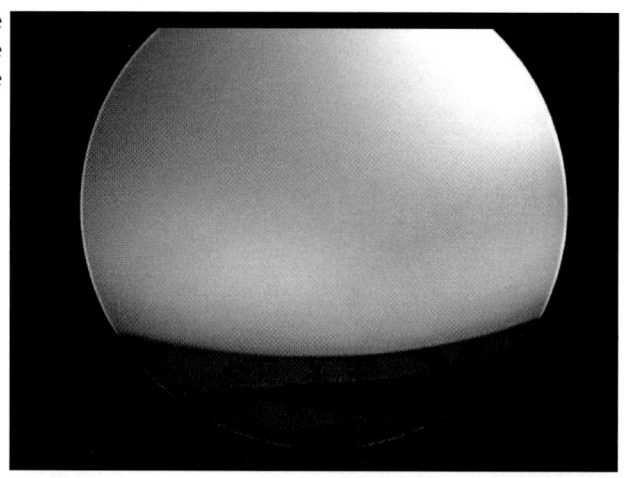

Figure 3-13. The ligamentum mucosum runs from the superior aspect of the intercondylar notch to the anterior compartment synovium.

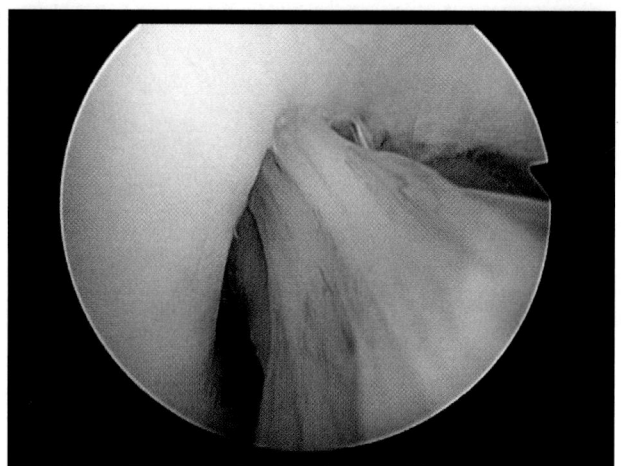

The femoral condyle is evaluated once the probe is removed from the back of the medial compartment to evaluate any pre-existing cartilaginous lesions as well as to ensure that no iatrogenic damage was done to the medial femoral condyle. This is best performed by rotating the arthroscope superiorly while taking the knee from extension into flexion in order to view the posterior aspect of the condyle (Figure 3-12).

INTERCONDYLAR NOTCH

Once the diagnostic examination of the medial compartment is complete, the arthroscope is withdrawn slightly and directed laterally. The camera should be aimed posteriorly, and the knee flexed to 90 degrees. The arthroscope should now be located in the intercondylar notch. The surgeon should first focus the arthroscope on the lateral border of the medial femoral condyle. It is helpful to then follow the arch of the notch in a sweeping fashion superiorly, then laterally down the medial border of the lateral femoral condyle. This will allow for complete evaluation of the notch while simultaneously avoiding the ligamentum mucosum (Figure 3-13).

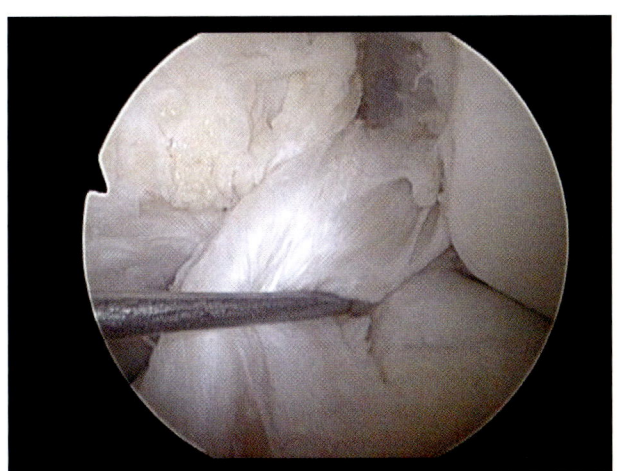

Figure 3-14. Left ACL with probe.

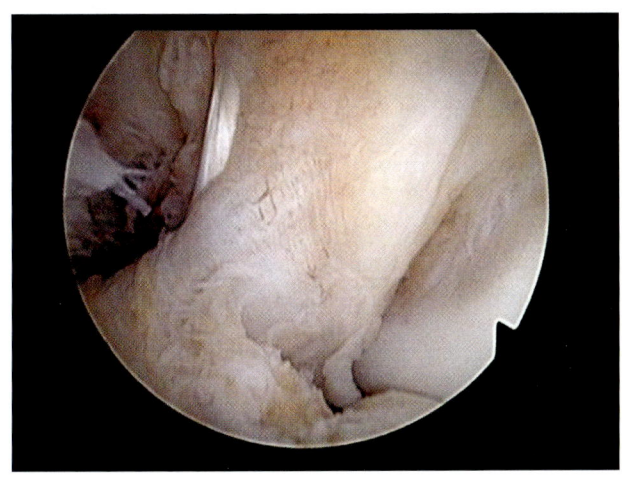

Figure 3-15. The right PCL is seen under a synovial veil as it broadly inserts onto the medial femoral condyle.

CRUCIATE LIGAMENTS

Once the arthroscope is on the lateral side of the intercondylar notch, the surgeon should have an excellent view of the anterior cruciate ligament (ACL) (Figure 3-14). This ligament should be inspected and probed to assess for attenuation or discontinuity (partial or complete). Occasionally, both of the ligament's 2 main fiber bundles—the anteromedial and posterolateral—can be distinguished. The surgeon may also want to perform an arthroscopic Lachman examination under direct visualization of the ligament while probing it to assess its tension.[5] The ACL should be seen originating deep in the notch on the medial border of the lateral femoral condyle. The presence of an "empty wall sign," meaning that there are no visualized ACL fibers attaching to the lateral femoral condyle, is indicative of an ACL tear, as is a "vertical strut sign" signifying adherence of the remaining ACL fibers to the posterior cruciate ligament (PCL).[6] The ACL's insertion onto the tibial eminence should also be visualized adjacent to the anterior horn of the lateral meniscus.

The ACL should then be retracted laterally with a probe to allow visualization of the PCL (Figure 3-15). A direct view of the PCL fiber bundles, including the anterolateral bundle, posteromedial (Figure 3-16) bundle, and variably present anterior meniscofemoral ligament of Humphrey (Figure 3-17), should be possible as the ligament attaches broadly onto the lateral border of the medial femoral condyle.[7] The PCL should also be probed to assess its tension, which

Figure 3-16. Posteromedial bundle of the right PCL outlined with probe.

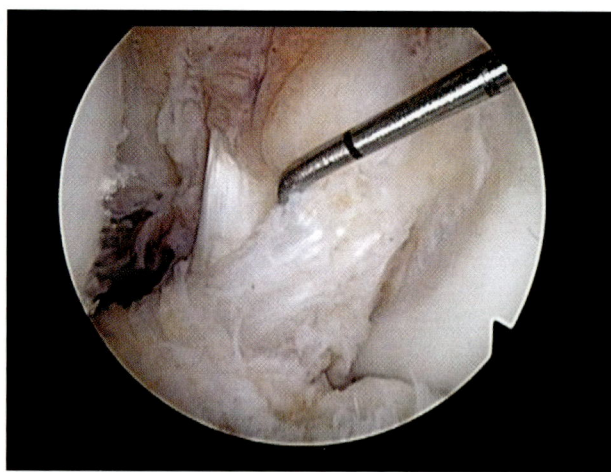

Figure 3-17. Ligament of Humphrey of the left PCL outlined with probe.

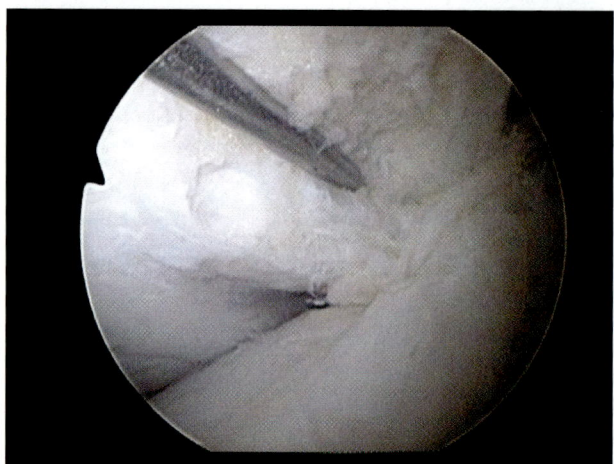

is enhanced with the knee at 90 degrees of flexion. Occasionally, loose bodies can be found in the intercondylar notch between or adjacent to the cruciate ligaments.

ANTERIOR INTERVAL

With the camera held steady, the arthroscope is rotated around to view anteriorly and inferiorly. This will allow further visualization of the fat pad, the anterior slope of the tibial plateau, and the inter-meniscal ligament. Depending on the circumstance, this area should be evaluated for loose bodies, tibial spine avulsion fractures, anteriorly displaced tears of the ACL, the so-called "cyclops" lesion following ACL reconstruction, and the integrity of the intermeniscal ligament.[8,9] The ligamentum mucosum can impair visualization of this area, but it may be pulled medially with a probe to facilitate the view.

LATERAL COMPARTMENT

Next, the arthroscope should be moved to the inferior aspect of the medial border of the lateral femoral condyle. The camera should be aimed posteriorly, and the probe placed just medially in the notch in the triangle formed by the lateral border of the ACL, the medial border of the lateral femoral condyle, and the anterior horn of the lateral meniscus. The knee should be brought out

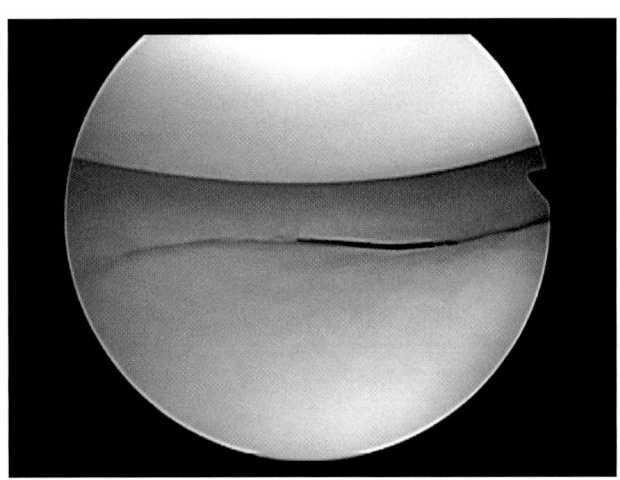

Diagnostic Arthroscopy of the Knee—The 10-Point Exam 37

Figure 3-18. Posterior horn of the lateral meniscus.

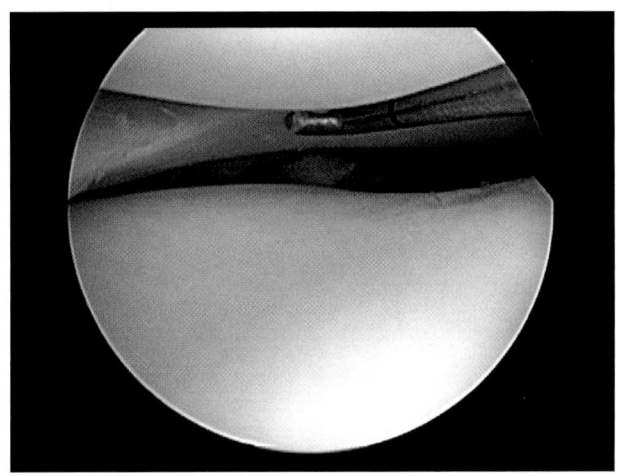

Figure 3-19. Popliteal hiatus seen under the posterior horn of the lateral meniscus.

to approximately 20 degrees of flexion with internal rotation and a varus load applied to open up this triangle and allow for entry into the lateral compartment. Once in the lateral compartment, the surgeon should carry out a systematic evaluation starting with the posterior horn of the lateral meniscus (Figure 3-18). The posterior horn is a common site for missed meniscal tears because it can be hard to visualize directly behind the ACL and tibial spine and is often overlooked on magnetic resonance imaging (MRI). This area should be probed and directly visualized while applying firm, but gentle, varus stress.

The popliteal hiatus should then be probed superiorly and inferiorly (Figure 3-19). Normally, there is more laxity to the posterior horn of the lateral meniscus compared to the medial meniscus; therefore, increased mobility to this meniscus should not be assumed to represent a tear. However, it is important to directly visualize this area because it is not uncommon to find a meniscal tear posterior to the popliteal hiatus overlooked by MRI.[10,11] The popliteus tendon should be probed to assess its degree of laxity, and the hiatus inspected for any occult loose bodies, especially under the synovial fold adjacent to the under-surface of the lateral meniscus.

Next, the mid-body of the lateral meniscus should be evaluated by moving the camera laterally and aiming the arthroscope inferiorly (Figure 3-20). This maneuver is facilitated by a rotating motion so as not to damage the articular surface of the lateral femoral condyle. Again, this part of the meniscus should be probed as it is visualized. The anterior horn is then viewed by holding the

Figure 3-20. Mid-body of the lateral meniscus.

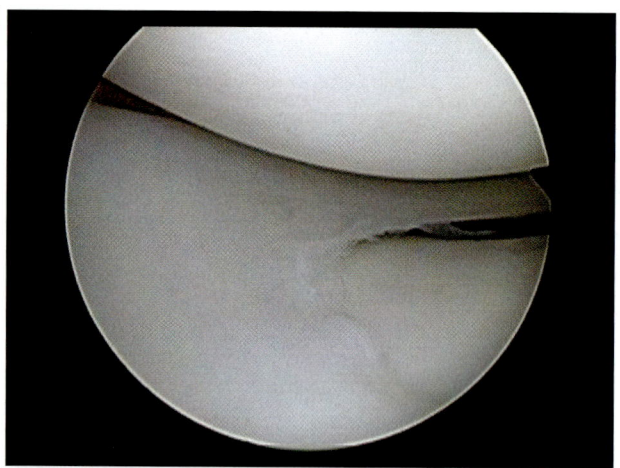

Figure 3-21. Anterior horn of the lateral meniscus.

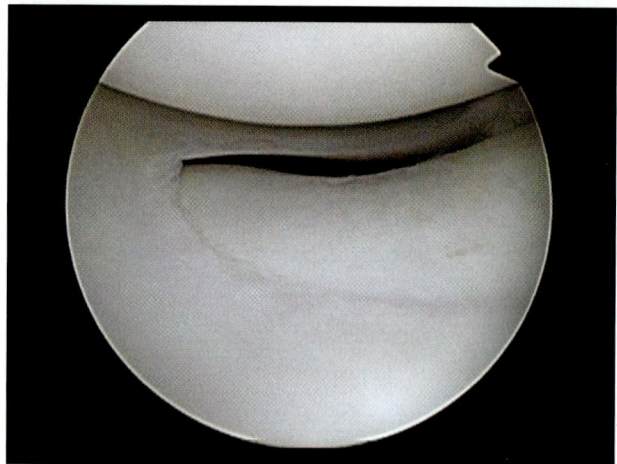

camera still, while aiming the arthroscope directly inferiorly and gently backing it out of the knee (Figure 3-21). This is one of the more difficult areas of the knee to visualize because it is directly beneath the arthroscope.

Finally, the articular surface of the femoral condyle and tibial plateau should be evaluated. This is done by holding the camera stationary and aiming the arthroscope superiorly while taking the knee from near-full extension to 100 degrees of flexion. It is imperative to remove the probe out of the lateral compartment when performing this maneuver to avoid inadvertent injury to the cartilage.

POSTERIOR COMPARTMENTS

The posteromedial and posterolateral compartments are best visualized from the contralateral anterior portals by traversing through the intercondylar notch with the knee at 90 degrees of flexion.[12] To view the posteromedial compartment, the 30-degree arthroscope and cannula are removed from the knee, and the 70-degree arthroscope is coupled to the camera. The blunt trocar is inserted into the arthroscopic cannula, which is then re-introduced through the anterolateral portal, under the PCL in the intercondylar notch, and into the posteromedial compartment.[13] In doing this, the lateral wall of the medial femoral condyle should be palpated with the trocar, and the surgeon should attempt to glide the trocar posteriorly and inferiorly along this wall. This is

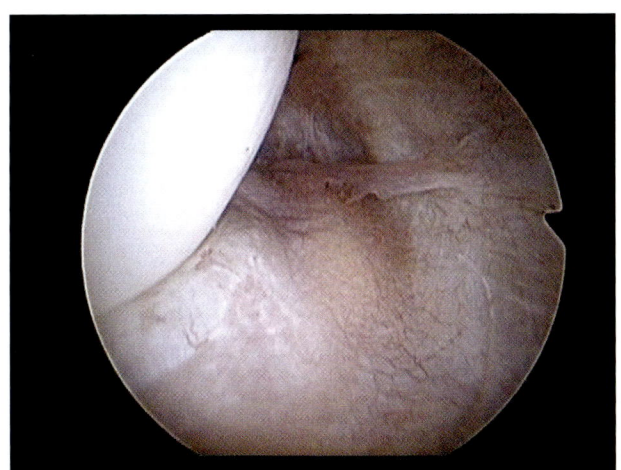

Diagnostic Arthroscopy of the Knee—The 10-Point Exam | 39

Figure 3-22. Posteromedial compartment viewed with a 70-degree arthroscope from the anterolateral portal.

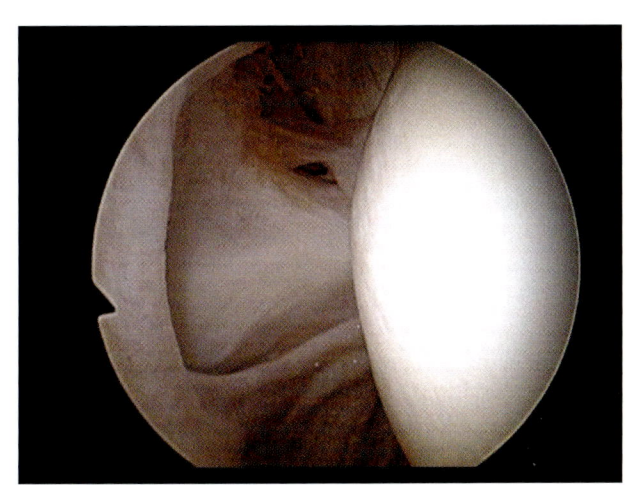

Figure 3-23. Aperture of the semimembranosus bursa seen in the superior aspect of the posteromedial compartment with a 70-degree arthroscope from the anterolateral portal.

facilitated by raising the camera superiorly while extending the knee approximately 20 degrees. Eventually, a palpable giving-way sensation is felt as the trocar is maneuvered past the PCL and into the posteromedial compartment. The trocar is then removed, and the 70-degree arthroscope is locked into the cannula. The inflow is turned on, and the arthroscope is rotated anteriorly and inferiorly. If the arthroscope has been correctly placed, an excellent view of the posterior aspect of the medial femoral condyle and the synovial attachment of the posterior horn of the medial meniscus will be obtained (Figure 3-22). This is an excellent way to view the integrity of the meniscus, assess how much of the meniscus remains following débridement, rule out the presence of a displaced meniscal flap, and look for any loose or, in some cases, foreign bodies. The intra-articular aperture of the semimembranosus bursa can be seen at the superior field of view (Figure 3-23). This is the entry site of joint fluid that can result in a popliteal or Baker's cyst in the presence of osteoarthritis or chronic meniscal tears.

If a loose body or other pathology is identified, the surgeon must be prepared to make an accessory posteromedial portal for access. This portal is created by first trans-illuminating the skin over the posteromedial corner of the knee with the light from the arthroscope. An 18-gauge spinal needle is then inserted into the compartment 2 cm above the medial joint line just posterior to the medial femoral condyle. A longitudinal skin incision is made with a #11 scalpel with care taken to avoid both the saphenous nerve and vein. A sharp trocar is then advanced through this incision

Figure 3-24. Posterolateral compartment viewed with a 70-degree arthroscope from the anteromedial portal showing the popliteal tendon, popliteal hiatus, posterior horn of the lateral meniscus, and posterior surface of the lateral femoral condyle.

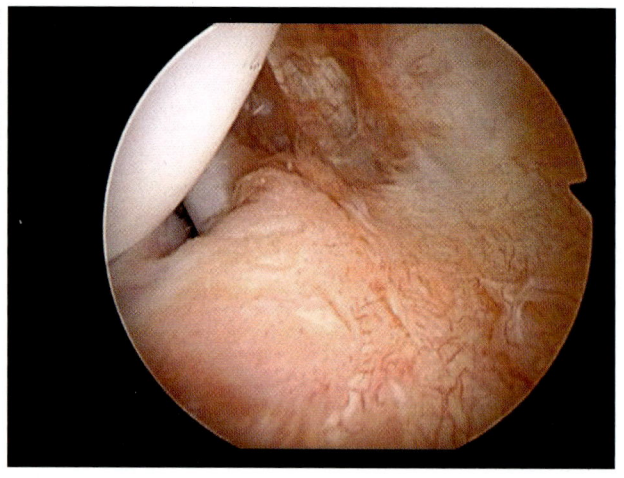

while puncturing the posteromedial capsule under direct visualization. Operating instruments can then be inserted as necessary. The arthroscope can also be inserted into this portal, if needed, to view along the width of the posterior tibial plateau.

The posterolateral compartment can be entered in the same fashion as the posteromedial compartment but is typically easier to reach. The surgeon starts with the knee in 90 degrees of flexion with the trocar placed in the anteromedial portal and directed posterolaterally along the medial wall of the lateral femoral condyle above the ACL. The trocar is moved posteriorly, with a twisting motion, until a giving-way sensation is perceived, indicating successful navigation of the intercondylar notch. From this view, the surgeon can inspect the posterior horn of the lateral meniscus, the extreme posterior aspect of the lateral femoral condyle, and the popliteal hiatus and tendon (Figure 3-24). In a subset of patients, the fabella can be visualized as it articulates with the femoral condyle. The posterolateral compartment is further evaluated for loose bodies or displaced meniscal fragments. If necessary, a posterolateral portal, created similarly to the posteromedial portal, can be made to facilitate loose body removal or meniscal débridement.

The portals may be closed with interrupted absorbable or non-absorbable sutures or staples at the surgeon's discretion. Local anesthetic (20 cc of 0.5% bupivacaine) is injected intra-articularly and into the portal sites, and a sterile dressing is applied with a compressive wrap. The dressing can be removed after 72 hours, when showering over the wound is allowed. However, underwater submersion should be avoided for at least 10 days or until the portals have healed.

TIPS AND PEARLS

- ✔ Several clues exist to the problem of an outflow portal being placed in an intra-synovial location: stagnant-appearing joint fluid, absence of flow through the outflow tubing, and lack of direct visualization of the outflow cannula. If the cannula is not immediately visualized, it must be replaced with the trocar before continuing with the diagnostic examination.

- ✔ Proper orientation of the assembled camera and arthroscope is present if the camera cord ("tail") is pointed toward the floor and the writing on the camera is directed toward the ceiling. This is a useful rule of thumb irrespective of the area of the knee being evaluated.

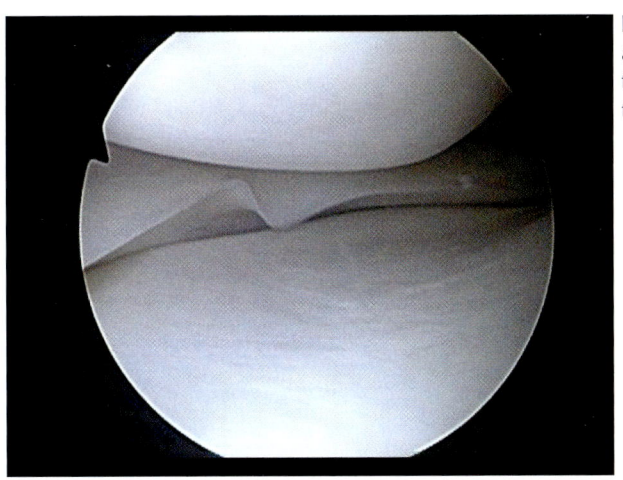

Diagnostic Arthroscopy of the Knee—The 10-Point Exam

Figure 3-25. "Meniscal flounce," seen as a wavy configuration of the inner edge of the medial meniscus, typically indicates the absence of a meniscal tear.

- ✔ It is our preference to have the fluid inflow through the arthroscopic cannula rather than through the suprapatellar cannula, so that joint debris is "blown" away from the viewing scope and out of the knee.
- ✔ With joint distention under fluid pressure, the patella may appear to be subluxed laterally with associated lateral tilt leading to an over-estimation of the tightness of the lateral retinaculum.
- ✔ When attempting to view the anterior interval, the 70-degree arthroscope may be placed through the superomedial portal viewing anteriorly to more thoroughly visualize the anterior compartment, though this is rarely necessary.
- ✔ Absence of "meniscal flounce," seen as a wavy configuration of the medial meniscus (Figure 3-25), is often indicative of an occult meniscal tear.[14]
- ✔ The probe should be used to pull the anterior horn of the lateral meniscus anteriorly to allow smooth advancement of the arthroscope into the lateral compartment over the probe. The probe can then be passed straight posteriorly into the field of view. If there is any question as to the integrity of the anterior horn of the lateral meniscus, the arthroscope should be switched to the anteromedial portal for more direct visualization. This also applies to any situation in which the entirety of the lateral meniscus cannot be thoroughly viewed or if a surgical procedure (ie, meniscectomy) cannot be completely performed through the anteromedial portal.
- ✔ As the lateral tibial plateau is convex from anterior to posterior, there is a corresponding concavity in the medial aspect of the lateral femoral condyle, known as the "condylopatellar sulcus," or "sulcus terminalis." This normal articular contour should not be mistaken for a compression fracture or cartilage defect.
- ✔ A good rule of thumb as to whether or not the surgeon has successfully navigated into the posteromedial or posterolateral compartment is that the hub of the cannula should rest approximately 3 to 4 cm from the portal.
- ✔ At the end of the arthroscopy, the knee should be copiously irrigated to facilitate the removal of any loose debris. The surgeon should cycle the knee from flexion to extension multiple times to free up debris that may be lodged in the back of the joint.

Pitfalls

✗ Inferior orientation of the scalpel blade while making the anteromedial and anterolateral portal incisions should be avoided because this may lead to inadvertent laceration of the anterior meniscal horn.

✗ Undue valgus strain upon the knee should be avoided, especially in older adults, to avoid iatrogenic rupture of the medial collateral ligament or fracture of the distal femur. Typically, there is no more than 6 mm of separation between the medial femoral condyle and tibial plateau.

✗ It is important to examine the full extent of the femoral condyle(s) because a far posterior or anterior condylar defect is not always readily apparent upon initial entry into the compartment(s).

✗ Failure to go "up and over" the ligamentum mucosum will lead to entrapment of the arthroscope within the retropatellar fat pad signified by a diffuse yellow appearance. If this occurs, the knee may be extended and the arthroscope placed in the patellofemoral joint. With gradual knee flexion, the arthroscope is aimed distally (downward) to descend down into the notch. Débridement of the ligamentum mucosum and fat pad will facilitate this maneuver in order to thoroughly view the cruciate ligaments.

References

1. Patel D. Arthroscopy of the plicae—synovial folds and their significance. *Am J Sports Med.* 1978;6(5):217-225.
2. Ogilvie-Harris DJ, Basinski A. Arthroscopic synovectomy of the knee for rheumatoid arthritis. *Arthroscopy.* 1991;7(1):91-97.
3. Bach BR Jr, Warren RF. "Empty wall" and "vertical strut" signs of ACL insufficiency. *Arthroscopy.* 1989;5(2):137-140.
4. Jackson RW. Current concepts review arthroscopic surgery. *J Bone Joint Surg Am.* 1983;65(3):416-420.
5. McGuire DA, Wolchok JC. Arthroscopic Lachman test: a new technique using anatomic references. *Arthroscopy.* 1998;14(6):641-642.
6. Dupont J. Synovial plicae of the knee: controversies and review. *Clin Sports Med.* 1997;16(1):87-122.
7. Lysholm J, Gillquist J. Arthroscopic examination of the posterior cruciate ligament. *J Bone Joint Surg Am.* 1981;63:363-366.
8. McMahon PJ, Dettling JR, Yocum LA, et al. The cyclops lesion: a cause of diminished knee extension after rupture of the anterior cruciate ligament. *Arthroscopy.* 1999;15(7):757-761.
9. Olson PN, Rud P, Griffiths HJ. Cyclops lesion. *Orthopedics.* 1995;18(10):1041-1045.
10. Kimura M, Shirakura K, Hasegawa A, et al. Anatomy and pathophysiology of the popliteal tendon area in the lateral meniscus: 1. arthroscopic and anatomical investigation. *Arthroscopy.* 1992;8(4):419-423.
11. Kimura M, Shirakura K, Hasegawa A, et al. Anatomy and pathophysiology of the popliteal tendon area in the lateral meniscus: 2. clinical investigation. *Arthroscopy.* 1992;8(4):424-427.
12. Morin WD, Steadman JR. Arthroscopic assessment of the posterior compartments of the knee via the intercondylar notch: the arthroscopist's field of view. *Arthroscopy.* 1993;9(3):284-290.
13. Gillquist J, Hagberg G, Oretorp N. Arthroscopic examination of the posteromedial compartment of the knee joint. *Int Orthop.* 1979;3(1):13-18.
14. Wright RW, Boyer DS. Significance of the arthroscopic meniscal flounce sign: a prospective study. *Am J Sports Med.* 2007;35:242-244.

Techniques of Meniscal Repair

Asheesh Bedi, MD and Russell F. Warren, MD

The crucial role of the medial and lateral menisci in load transmission, shock absorption, and secondary stabilization of the knee has been increasingly recognized during the past several years. Total meniscectomy was the historical treatment of choice for a torn meniscus. Several long-term studies have subsequently demonstrated complete or partial meniscectomy to be deleterious to the chondral surface. Degenerative changes have been reported in 38% of patients after medial meniscectomy and 24% of patients after lateral meniscectomy at an mean duration of 5 years postoperatively.[1] Furthermore, knee function has been shown to inversely correlate with the volume of meniscus that is resected.[2]

With this increased appreciation of meniscal function, surgical techniques have focused on preservation and repair whenever possible. Arthroscopy has allowed for various repair strategies with minimal invasion and excellent visualization. This chapter will present our preferred approach to the evaluation and management of repairable meniscal tears.

"TIPS AND PEARLS" FOR MENISCAL REPAIR PATIENT SELECTION

Tear selection is the most important factor for success with meniscal repair surgery. The decision to repair a meniscus tear is based on several factors, including the location of the tear, pattern of tear, length of tear, chronicity, ligamentous stability of the knee, and patient age. While each case must be evaluated on an individual basis, we have found the following principles to be useful in guiding our decision-making process:

* Rim width is the most important prognostic criteria for healing after meniscal repair. Therefore, peripheral, longitudinal tears within 3 mm (red-red zone) of the meniscocapsular junction should be repaired. Longitudinal tears within 3 to 6 mm width (red-white zone) have less predictable success, but should still be considered for repair in younger patients. Tears more than 6 mm from the peripheral blood supply are generally avascular and are not suitable for repair (Figure 4-1).

* Acute, traumatic tears have an improved prognosis for healing compared to chronic, degenerative lesions.

* Atraumatic tears, even in younger patients, are usually degenerative and are typically poor candidates for operative repair.

Figure 4-1. Sagittal section demonstrating peripheral vascular zone and peripheral capillary plexus (PCP) of the meniscus in a canine model. Healing is predictably improved after meniscal repair in the vascular zone. F=femur, T=tibia. (Reprinted with permission from Arnoczky SP, Warren RF. Microvasculature of the human meniscus. *Am J Sports Med.* 1982;10(2):90-95. © 1982 by *Am J Sports Med.* Reprinted with permission of SAGE Publications.)

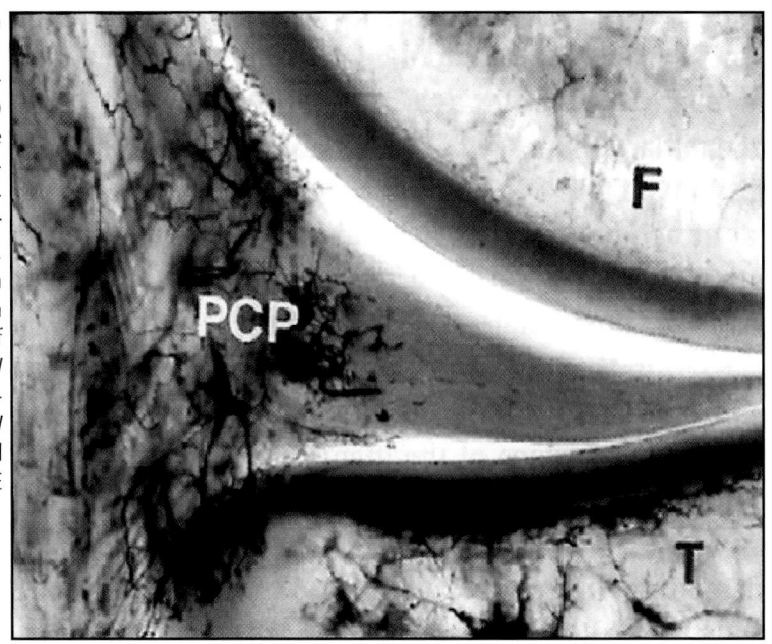

* Longitudinal tears are more amenable to repair than the flap, horizontal cleavage, or complex degenerative patterns (Figure 4-2).
* The management of the radial tear is controversial. Large radial tears extending to the periphery are technically easy to repair and should be considered for repair in young patients to restore hoop stresses and load transmission function of the meniscus. Tears that extend up to half the width of the meniscus or less are more difficult to repair and are of questionable benefit (Figure 4-3).
* Age should not be used as an absolute criteria for determining the feasibility of repair. While younger patients have a more favorable prognosis, successful healing has been reported in older patients. Therefore, the decision should be guided by the patient's activity level, functional expectations, and quality of the tissues.
* Higher rates of failure have been noted in the setting of unstable knees secondary to excessive shear forces that prevent healing. Therefore, an insufficient anterior cruciate ligament (ACL) should be reconstructed at the time of meniscal repair.
* Partial-thickness tears that are shallow and stable (<3 mm depth and <1 cm length) generally heal spontaneously. Unstable partial-thickness tears, however, should be repaired. The eyelid sign, defined by the meniscus, which may be lifted and everted at the tear with probing, is a sign of instability and should prompt a repair (Figure 4-4).

SURGERY

PEARLS FOR PATIENT POSITIONING

Careful attention to patient positioning is critical to ensure that the knee is accessible circumferentially. The tourniquet is positioned on the proximal thigh at least 14 cm above the joint line. The patient is placed supine on the table such that the break in the table is at the distal thigh to

Techniques of Meniscal Repair | 47

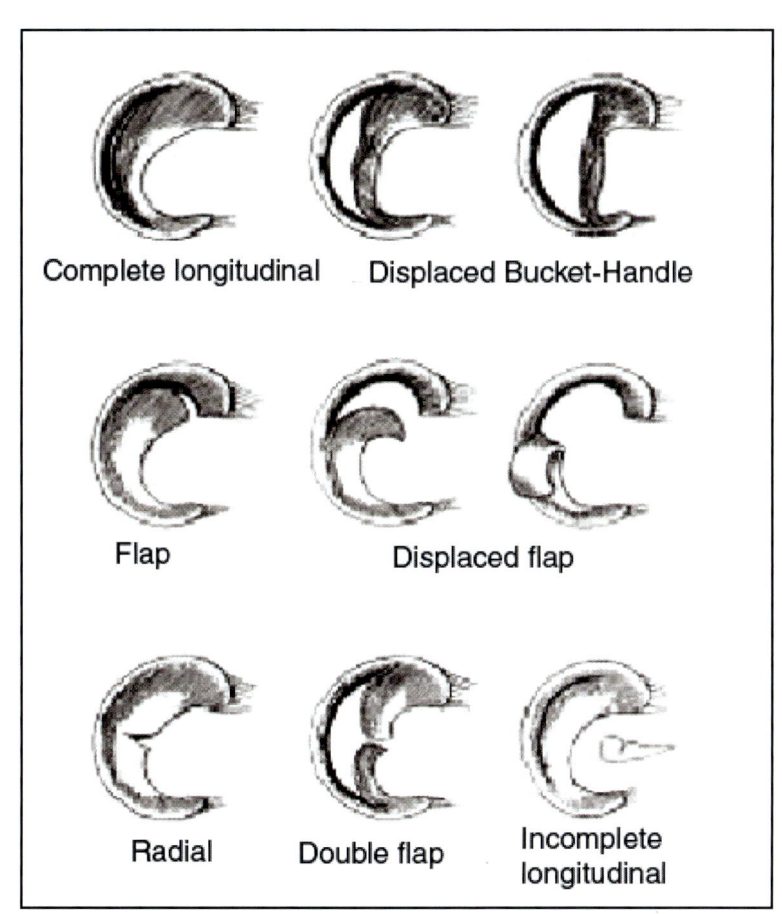

Figure 4-2. Variable patterns of meniscal tears.

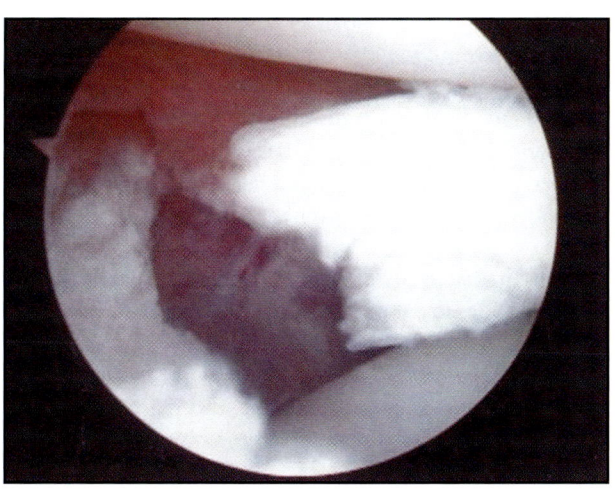

Figure 4-3. Arthroscopic photo of a complete radial tear at the middle and posterior body junction of the lateral meniscus.

allow for full flexion and extension of the knee as necessary. A well-padded post is positioned at the level of the tourniquet to allow for valgus stress and access to the medial compartment. Circumferential access to the knee is ensured before arthroscopy, such that a posteromedial or posterolateral exposure for suture passage and capture can be easily performed if an inside-out technique is selected.

Figure 4-4. Eyelid sign—this partial-thickness meniscal tear can be everted at the tear with gentle probing and is a sign of instability.

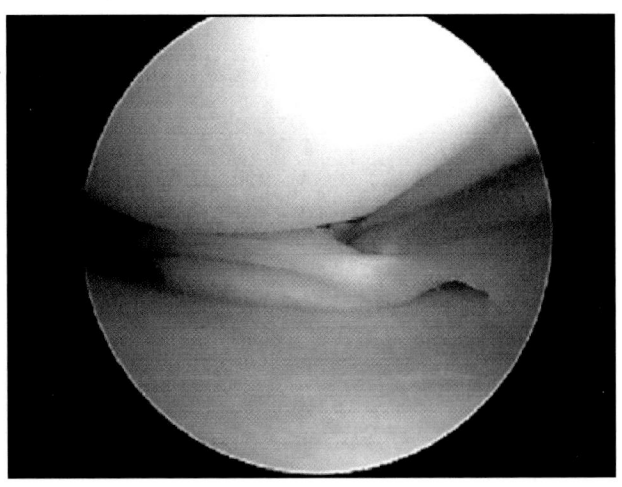

SURGICAL TECHNIQUE TIPS

Evaluate the medial and lateral meniscus with a 30-degree arthroscope as part of standard, comprehensive arthroscopy of the knee. Probe the anterior horn, body, and posterior horns on both superior and inferior surfaces. Place the nerve hook in the popliteal hiatus, and confirm a secure lateral meniscocapsular junction by attempting to sublux the lateral meniscus into the joint. An injury to the lateral meniscocapsular tissues can render the meniscus completely unstable and requires repair. Pass the arthroscope from the anterolateral portal into the notch between the medial femoral condyle and posterior cruciate ligament (PCL) to visualize the posterior horn of the medial meniscus. A very peripheral, posterior horn longitudinal tear can be missed without viewing from this position. A 70-degree arthroscope may also be used improve visualization. Advance the arthroscope from the anteromedial portal underneath the ACL to visualize the posterolateral compartment and examine for any occult posterior horn lateral meniscal tears.

If a repairable posterior tear is visualized, a posteromedial or posterolateral portal can be created to improve visualization and to provide access for tear preparation. The posteromedial portal is created with the knee at 90 degrees of flexion. Place a spinal needle about 1 cm above the medial joint line and anterior to the hamstring tendons under direct visualization. Placing the portal above the hamstring tendons with a flexed knee protects the saphenous nerve running along the inferior border of the sartorius. After satisfactory positioning, remove the spinal needle, and make a small incision along the same trajectory.

Access to the posterior horn of the medial meniscus from a posteromedial portal can be improved by applying an internal rotation force on the flexed knee, which acts to move the meniscus posteriorly. The posterolateral portal is created in a similar fashion with the knee at 90 degrees of flexion. This is critical to decrease tension on the peroneal nerve and allow it to translate posterior to the biceps tendon. Under direct visualization, a spinal needle is advanced anterior to the biceps tendon and posterior to the iliotibial band (ITB) approximately 1 cm above the joint line. Make an incision along the same path after a satisfactory trajectory is achieved.

TEAR PREPARATION

Use a full-radius, motorized arthroscopic shaver or rasp to prepare the apposing edges of the meniscal tear. We use a small 3.5-mm radius cutting head due to its small size and easy maneuverability into the tear. Complete tear débridement and rasping is essential to promote a potent healing response (Figure 4-5). Rasp the synovial fringes at the meniscocapsular junction in the zone

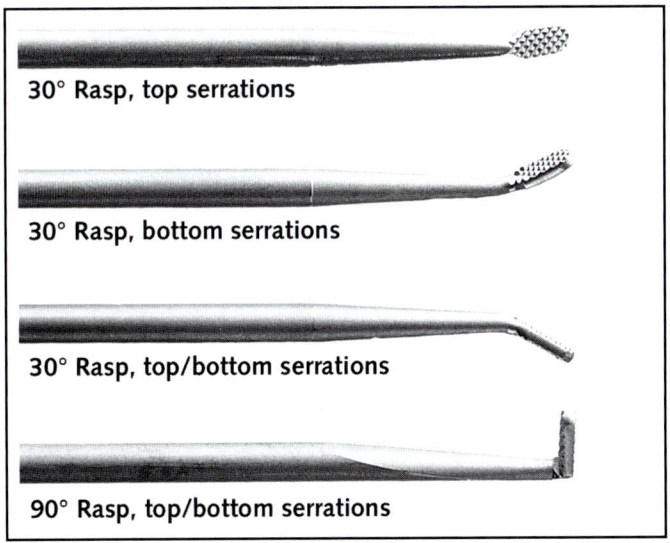

Figure 4-5. Different angle rasps that can be used to prepare the meniscal tear and stimulate mesenchymal stem cells and a healing response. (Reprinted with permission from Conmed-Linvatec Inc, Largo, FL.)

of the tear to incite a vascular healing response and stimulate mesenchymal stem cells. Posterior longitudinal tears of the medial meniscus may require instrumentation through a posteromedial portal (see above).

REPAIR TECHNIQUES

Outside-In Repair

Advantages/Indications

Outside-in repair is particular well-suited for anterior horn tears that cannot be approached from a desirable angle with all-inside or inside-out techniques. Needles can be safely placed anteriorly using the topographic anatomy of the joint line (Figure 4-6). Outside-in repair is often useful for the middle and anterior zone fixation of meniscus allografts in which secure, circumferential sutures are necessary. This technique is simple and can be performed with 2 18-gauge spinal needles, a suture grasper, and nonabsorbable suture. This method affords increased flexibility and varied angle of approaches to the meniscus tear relative to the more restricted access afforded by rigid cannulas used with an inside-out technique (see Figure 4-6). The smaller instrumentation may also have less risk of iatrogenic chondral injury compared to the instrumentation required for all-inside or inside-out repair. Fibrin clot fixation for augmentation of healing is technically easy with this technique.

Limitations

Far posterior horn tears of the meniscus that approach the midline are difficult to safely access, due to the danger of injury to the neurovascular structures with spinal needle placement. The angle of needle entry is sometimes limited and can preclude anatomic reduction and closure of the tear with suture tensioning and fixation.

Technique

Visualize the pattern and extent of the tear to determine optimal suture configuration. Plan the external entry site for the spinal needles by finger palpation along the joint line (Figure 4-7). A probe may be placed through an anterior portal and pushed against the capsule to facilitate localizing the joint line.

Figure 4-6. Principles of outside-in repair. Spinal needles are placed to pass sutures and perform a mattress suture repair of the tear. This technique is particularly useful for anterior horn tears that cannot be approached via all-inside or inside-out techniques. (Reprinted with permission from Rodeo SA, Warren RF. Meniscal repair using the outside-to-inside technique. *Clin Sports Med.* 1996;15:469-481 © Elsevier 1996.)

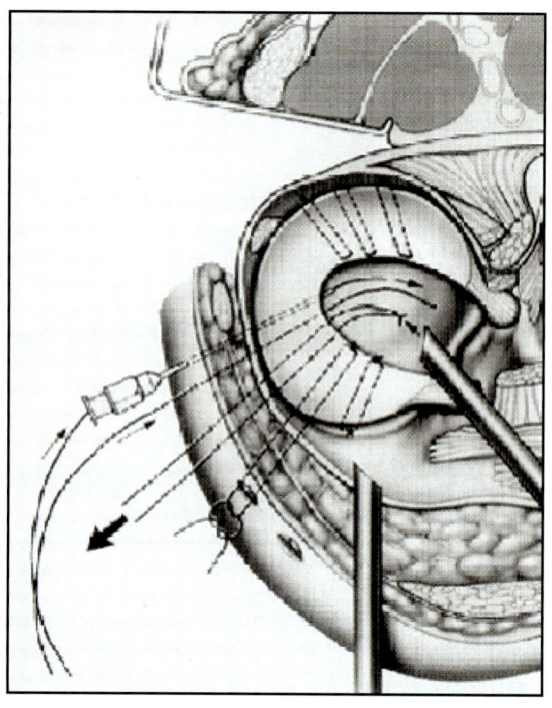

Figure 4-7. Photograph demonstrating spinal needle insertion at the joint line and through meniscus for outside-in repair. The light from the arthroscope or a probe within the joint can help to localize the joint line.

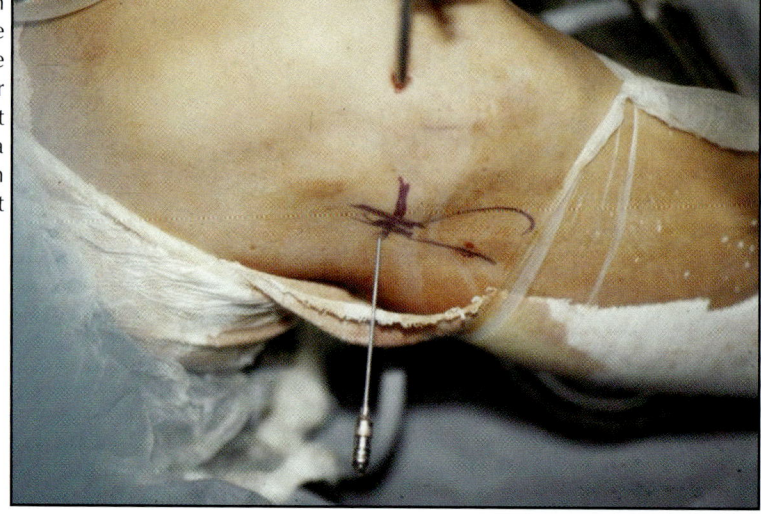

Trans-illumination with the arthroscope can facilitate visualization and avoidance of the saphenous nerve and vein with needle passage. Insert an 18-gauge spinal needle, and impale the meniscus at the desired location as it passes into the joint (Figure 4-8).

Insert a 2-0 PDS (polydioxanone) suture into the spinal needle until it is clearly visualized within the joint. Retrieve the PDS suture with a grasper, and pull out the anterior portal. Make sure that the needle is withdrawn as the suture is retrieved to avoid cutting the suture on the sharp needle tip. Replace the spinal needle to allow penetration of the meniscus 3 to 4 mm from the prior location, creating a mattress suture configuration across the tear. Ideal needle orientation for repair of a peripheral longitudinal tear is shown (Figure 4-9).

Techniques of Meniscal Repair 51

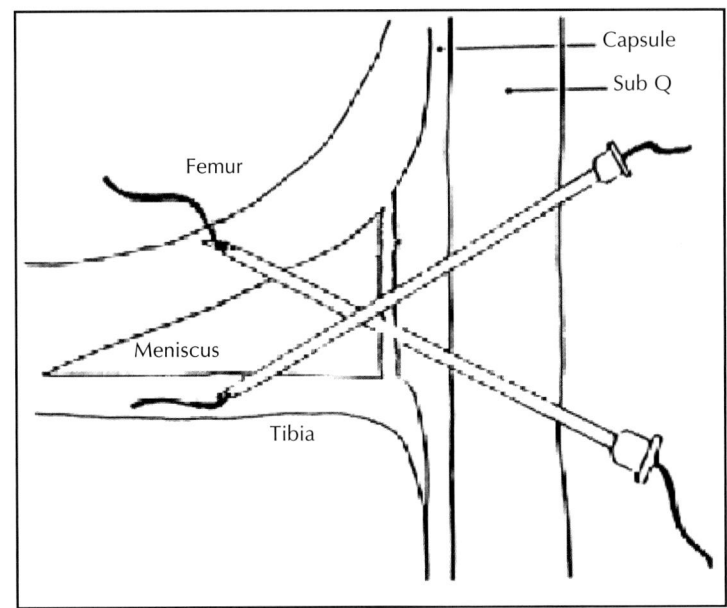

Figure 4-8. Ideal spinal needle orientation for outside-in repair of a peripheral, longitudinal meniscal tear. (Reprinted with permission from Cohen DB, Wickiewicz TL. The outside-in technique for arthroscopic meniscal repair. *Operative Techniques in Sports Medicine.* 2003;11(2):91-103. © 2003 with permission from Elsevier.)

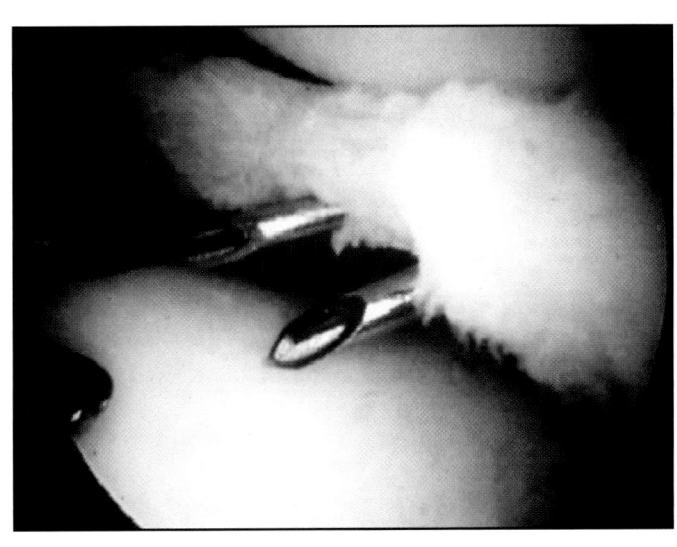

Figure 4-9. Arthroscopic photo demonstrating 2 spinal needles in place to allow for outside-in mattress suture repair of a radial tear.

Insert and retrieve another 2-0 PDS suture from the anterior portal as above.

Tie the 2 PDS sutures together with a simple knot outside of the anterior portal. Make sure the knot is secure, as a loose knot will unravel during suture shuttling through the meniscus. A small "dilator" knot can be placed in front of this knot on the shuttle limb to facilitate passage through the meniscus.

Pull 1 of the 2 sutures at the external entry site to allow shuttling of a single suture across the meniscus, creating a mattress repair (Figure 4-10). Alternatively, the end of each separate suture can be tied in a standard square (so-called "Mulberry") knot. The knots are then pulled back into the joint from the anterior portal, such that they reduce the tear and rest firmly against the femoral or tibial surface of the meniscus (Figure 4-11). Create a small skin incision connecting the suture limbs at the external entry sites. Retrieve the suture through the incision, and apply light

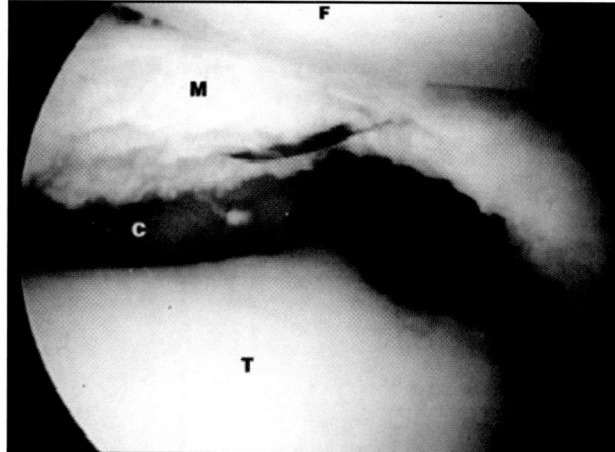

Figure 4-10. Horizontal mattress suture placed via outside-in technique for repair of peripheral zone of a radial tear. F = femur, T = tibia, C = capsule, M = meniscus. (Reprinted with permission from Cohen DB, Wickiewicz TL. The outside-in technique for arthroscopic meniscal repair. *Operative Techniques in Sports Medicine.* 2003;11(2):91-103. © 2003 with permission from Elsevier.)

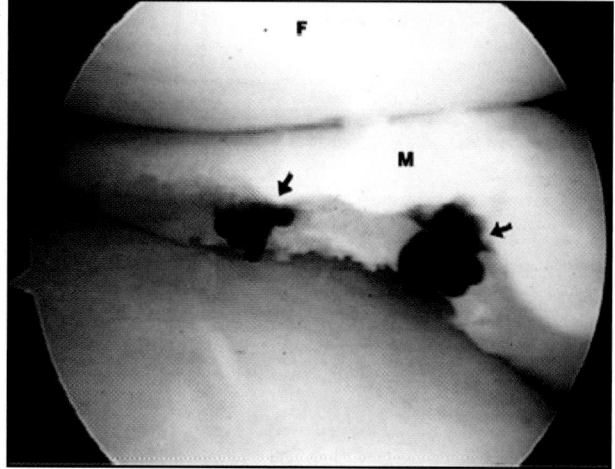

Figure 4-11. Alternative "Mulberry" knot technique to reduce and repair meniscus tear via outside-in technique. Arrows point to knots that have been tied and pulled back into the joint to rest firmly against the meniscal surface and secure the repair. F = femur, M = meniscus. (Reprinted with permission from Cohen DB, Wickiewicz TL. The outside-in technique for arthroscopic meniscal repair. *Operative Techniques in Sports Medicine.* 2003;11(2):91-103. © 2003 with permission from Elsevier.)

traction, confirming reduction of the tear arthroscopically. Clamp but do not tie paired sutures until all sutures are placed.

Bluntly dissect through subcutaneous fat to the capsule, retracting and protecting the cutaneous nerves. Tie paired sutures down directly on the capsule.

Beware of the inferior lateral genicular artery, which courses along the joint line and is at particular risk during outside-in repair of lateral meniscal tears.

Close the small incisions in standard, layered fashion. The procedure can alternatively be performed with spinal needles and wire cable loop that is passed through the spinal needle to facilitate suture shuttling. For repairable bucket handle tears, the fragment should be reduced and secured first with a suture at the mid-portion of the tear. Traction on this suture will reduce the tear and facilitate the placement of remaining stitches. Subsequent stitches should be alternated anterior and posterior to the middle stitch to achieve anatomic reduction of the tear.

Inside-Out Repair

Advantages/Indications

This is the historical "gold standard" of meniscal repair techniques. It allows repair of extensive tears that would otherwise require both anterior and posterior approaches with outside-in techniques, and it allows for biomechanically favorable, vertical mattress suture configuration.

Limitations

The approach is difficult for far posterior horn tears that approach the midline, due to the risk of neurovascular injury with needle passage. This technique is difficult for anterior zone tears, due to suboptimal trajectory afforded by portals and rigid cannulas, and it requires open posterolateral or posteromedial exposure with the associated risks of wound complication and neurovascular injury.

Technique—Medial Meniscus

The position of the anteromedial portal is critical to allow adequate access to the posterior horn. Confirm the trajectory prior to creating the portal with a spinal needle; it should enter just superior to the anterior horn of the medial meniscus at a trajectory that is tangential to the plateau. Portals that are too high cannot access the posterior horn due to obstruction from the medial femoral condyle.

Create a posteromedial extracapsular exposure. With the knee in 70 to 80 degrees of flexion, create a 4-cm incision parallel and posterior to the medial collateral ligament. The incision is centered with one third above and two thirds below the joint line. Localization of the joint line can be facilitated by pressing the arthroscopic probe against the capsule (Figure 4-12).

Sharp dissection is performed down the sartorial fascia. The fascia is divided along the anterior border of the sartorius. The sartorius and the saphenous nerve run along its inferior border and are protected by retracting the pes tendons posteriorly. Blunt finger dissection subsequently exposes an extracapsular plane anterior to the medial head of the gastrocnemius and semimembranosus tendon. The joint line sulcus can be palpated if the appropriate surgical plane has been identified (see Figure 4-12). Place a Henning retractor in this space to protect posterior neurovascular structures during suture passage and retrieval.

Place the knee in 10 to 20 degrees of flexion. This helps to reduce longitudinal tear edges and further avoids risk of creating a flexion contracture from posterior capsular plication. Visualize the tear, and determine the appropriate angle of approach for vertical mattress suture placement. Posterior horn tears are frequently best approached directly with a cannula in the anteromedial portal, while body tears may be better approached from the anterolateral portal.

Various single- and double-lumen cannula systems are available for suture passage. We prefer using single- and double-lumen zone-specific cannula systems (Linvatec Inc, Largo, FL) (Figure 4-13). We typically use 2-0 nonabsorbable Ethibond (Ethicon Endo-Surgery, Inc, Cincinnati, OH) suture for our inside-out repairs.

The configuration and number of sutures are determined by the tissue quality and tear pattern. Ideally, vertical mattress sutures are placed at 3- to 4-mm intervals along the entire length of the tear. Sutures should be inserted from both the superior and inferior surfaces of the meniscus to reduce and oppose the torn surfaces (Figure 4-14).

The appropriate zone-specific cannula is selected and introduced into the medial compartment. The cannula is rigid and pre-bent with curves to approach the anterior, middle, or posterior zones of the meniscus (see Figure 4-13).

With the cannula in position, the 10-inch flexible needle of a double-arm 2-0 Ethibond suture is advanced until the tip is exposed. The tip can be used with the cannula to harpoon, oppose, and reduce the torn edges. The needle is then advanced across the tear.

The cannula must be held securely during needle passage to avoid skiving the needle off the meniscus surface with passage.

The tip of the cannula should always be directed away from the midline and toward the Henning retractor. Tactile feedback of resistance of the needle against the retractor after 1- to 2-cm of advancement confirms appropriate trajectory.

The needles have a tendency to exit inferior to the popliteal retractor. The assistant should hold and "toe-in" the retractor to facilitate proper needle capture with passage.

Figure 4-12. Posteromedial approach for inside-out meniscal repair. The fascia is divided along the anterior border of the Sartorius, and the pes tendons are retracted posteriorly. The extracapsular plane anterior to the medial head of the gastrocnemius and semimembranosus tendons is exploited to create space for the Henning retractor. (© 2005 American Academy of Orthopaedic Surgeons. Reprinted from the *Journal of the American Academy of Orthopaedic Surgeons*, Volume 13(2), pp. 121-128 with permission.)

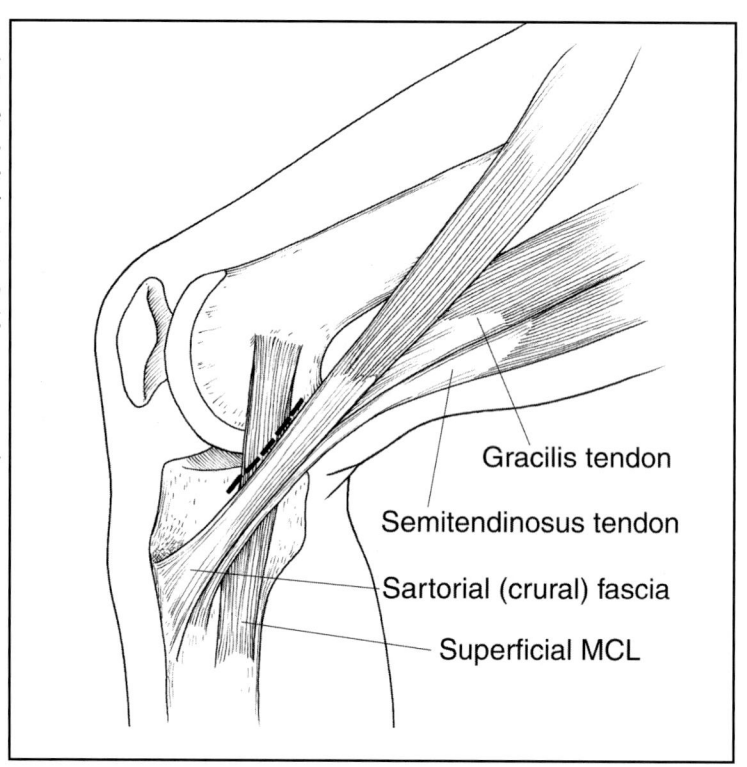

Figure 4-13. Zone-specific cannula systems to facilitate suture passage and repair in a mattress configuration. (Reprinted with permission from Conmed-Linvatec Inc, Largo, FL).

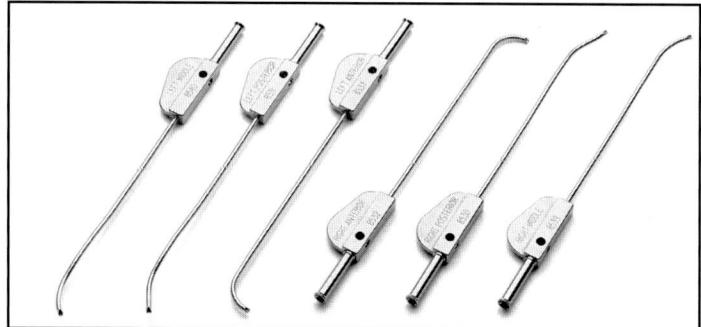

The needle with the attached suture is visualized and retrieved by an assistant with a needle driver. The needle is cut and safely disposed. Advance the companion needle in a similar fashion at a position 3 to 4 mm from the prior pass to create a vertical or horizontal suture configuration. The paired sutures are clamped but not tied until all sutures have been passed.

Repeat the above steps until an appropriate number of stitches have been placed for a secure repair.

Peripheral radial tears may be repaired using a horizontal mattress configuration, with sutures placed on either side of the tear. Multiple sutures may be placed based on the depth of tear and tissue quality.

After all sutures have been placed, probe the meniscus, and repair while light traction is applied to the sutures. After satisfactory reduction is visibly confirmed, separate each suture pair, and clear any extraneous tissue. Tie sutures securely to the capsule, progressing from posterior to anterior with the knee held in 0 to 10 degrees of flexion. Do not tie the sutures with the knee in

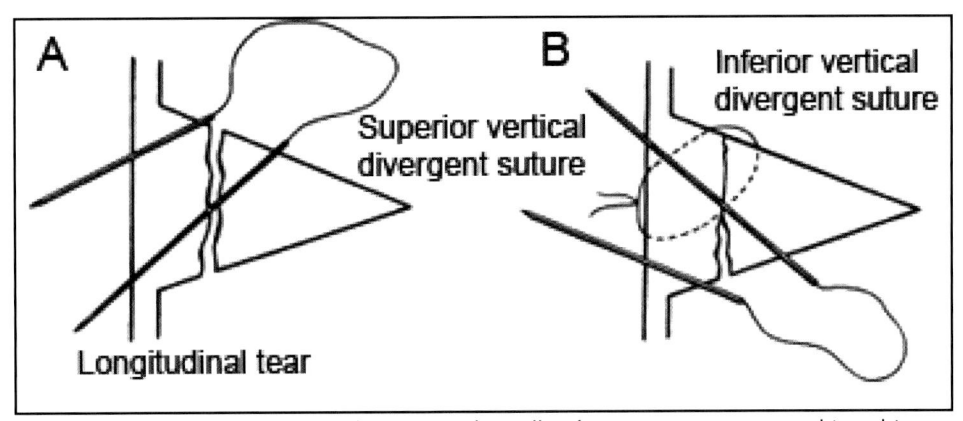

Figure 4-14. Ideal, divergent configuration of needles for suture passage to achieve biomechanically superior vertical mattress repair with inside-out technique. (*American Journal of Sports Medicine* by Noyes FR, Barber-Westin SD. Copyright 2002 by SAGE Publications Inc. Permission conveyed through Copyright Clearance Center, Inc.)

significant flexion, as posterior capsular plication and a secondary flexion contracture can result. Irrigate and close the posteromedial exposure in a standard, layered fashion.

Technique—Lateral Meniscus

Create a posterolateral knee exposure. Place the knee in 70 degrees of flexion to allow the peroneal nerve to translate posteriorly and inferiorly to the biceps tendon (Figure 4-15). Make a 4-cm incision along the posterior margin of the ITB with one third centered above and two thirds centered below the joint line. Typically, the skin incision will extend from the fibular styloid proximally. Localization of the joint line can be facilitated by pressing the arthroscopic probe against the capsule.

Sharp dissection is undertaken down to the ITB and biceps fascia. Divide the fascia along the anterior margin of the biceps and the posterior border of the ITB. The peroneal nerve is medial and posterior to the biceps, such that dissection should never be directed posterior to the biceps tendon (see Figure 4-15). Blunt finger dissection will develop the deeper plane between the posterolateral knee capsule and the lateral head of the gastrocnemius tendon. The retracted gastrocnemius tendon and biceps tendon will both serve to protect the peroneal nerve. The lateral gastrocnemius is proximally more adherent to the capsule relative to the medial side. Identification of the plane may be facilitated by dissecting distally where the layers are more separable. Passive ankle dorsiflexion may also relax the gastrocnemius and facilitate retraction.

Place the Henning retractor into this interval just posterior to the capsule at the joint line. Place the knee in the figure-of-four position with 50 to 70 degrees of flexion for lateral meniscus repair.

With the zone-specific cannulas placed via the anterolateral portal and the camera positioned anteromedially, the tear is visualized and repaired with mattress sutures. The steps of suture passage and fixation are similar to that of medical meniscus repair and are described above.

While every attempt is made to avoid the popliteus tendon with needle passage, it can be incorporated into the repair if necessary for optimal suture configuration and repair.

Exercise particular caution with needle trajectory at the posterior horn of the lateral meniscus given the proximity of the popliteal artery. Never pass needles from the anterolateral portal for a lateral posterior horn tear, given the risk of midline needle passage and neurovascular injury.

Figure 4-15. Posterolateral approach for inside-out meniscal repair. The fascia is divided in the interval anterior to the biceps tendon and posterior to the ITB. Blunt dissection can subsequently develop the plane between the capsule anteriorly and the lateral head of the gastrocnemius posteriorly. The Henning retractor can be placed in this interval. Dissection should never proceed posterior to the biceps tendon in the region of the peroneal nerve. (© 2005 American Academy of Orthopaedic Surgeons. Reprinted from the *Journal of the American Academy of Orthopaedic Surgeons*, Volume 13(2), pp. 121-128 with permission.)

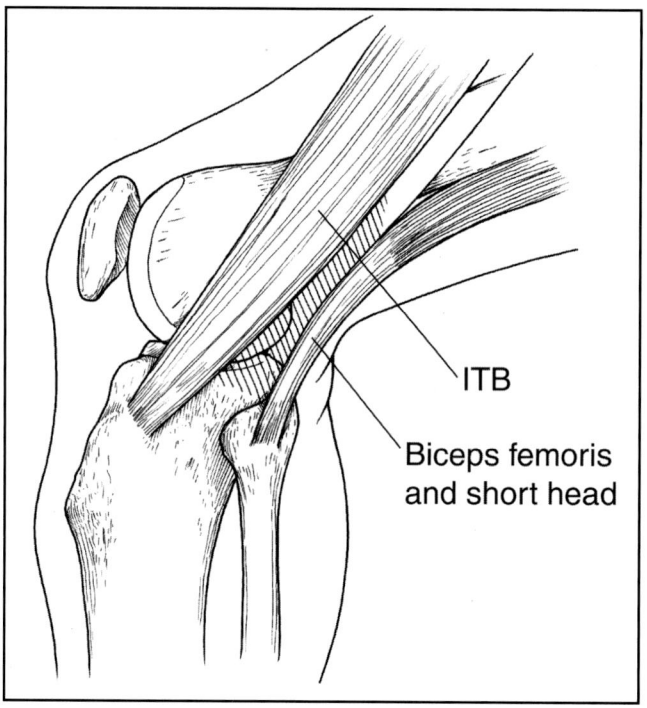

All-Inside Repair

Advantages/Indications

All-inside repair is particularly useful for repairable posterior horn tears approaching the midline, in which it is difficult to expose and protect neurovascular structures using inside-out or outside-in techniques. No open posterior capsular exposure is required. There is no risk of flexion contracture from posterior capsular plication that can occur with inside-out or outside-in techniques. Improved devices are versatile and allow for mattress suture configuration in most zones (Figure 4-16).[3-10] Biomechanically equivalent outcomes to standard vertical mattress repairs have been reported with later-generation devices. Fourth-generation devices can deform and translate with the meniscus during weightbearing, thereby reducing the risk of iatrogenic chondral injury.

Limitations

The stability of these repair devices requires an intact meniscocapsular junction. Therefore, frank meniscocapsular separation is a contraindication to their use. Access for anterior zone repairs is extremely difficult and is better suited for repair with outside-in techniques.

Technique (FasT-Fix)

While various devices are available, we prefer the FasT-Fix (Smith & Nephew, London, United Kingdom) for all-inside repair. This is a fourth-generation device that can be inserted using standard anterior arthroscopic portals (Figure 4-17). The device uses 2 peripheral T-fix anchors on a single inserter. The anchors are separately placed extracapsular or at the meniscocapsular junction across the tear and secured with an O-polyester suture and a tensioned slip knot.

Select the straight or curved delivery needle for optimal trajectory and suture placement across the tear. Cut the depth penetration limiter to 13 mm. This preset depth helps to avoid potential

Techniques of Meniscal Repair 57

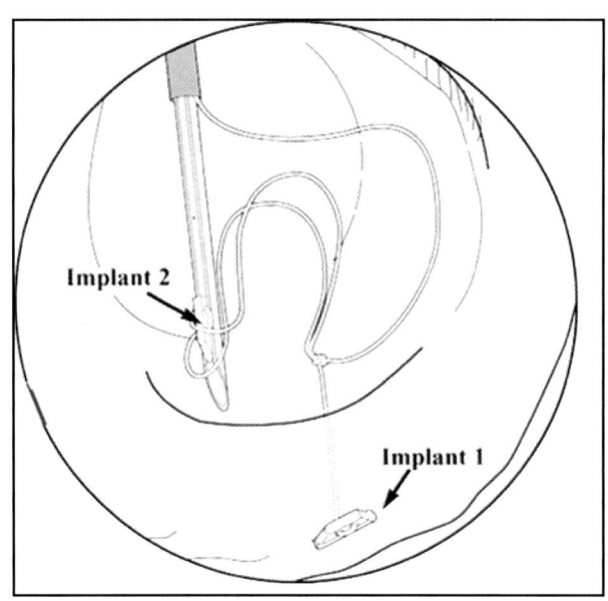

Figure 4-16. Concept of all-inside meniscal repair. Two peripheral anchors are loaded on a single inserter. The anchors are deployed separately at different extracapsular locations to create a mattress configuration across the tear. The repair is secured with a tensioned slip knot. (Reprinted with permission from Smith & Nephew Inc, London, United Kingdom).

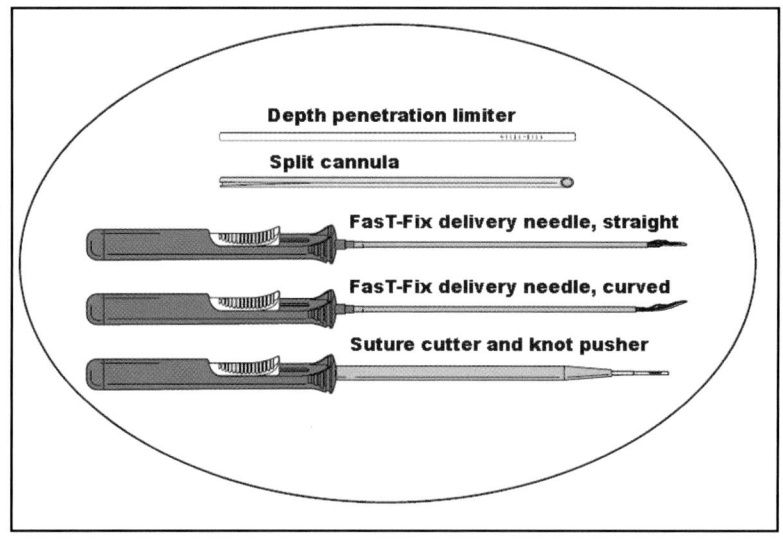

Figure 4-17. Equipment provided for the FasT-Fix All-inside Repair System. (Reprinted with permission from Smith & Nephew Inc, London, United Kingdom).

neurovascular injury from the delivery needle. Advance the delivery needle and penetration limiter through the split cannula via an anterior arthroscopic portal. The split in the cannula should be oriented 90 degrees relative to the delivery needle (Figure 4-18). Remove the split cannula after introducing the device.

Push the delivery needle and first implant through the meniscus at the desired position (Figure 4-19). Rotate the device 5 degrees internally and externally to deploy the first implant. Retract the needle into the joint but not outside the portal. Advance the second implant to deployment position by sliding the handle button forward. An audible click is heard when the device is in the correct position. This often requires considerable force to engage fully (Figure 4-20).

Advance the needle and second implant into the desired position. Superior or inferior translation can allow for vertical or oblique mattress configuration (Figure 4-21).

Figure 4-18. Split cannula for FasT-Fix device is positioned 90 degrees relative to the curve of the delivery needle. (Reprinted with permission from Smith & Nephew Inc, London, United Kingdom.)

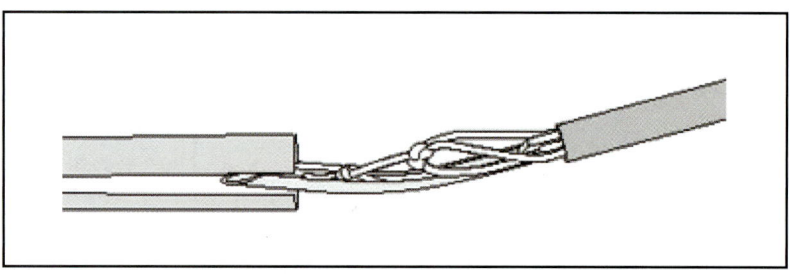

Figure 4-19. FasT-Fix Delivery needle is advanced after split cannula is removed to deploy the first anchor at desired location. (Reprinted with permission from Smith & Nephew Inc, London, United Kingdom.)

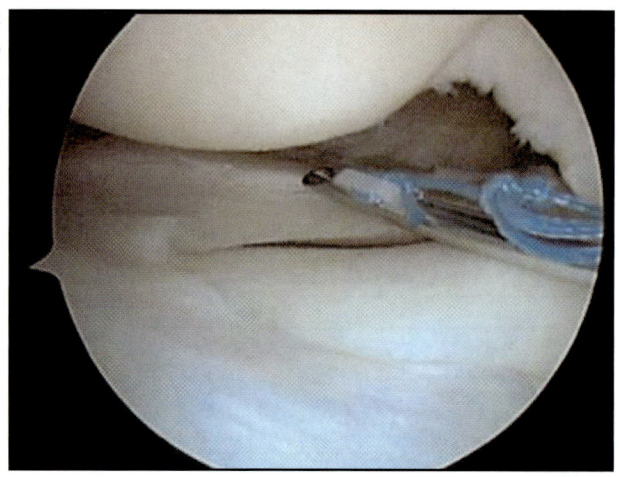

Withdraw the delivery device with the free suture end exiting the arthroscopic portal. Load the suture on the knot pusher/cutter device, and tension appropriately to reduce and compress the tear. Cut the suture by sliding the handle button on the knot pusher forward.

TIPS ON REPAIR AUGMENTATION—FIBRIN CLOT

Exogenous fibrin clot is used to augment meniscal tear healing, particularly in cases of marginal vascularity. The clot provides an inflammatory stimulus and a scaffold for healing (Figure 4-22).

Longitudinal tears in red-white zones, white-white zones, and deep radial tears may be particularly suitable for clot augmentation. Obtain 30 to 40 cc of blood from the patient through standard phlebotomy. Mix the blood in a sterile glass container with a sintered glass rod. The glass rod promotes clot formation.

Gently rinse the clot with normal saline and dry between gauze sponges. Contour 1 to 2 cc of the clot to match the tear pattern and configuration. For inside-out repair, suture the clot with Bunnell stitches using 2-0 absorbable sutures. Load the free ends onto Keith needles, and pass them in a routine fashion for inside-out meniscal repair. Tie the clot sutures over the capsule in standard fashion.

For outside-in technique, simply introduce the clot via the anterior portal, and wedge it between the tibial surface of the meniscus and tibia. Positioning can be adjusted with a Freer elevator. Incorporate the clot into the meniscal repair stitches that are placed with the spinal needles.

Techniques of Meniscal Repair 59

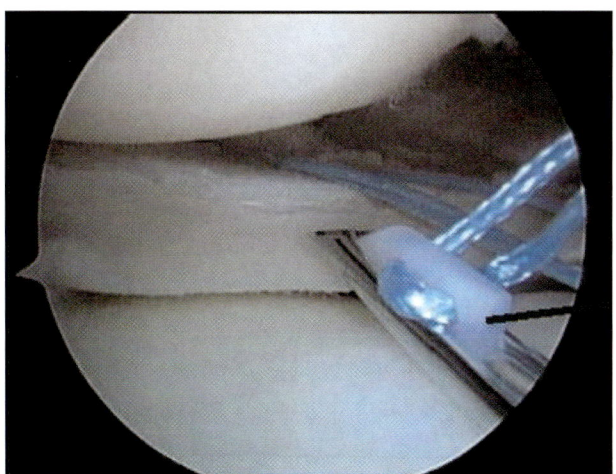

Figure 4-20. The second anchor is advanced into the loaded position and positioned at the desired location to create a mattress suture configuration across the repair. (Reprinted with permission from Smith & Nephew Inc, London, United Kingdom).

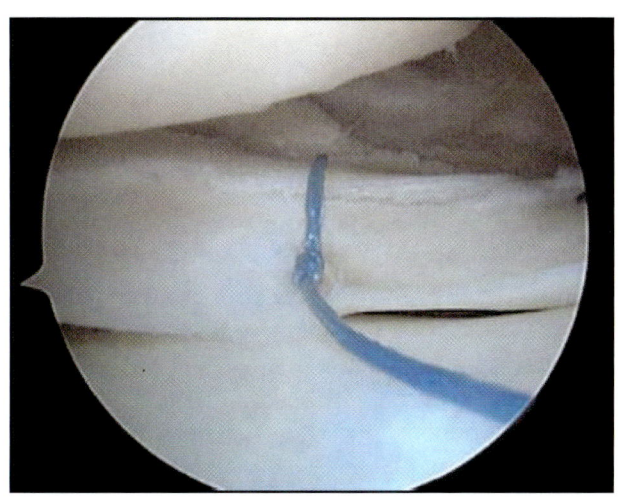

Figure 4-21. Vertical mattress repair of peripheral longitudinal tear after tightening of the slip knot. (Reprinted with permission from Smith & Nephew Inc, London, United Kingdom).

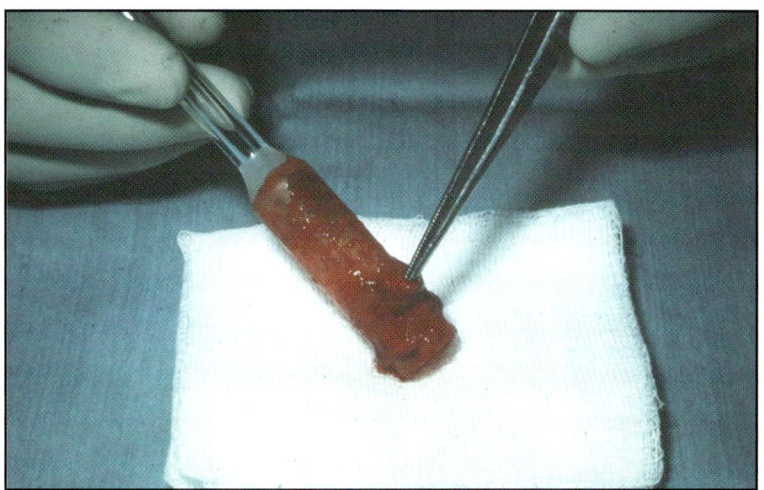

Figure 4-22. Example of fibrin clot specimen that is prepared for repair augmentation using sintered glass rod and autologous blood.

Rehabilitation

The effect of tear configuration and knee range of motion on meniscal healing can guide rehabilitation. Compressive loads on peripheral longitudinal tears with knee in extension typically reduce the tear edges. Compressive loads on peripheral longitudinal tears in flexion displace the posterior horn and tear edges. Radial tears are unfavorably stressed with compressive loads at all positions of flexion.

The menisci translates posteriorly with knee flexion, but minimally from 0 to 60 degrees. The lateral demonstrates more translation than the medial meniscus.

Our current evidence-based protocol is:

* Peripheral, longitudinal tears: Hinged knee brace postoperatively locked in extension for 3 to 4 weeks. Partial weightbearing for 4 weeks with the brace locked in extension. Advance range of motion and weightbearing over 3 to 6 weeks. Sport-specific training and strengthening at 6 to 8 weeks. No running for 4 months.
* Radial tears/Complex tears: Hinged knee brace postoperatively is locked in extension for 3 to 4 weeks. Toe-touch weightbearing for 4 weeks with the brace locked in extension. Range of motion and weightbearing are gradually advanced in the brace at 4 to 6 weeks.

Tips and Pearls

- ✔ Traumatic longitudinal tears, particularly in the setting of a concomitant ACL reconstruction, have a favorable prognosis and should be repaired when technically feasible.
- ✔ Partial-thickness meniscal tears that can be everted with probing are unstable and should prompt a repair.
- ✔ Complete tear débridement and rasping is essential to promote a potent healing response with meniscal repair. Rasp the synovial fringes at the meniscocapsular junction in the zone of the tear to incite a vascular healing response and stimulate mesenchymal stem cells.
- ✔ Outside-in repair is particularly well-suited for anterior horn tears that cannot be approached from a desirable angle with all-inside or inside-out techniques.
- ✔ Avoid an outside-in technique for far posterior horn tears of the meniscus due to the increased risk of injury to critical neurovascular structures.
- ✔ Determine an optimal suture configuration for repair based on tear pattern and severity. Vertical mattress sutures offer the best fixation for longitudinal tear patterns. Sutures should be placed to both reduce and oppose torn surfaces.
- ✔ "Inside-out" repair remains the gold standard of meniscal repair techniques but requires an open posterolateral or posteromedial exposure for safe suture retrieval and fixation.
- ✔ Posteromedial exposure for inside-out repair is best performed through an extracapsular plane between the medial head of the gastrocnemius and semimembranosus tendons.
- ✔ Posterolateral exposure for inside-out repair utilizes a superficial interval between the iliotibial band and biceps tendon followed by a deeper interval between the lateral head of the gastrocnemius and posterolateral joint capsule. The retracted biceps and lateral head of the gastrocnemius protect the peroneal nerve.
- ✔ All-inside repairs are particularly useful for repairable posterior horn tears that approach the midline, in which inside-out techniques may render the neurovascular structures at increased risk of injury.

- ✔ Consider the use of exogenous fibrin clot to augment meniscal repair healing, particular in the setting of marginal vascularity at red-white zones.
- ✔ Postoperative rehabilitation should be individualized based on the tear pattern and repair configuration.

REFERENCES

1. Rangger C, Klestil T, Gloetzer W, Kemmler G, Benedetto KP. Osteoarthritis after arthroscopic partial meniscectomy. *Am J Sports Med.* 1995;23:240-244.
2. Hede A, Larsen E, Sandberg H. The long-term outcome of open total and partial meniscectomy related to the quantity and site of the meniscus removed. *Int Orthop.* 1992;16:122-125.
3. Diduch DR, Poelstra KA. The evolution of all-inside meniscal repair. *Operative Techniques in Sports Medicine.* 2003;11:83-90.
4. King DJ, Matava MJ. All-inside meniscal repair devices. *Operative Techniques in Sports Medicine.* 2004;12:161-169.
5. Medvecky MJ, Noyes FR. Surgical approaches to the posteromedial and posterolateral aspects of the knee. *J Am Acad Orthop Surg.* 2005;13:121-128.
6. Cohen DB, Wickiewicz TL. The outside-in technique for arthroscopic meniscal repair. *Operative Techniques in Sports Medicine.* 2003;11:91-103.
7. Watson FJ, Arciero RA. Inside-out meniscus repair. *Operative Techniques in Sports Medicine.* 2003;11:104-126.
8. Mooney MF, Rosenberg TD. Meniscus repair: the inside-out technique. In: Jackson DW, ed. *Master Techniques in Orthopaedic Surgery: Reconstructive Surgery.* 3rd ed. Philadelphia, PA: Lippincott, Williams & Wilkins; 2008.
9. Johnson LL. Meniscus repair: the outside-in technique. In: Jackson DW, ed. *Master Techniques in Orthopaedic Surgery: Reconstructive Surgery.* 3rd ed. Philadelphia, PA: Lippincott, Williams & Wilkins; 2008.
10. Morgan CD, Leitman EH. Meniscus repair: the all-inside arthroscopic technique. In: Jackson DW, ed. *Master Techniques in Orthopaedic Surgery: Reconstructive Surgery.* 3rd ed. Philadelphia, PA: Lippincott, Williams & Wilkins; 2008.

Microfracture

Luke S. Oh, MD and Thomas J. Gill, MD

Microfracture is used for the treatment of chondral defects. The goal of the microfracture technique is to penetrate the subchondral bone at the site of articular cartilage injury and allow marrow blood to fill the chondral defect (Figure 5-1) and provide the necessary mesenchymal stem cells for extrinsic repair. The underlying marrow is an excellent source of new blood vessels and primitive cells for differentiation and modulation to fibroblasts, which produce a reparative granulation tissue.

INDICATIONS

Microfracture may be useful for both focal traumatic chondral defects as well as degenerative lesions. This differentiates microfracture from "cell-based" or "biologic" treatments. Furthermore, microfracture is not limited to unipolar defects. Unipolar defects are lesions that are found on only one side of the joint (either the femoral condyle or tibial plateau). Microfracture may be used in the presence of bipolar or "kissing" lesions. Bipolar lesions are found on both sides of the joint at adjacent locations.

The microfracture technique is safe and technically straightforward and has an extremely low rate of associated patient morbidity. Thus, it is very useful as a first-line treatment for almost all focal, traumatic chondral defects in the knee, regardless of the location or size. The defect location and size do not reveal a statistical difference in the patient's clinical outcome. Another advantage of the microfracture technique is that it does not burn any bridges with regard to future surgical procedures should the microfracture fail.

Microfracture has several other advantages over other surgical treatments for chondral defects in the knee. Initial reports on autologous chondrocyte transplantation demonstrated inferior results in the patellofemoral joint, although these inferior results may be related to patellar maltracking. Techniques such as osteoarticular transplantation might have limited indications for larger lesions due to the potential for graft site morbidity. Such techniques also limit the availability of potential future surgical options in the event of initial clinical failure.

Figure 5-1. The goal of the microfracture technique is to penetrate the subchondral bone at the site of articular cartilage injury and allow marrow blood to fill the chondral defect and provide the necessary mesenchymal stem cells for extrinsic repair.

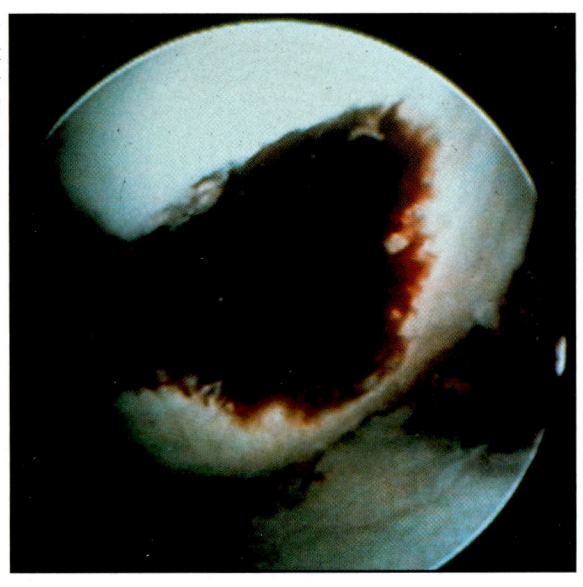

CONTRAINDICATIONS

SIZE OF DEFECT

While there is no statistically significant difference in the outcome of microfracture based on size alone, lesions smaller than 400 mm^2 tend to have less postoperative pain than larger lesions. In the setting of a larger lesion (>3 cm diameter), second-look arthroscopy may be helpful after microfracture. If healing is judged to be incomplete when evaluated arthroscopically, a repeat microfracture to the unhealed area can be performed, or a different resurfacing technique can be considered.

DURATION OF INJURY

The amount of time elapsed from the date of injury is also a consideration in the treatment of chondral defects. Lesions treated by microfracture within 12 weeks of injury have significantly better outcomes than more chronic lesions. However, even degenerative lesions can have excellent outcomes following microfracture.

LOCATION OF LESION

While there is no statistical difference in the outcome of microfracture based purely on location in the knee, femoral and trochlear lesions seem to have a more predictable "fill" than tibial or patellar lesions. This seems particularly important when the microfracture is performed on an arthritic knee. Our experience with second-look arthroscopy following microfracture of the medial compartment performed in conjunction with a high tibial osteotomy typically reveals a good healing response on the medial femoral condyle, but more patchy coverage on the tibial plateau. This finding may be secondary to the dense, sclerotic bone present in the tibial plateau in the setting of varus gonarthrosis.

Depth of Lesion

Microfracture has limited indications for lesions with a depth greater than 5 mm and should generally not be used for defects more than 10 mm in depth. Deep lesions must be evaluated individually in order to choose the appropriate procedure. In these situations, we would typically débride and bone graft the defects. Depending on the size and location of the lesion, a mosaicplasty or autologous chondrocyte transplantation may be preferred. Osteochondritis dissecans is not an absolute contraindication to microfracture unless marrow bleeding cannot be produced from the base of the defect after debridement or the depth of the lesion is greater than 10 mm.

Knee Alignment

The most significant contraindication to the microfracture technique is a malaligned knee. While there are no specific criteria regarding the degree of deformity, any attempt at resurfacing the medial compartment in the setting of varus alignment will almost routinely fail because the stress pattern of the underlying pathologic malalignment will continue to destroy the medial compartment. In this situation, a microfracture should be performed in conjunction with a high tibial osteotomy to re-establish a neutral mechanical axis. Similarly, lateral patellofemoral chondral lesions have a worse prognosis in the setting of patellar maltracking. In this situation, consideration should be given to correcting the patellar-tracking problem at the same time as the treatment of the chondral injury.

Operative Technique

- First, perform a routine diagnostic arthroscopy in order to evaluate every compartment of the knee. Prior to performing the microfracture, address any associated intra-articular pathology (ie, meniscus tear).
- If any damage is noted on the articular surfaces, use a probe to assess the quality of the cartilage as well as the location, size, and depth of the lesion (Figure 5-2).
- Débride any unstable flaps sharply with an arthroscopic shaver or curette (Figure 5-3).
- Then, use a curette to débride the calcified cartilage layer from the base of the full-thickness defect (Figure 5-4). This is an important step because removal of the calcified cartilage layer can greatly enhance the potential to fill the defect.
- Use a surgical awl to create multiple small holes ("microfractures") spaced 1 to 2 mm apart in the exposed bone of the chondral defect (Figure 5-5). Be careful to leave an adequate bone bridge between the holes. An inadequate bone bridge may destabilize the bony compartment and result in malalignment.
- After the microfracture technique has been completed, turn off the arthroscopic pump and observe—as well as document with arthroscopic photographs—the marrow bleeding from each microfracture hole (Figure 5-6).

Tips and Pearls

- ✔ When débriding the calcified cartilage layer, use a curette instead of an arthroscopic shaver (Figure 5-7). With a shaver, it is difficult to control the amount of bone removed, and the subchondral bone is more likely to be violated.

Figure 5-2. Use a probe to assess the quality of the cartilage as well as the location, size, and depth of the lesion.

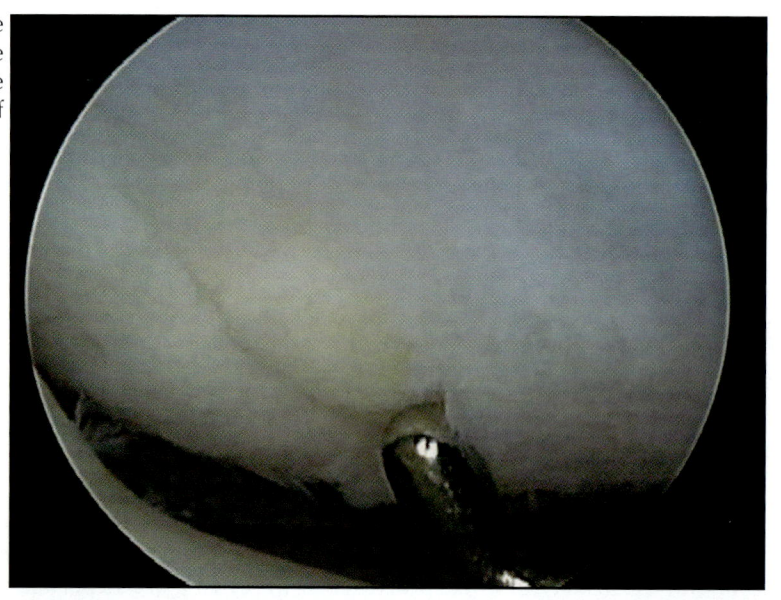

Figure 5-3. Débride the chondral lesion to a stable rim.

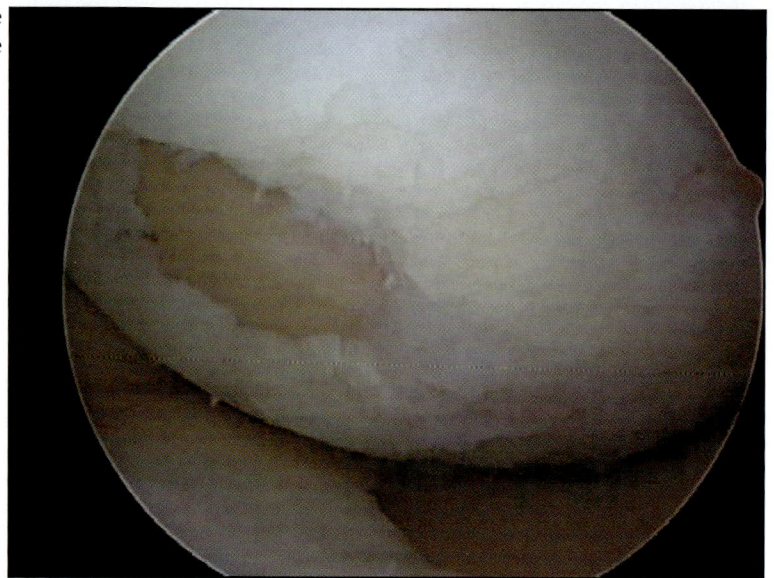

✔ Ensure that microfracture holes are created in the most peripheral aspects of the chondral defect (Figure 5-8) in order to increase the probability of healing of the repair tissue to the adjacent healthy articular cartilage.

✔ If there are any microfracture holes that do not demonstrate marrow bleeding after the arthroscopic pump has been turned off, then carefully place the awl in those pre-existing holes to penetrate the subchondral bone deeper.

Microfracture | **67**

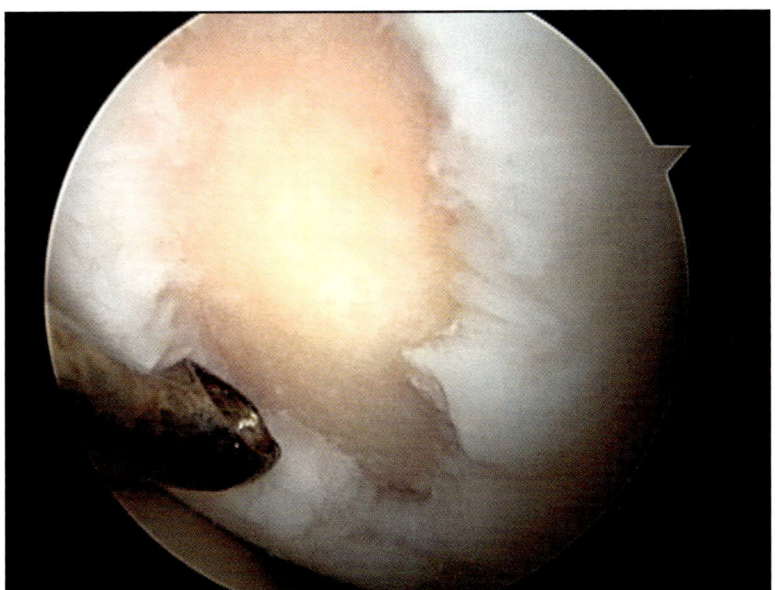

Figure 5-4. De-bridement of the calcified cartilage layer from the base of the chondral lesion is a very important step that greatly enhances the potential to fill the defect.

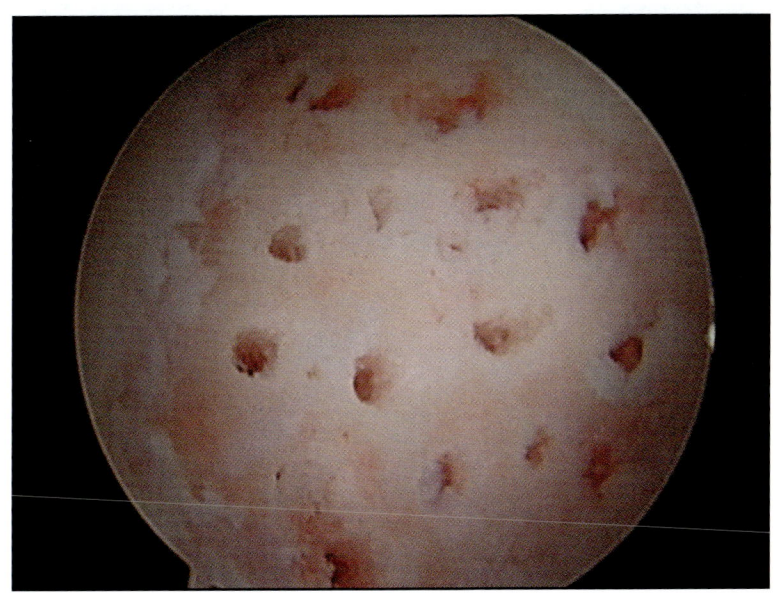

Figure 5-5. Multiple small holes ("microfractures") are created in the exposed bone of the chondral lesion using a surgical awl.

PITFALLS

✘ In order to minimize the risk of fracturing the bone bridges between microfracture holes, ensure that the awl is placed perpendicular to the subchondral bone (Figure 5-9).

✘ In addition to aiming with the most appropriately angled awl (Figure 5-10), changing the position of the knee may improve visualization and also help obtain the optimal angle for penetration of subchondral bone.

Figure 5-6. After the microfracture technique has been performed, marrow bleeding can be visualized by turning off the arthroscopic pump. (A) Before turning off the arthroscopic pump. (B) After turning off the arthroscopic pump.

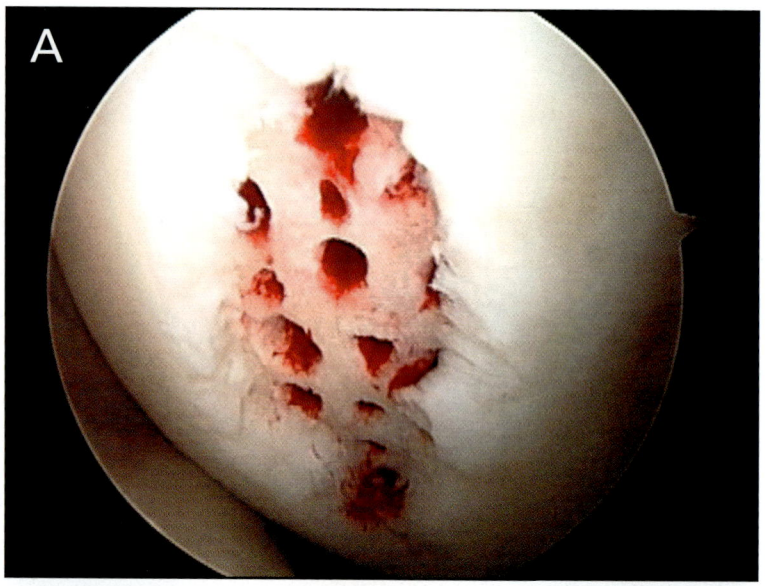

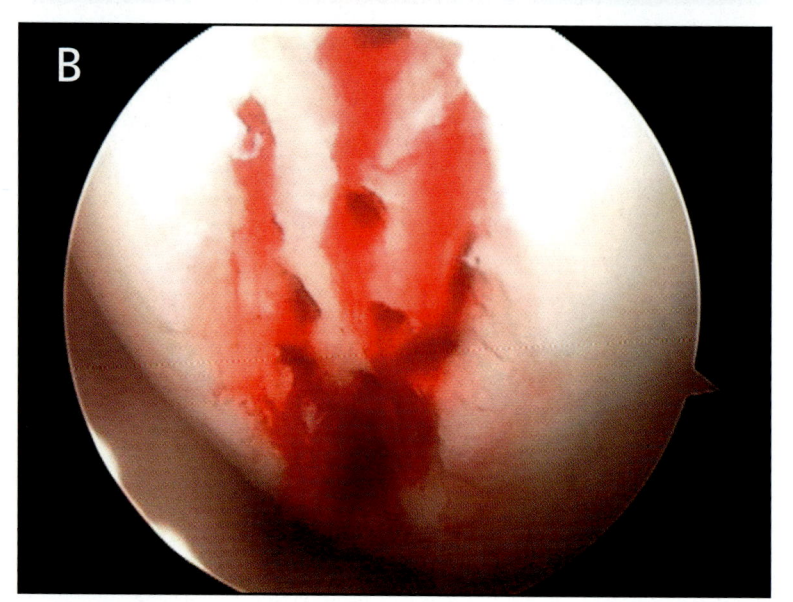

POSTOPERATIVE PROTOCOL

With regard to the microfracture technique, the postoperative management is critical.

LESIONS IN PATELLA OR TROCHLEAR GROOVE

Patients with lesions involving the articular surface of the patella and trochlear groove may be weightbearing as tolerated in a hinged knee brace, with a 30-degree flexion stop. The patella begins to engage the trochlear groove at 30 degrees of flexion; therefore, limiting knee range of motion from 0 to 30 degrees of flexion prevents excessive pressure in the patellofemoral joint. Patients may remove their brace when they are not weightbearing, at which time they should use

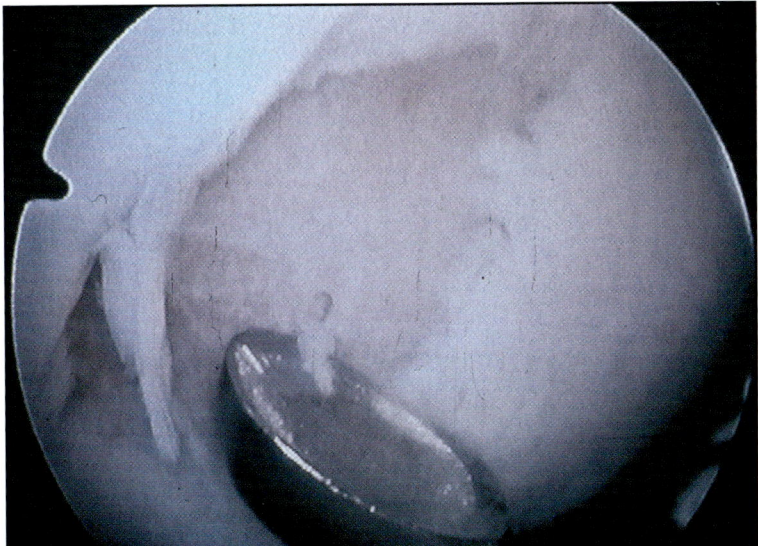

Figure 5-7. When débriding the calcified cartilage layer, use a curette instead of an arthroscopic shaver. With a shaver, it is difficult to control the amount of bone removed, and the subchondral bone is more likely to be violated.

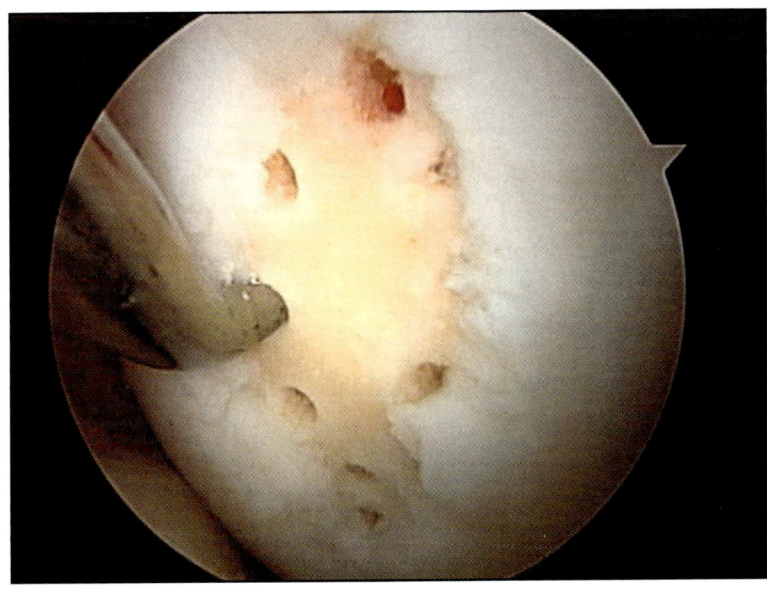

Figure 5-8. Ensure that microfracture holes are created in the most peripheral aspects of the chondral defect in order to increase the probability of healing of the repair tissue to the adjacent healthy articular cartilage.

a continuous passive motion (CPM) machine from 10 to 90 degrees. The CPM machine should be used for at least 8 hours per day.

LESIONS IN THE MEDIAL OR LATERAL COMPARTMENT

If the chondral defect is located in a weightbearing region in the medial or lateral compartment of the knee, then the patient should maintain touch-down weightbearing (15% weightbearing) for the first 6 weeks after surgery. The CPM machine should be set to 1 cycle per minute and the greatest range of motion that the patient can tolerate. Following the initial 6-week period of protected weightbearing, patients may progress to full weightbearing as tolerated and begin active range of motion exercises.

Figure 5-9. To minimize the risk of fracturing the bone bridges between microfracture holes, ensure that the awl is placed perpendicular to the subchondral bone.

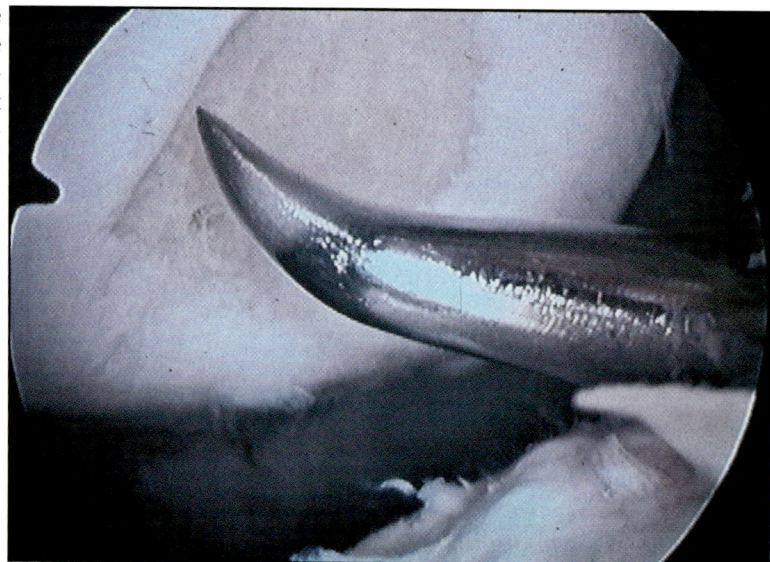

Figure 5-10. Selecting the most appropriately angled awl helps to obtain the optimal angle for penetration of subchondral bone.

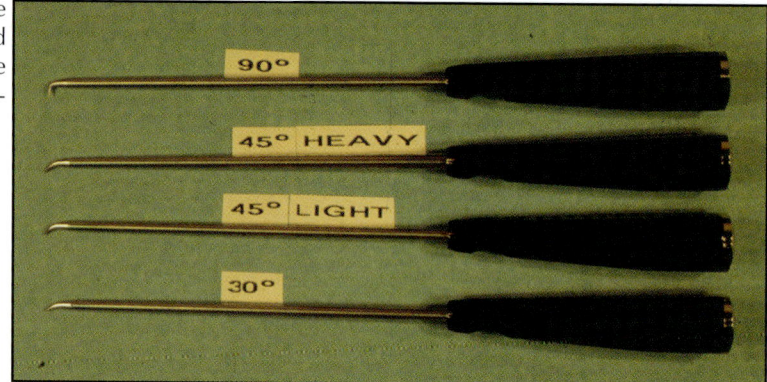

Osteochondral Transplantation

Michael J. DeFranco, MD; Allison G. McNickle, MS; and Brian J. Cole, MD, MBA

Osteochondral autograft (OAT) indications include symptomatic, focal, Outerbridge Grade III or IV chondral lesions of the weightbearing femoral condyles; well-contained lesions of 1 to 4 cm^2; lower demand patients younger than 50 years of age; and lesions associated with limited bone loss.

Osteochondral allograft indications include symptomatic, focal, Outerbridge Grade III or IV chondral lesions of the femoral condyle, trochlea, and patella; larger, well-contained lesions of 2 to 10 cm^2; defects due to trauma, osteochondritis dissecans, avascular necrosis, or intra-articular tibial plateau fractures; young, high-demand patients who are not candidates for joint replacement; and pain and symptoms localized and due to the damaged regions.

Relative contraindications include a body mass index greater than 30 kg/m^2; age greater than 50 years; bipolar lesions; and uncorrected malalignment, ligament insufficiency, or meniscus deficiency.

Absolute contraindications include rheumatoid or osteoarthritis, tumor or infection, and medical conditions that may affect graft incorporation (ie, insulin-dependent diabetes mellitus).

SURGICAL GOALS

Osteochondral grafting involves implanting a healthy plug of hyaline cartilage and subchondral bone to replace a damaged region. Both OAT and osteochondral allografting are indicated in patients with localized, symptomatic Grade III or IV cartilage damage. Deciding between autografting and allografting is usually dependent upon the size of the lesion.

OAT transfers a healthy chondral plug from a low weightbearing area (lateral trochlea or intercondylar notch) to a damaged region of the weightbearing femoral condyle. For large or irregularly shaped lesions, multiple plugs (called "mosaicplasty") can be used to resurface the region. In general, the OAT procedure involves 4 steps: diagnostic arthroscopy, graft procurement, recipient socket preparation, and implantation of the osteochondral plug. Several commercially available systems are available to perform this procedure. Advantages of the OAT procedure include the reconstitution of hyaline-like cartilage at the defect site and a minimal risk of disease transmission. However, the procedure is technically demanding, and donor site morbidity is a significant concern.

During osteochondral allografting, a "prolonged fresh" graft from a deceased donor is implanted into the defect. The tissue is generally provided as an entire hemicondyle, so large

Figure 6-1. The appropriate size of the OAT plug is determined with a sizing cylinder.

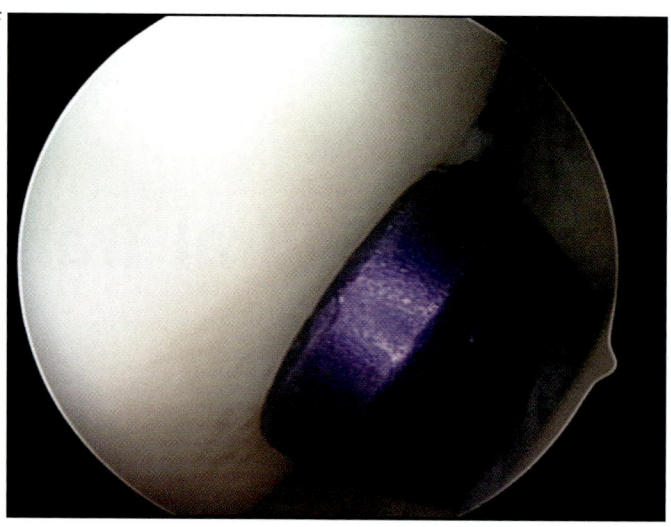

diameter plugs (up to 35 mm in diameter) or irregularly shaped "shell" grafts may be fashioned to match the lesion. The procedure for osteochondral allografting includes preparation of the recipient socket and harvesting of the osteochondral plug from the donor tissue. Prior to surgery, sizing radiographs are necessary to obtain a side- and size-matched donor graft. On the positive side, osteochondral allografting is amenable to large chondral defects with significant bone loss and avoids the donor site morbidity of the OAT procedure. Conversely, the use of a fresh graft increases the expense of the procedure and carries a risk of disease transmission.

Osteochondral Autograft Technique

* The patient is placed supine on operating room table. A tourniquet is place on the thigh of the operative extremity, and the knee should be free to flex as much as 120 degrees. The contralateral extremity is placed in a stirrup. The patient is given general or regional anesthetic as well as prophylactic antibiotics.
* A diagnostic knee arthroscopy is performed through medial and lateral anteroinferior portals to define the size, depth, and location of the lesion. A decision is made to proceed through an all-arthroscopic technique or mini-arthrotomy, which may be medial or lateral depending on the location of the lesion.
* Use the sizer to determine the diameter of the graft(s) that will be needed (Figure 6-1).
* The graft is harvested through the use of standardized, commercially available instrumentation. The senior author prefers to perform this step through a small lateral arthrotomy directly through the lateral retinaculum.
* The properly sized harvester with collared pin is introduced perpendicular to the donor site (Figure 6-2). The harvester is then gently advanced 12 to 15 mm into the cartilage and underlying subchondral bone.
* For removal, the harvester is twisted abruptly 90 degrees clockwise and counterclockwise with a parallel pull to remove the donor plug. The empty donor site may be backfilled to facilitate healing.

Osteochondral Transplantation

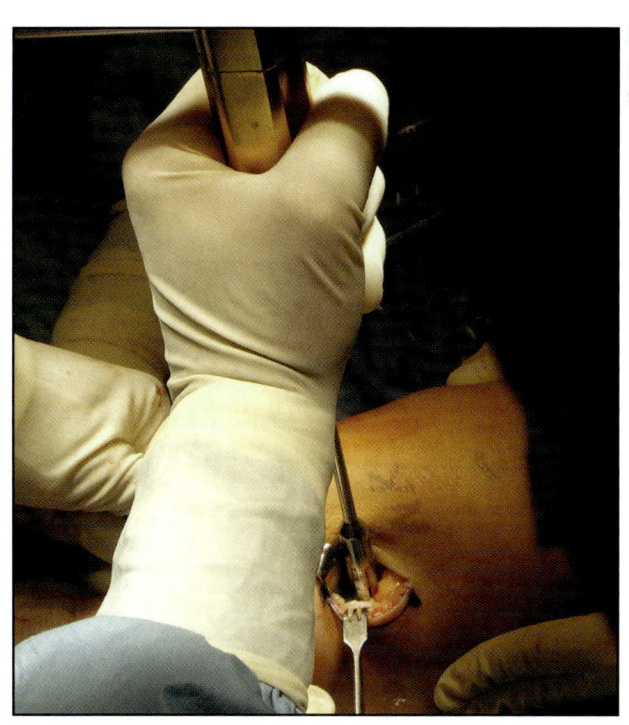

Figure 6-2. The harvester is positioned perpendicular to the surface of the donor site and advanced 12 to 15 mm.

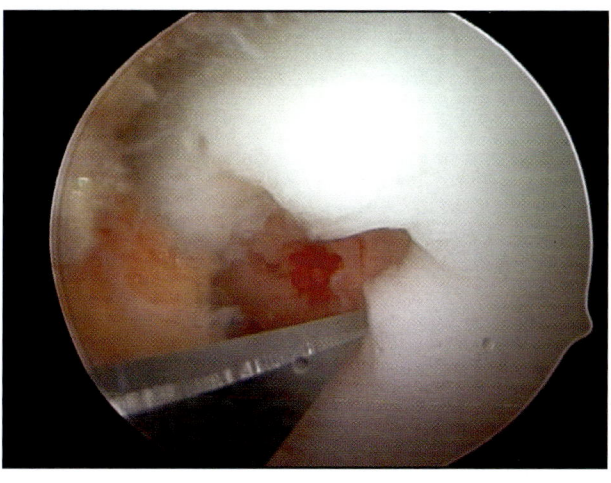

Figure 6-3. Recipient site preparation. Cartilage and fibrous tissue are excised to the subchondral bone.

* After the chondral or osteochondral defect is identified, all fibrous tissue is excised, and the lesion is curetted or abraded down to a bleeding base to promote fibrocartilage ingrowth between the grafts (Figure 6-3).
* The recipient socket(s) is created at the same depth as the donor graft and extracted in the same manner as the donor core (Figure 6-4). Maintaining the recipient corer perpendicular to the articular surface creates well-defined vertical walls and facilitates congruent plug placement. This requires a constant knee flexion angle and may require the use of accessory portals.
* Implanting the graft plug immediately after harvesting will facilitate maintaining the proper insertion angle. The donor tube harvester is placed over the recipient site, taking care to maintain perpendicular orientation and constant flexion angle (Figure 6-5). The donor

Figure 6-4. A prepared recipient socket. The bone core was removed with a tube harvester to a depth 2 mm less than the donor plug.

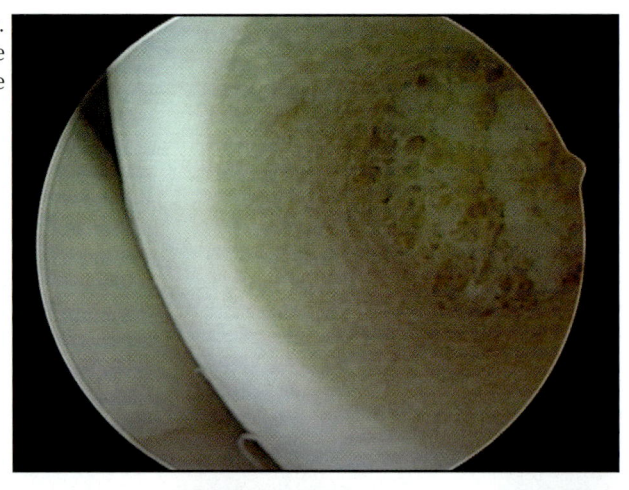

Figure 6-5. The beveled edge of the donor harvester is fully inserted into the recipient site to facilitate graft insertion.

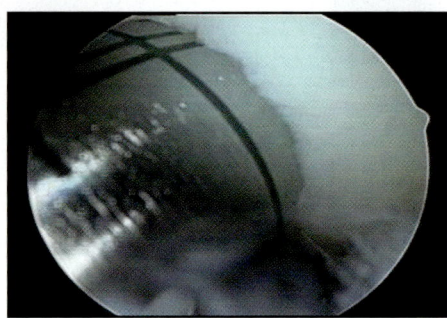

Figure 6-6. After removal of the donor harvester, the autograft remains slightly proud (1 mm) to the surrounding cartilage.

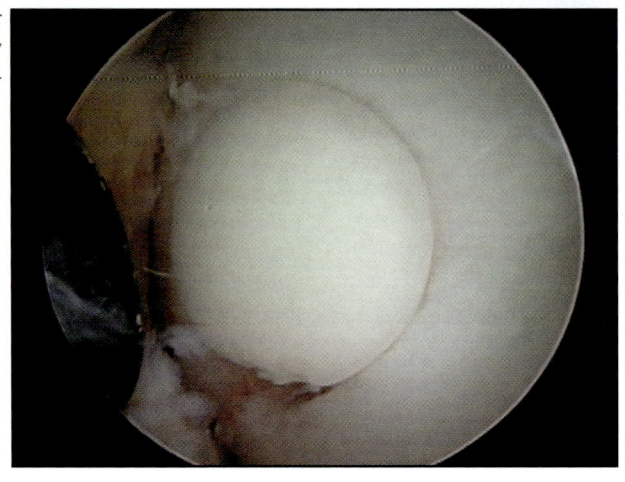

harvester has a tendency to "back off" the articular surface and should be held securely as the donor plug is advanced.

* The donor graft is then press-fit atraumatically and initially left proud (Figure 6-6). Premature advancement of the graft before it is well seated in the recipient tunnel may result in plug fracture or even escape of the plug, requiring collection using loose body retrieval techniques.

Osteochondral Transplantation

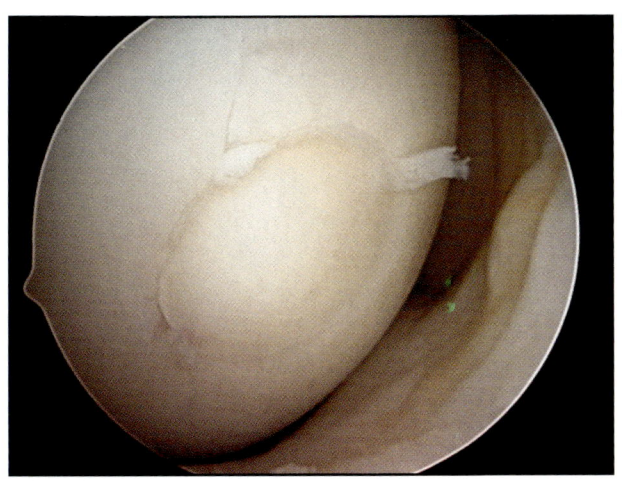

Figure 6-7. A completed autograft to the femoral condyle—flush with the surrounding cartilage and has a similar radius of curvature.

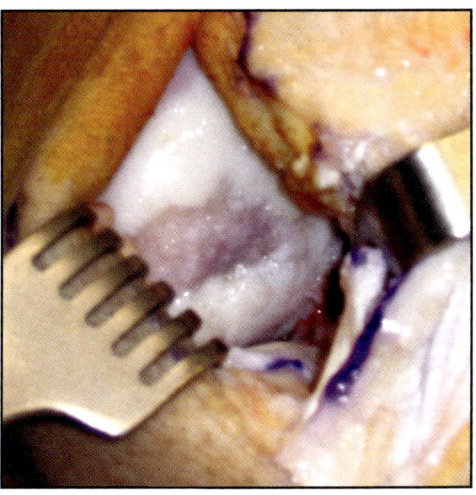

Figure 6-8. Grade IV osteochondral defect to the lateral femoral condyle, which has been exposed via a lateral parapatellar arthrotomy.

* To finalize placement, the plug is gently seated with an oversized tamp until flush with the surrounding articular cartilage (Figure 6-7). Graft congruence is key to minimize shear. When all of the holes are filled, the knee is put through a range of motion with varus and valgus stress to verify its stability and seating.

OSTEOCHONDRAL ALLOGRAFT TECHNIQUE

* The patient is placed supine on the operating room table. A tourniquet is placed on the proximal thigh, and the knee is positioned to be free to obtain up to 135 degrees of flexion. The contralateral limb is placed in a padded obstetric/gynecology leg holder. The patient is administered general or regional anesthesia as well as prophylactic antibiotics. The leg is prepped and draped per standard protocols.

* The site of the lesion is exposed via a medial or lateral parapatellar mini-arthrotomy. To better visualize the site, a Z-retractor or a Hohmann retractor is placed in the intracondylar notch to maintain a distraction force on the patella (Figure 6-8).

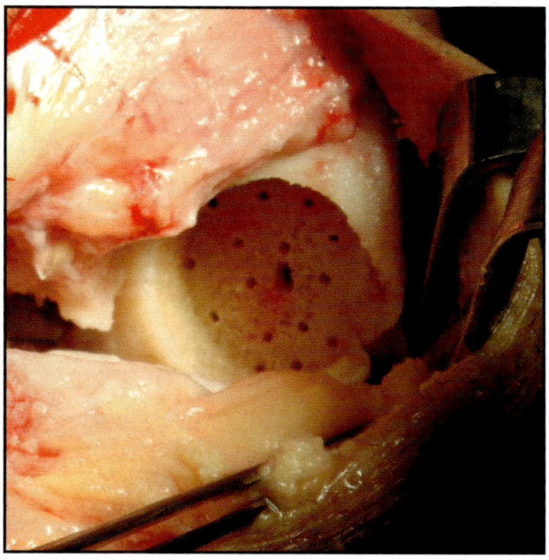

Figure 6-9. A recipient socket of 6 to 8 mm in depth. Multiple holes are drilled in the base to vascularize the osteochondral graft.

* Sizing cylinders, available in several diameters, are used to determine the appropriate diameter of the graft. If the lesion is oblong, 2 grafts could be placed in a "snowman" configuration.
* With the sizing cylinder in place, a guidepin is drilled through the center of the lesion to a depth of 2 to 3 cm. The guidepin must be oriented perpendicular to the surface of the cartilage to create an orthogonal recipient socket.
* A cannulated reamer of the same diameter is placed over the guidepin and drilled to a depth of 6 to 8 mm. This depth permits secure fixation of the graft, but minimizes the amount of donor subchondral bone—the most immunogenic graft component (Figure 6-9).
* The guidepin is removed, and the socket is lavaged to remove bone fragments. If necessary, the margins are débrided to a clean, sharp edge. The 12 o'clock position of the socket is marked for orientation, and a calibrator dilator is inserted to enlarge the socket by 0.5 mm.
* The depth of the recipient socket is measured in 4 quadrants (3, 6, 9, 12 o'clock).
* If provided as an entire hemicondyle, the graft is trimmed with a sagittal saw to create a flat base and is placed in the allograft workstation. The positioning pins are tightened to firmly secure the tissue (Figure 6-10). The bushing of the matching size is secured to the workstation, positioned to match the location and curvature of the recipient socket. A 12 o'clock position is marked for orientation within the socket.
* The graft is drilled perpendicularly through the full thickness of the hemicondyle and carefully extracted to avoid damaging the articular surface (Figure 6-11).
* The osteochondral plug is gripped with holding forceps and trimmed to match the depth of the recipient socket with a sagittal saw. The bony corners of plug are rounded slightly with a rongeur to facilitate insertion. Prior to placement, the plug is rinsed with pulsatile lavage including antibiotics to remove any residual marrow elements (Figure 6-12).
* The allograft is press-fit into the socket, paying attention to aligning the 12 o'clock markings. Once a preliminary fit is obtained, the graft is impacted with an oversized tamp to completely seat the graft (Figure 6-13). If the graft is large or at the edge of the condyle, fixation is obtained with a headless, bioabsorbable screw placed in the center of the graft.

Osteochondral Transplantation

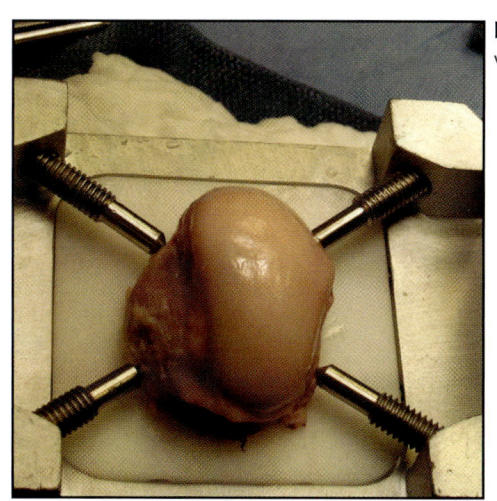

Figure 6-10. A hemicondyle secured in the allograft workstation prior to graft harvesting.

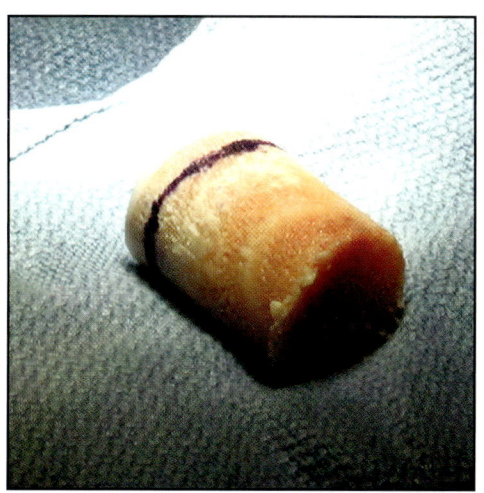

Figure 6-11. A full-thickness osteochondral plug, marked to match the depth of the recipient socket.

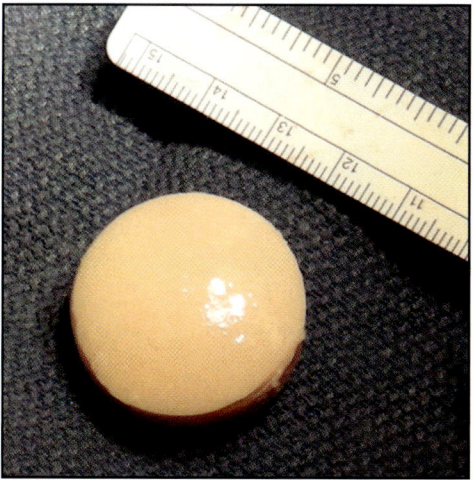

Figure 6-12. An osteochondral allograft plug prior to implantation.

Figure 6-13. An osteochondral allograft seated within the recipient socket.

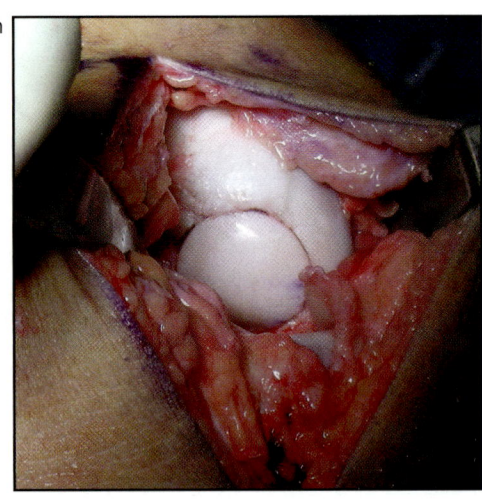

TIPS AND PEARLS

- ✔ Identify and address other pathological factors such as instability, malalignment, and meniscal deficiency.
- ✔ Plan all plugs (size and depth) before placement.
- ✔ During harvesting and implanting grafts, maintain a perpendicular orientation to the articular cartilage surface. These factors are also important to re-establishing convexity and smooth transition with the rest of the knee cartilage.
- ✔ Graft protuberance should always be avoided. Less than 1 mm of depression may fill with fibrocartilaginous tissue and do well clinically.
- ✔ Protective weightbearing is advised for 6 weeks. Graft healing is assessed through clinical and radiographic evaluation. Cartilage-specific magnetic resonance image scans are helpful at 3-month intervals. With evidence of full integration on plain radiographs, the patient is advanced to full weightbearing and weightbearing exercises at 6 to 8 weeks. Closed chain strengthening only is allowed for 3 months to prevent undo shear on the articular cartilage.
- ✔ Postoperatively, both passive and active motion are used to augment graft incorporation.

OSTEOCHONDRAL AUTOGRAFTING

- ✔ The senior author has seen a number of patients whose smaller plugs have delaminated over relatively short periods of time postoperatively. Based on this finding, preference is to use the smallest number of large-diameter plugs possible (ie, 10 mm).
- ✔ If performing several core transfers, each should be completed prior to proceeding with further recipient socket creation.
- ✔ Tibial implantations are more technically difficult in terms of reaching the recipient site. Careful preoperative planning is required to determine the appropriate approach for graft implantation. This can, in some circumstances, be performed in a retrograde fashion.

Osteochondral Allografting

✔ Securing the graft into the allograft workstation is facilitated by trimming the bone with a sagittal saw.

✔ To decrease the risk of disease transmission and immune response, the amount of donor subchondral bone should be minimized and residual marrow elements thoroughly removed with pulsatile lavage.

✔ Expanding the recipient socket with the calibrated dilator permits the press-fitting of the graft.

Pitfalls

✘ Non-perpendicular harvest and insertion may result in step-offs on the surface. Close monitoring with the use of the arthroscope and varied viewing angles helps to avoid such problems.

✘ Graft sinkage below the host surface should be avoided. Regular use of the oversized tamp can help to avoid insertion of the grafts too deeply by avoiding inadvertent over-impaction.

✘ Graft protuberance will lead to shearing and early failure.

✘ The larger the defect, the higher the rate of donor-site morbidity and the greater the difficulty of forming a congruent surface.

✘ Supported grafts heal well, but unsupported grafts tend to subside, eventually becoming covered by fibrous tissue.

✘ Early weightbearing can cause the grafts to sink. Therefore, proper patient selection, regular follow-up, and well-trained therapists help the patient to adhere to the postoperative protocol.

Autologous Chondrocyte Implantation

Andreas H. Gomoll, MD and Tom Minas, MD, MS

Lesions of the articular cartilage can result in activity-related pain, swelling, and mechanical symptoms such as locking and catching. Cartilage lesions that do not penetrate into the subchondral bone are avascular, do not heal, and may enlarge over time. Osteochondral defects have the potential to fill with a fibrocartilaginous scar because the injury extends to the underlying vascular bone. However, this reparative tissue is of unpredictable mechanical properties compared to the type II collagen-rich hyaline cartilage. Due to the limitations of intrinsic healing, various techniques have been developed to repair these defects. Conventional procedures, such as abrasion arthroplasty, drilling, or microfracture, attempt to fill the defect with a fibrocartilaginous repair tissue produced by marrow-derived mesenchymal cells. This tissue, however, is of unpredictable biological and mechanical quality, and clinical improvement, especially in larger defects, is often only transient. Autologous chondrocyte implantation (ACI) was developed in the late 1980s[1,2] and has been used in the United States to treat more than 10,000 patients since its approval by the Food and Drug Administration in 1997. This technique introduces chondrogenic cells into the defect area, resulting in the formation of a repair tissue that more closely resembles articular (hyaline) cartilage. Several studies with follow-up periods of up to 9 years[3-6] have shown promising results with ACI for the treatment of chondral defects of the femoral condyles and, more recently, also the patellofemoral joint.[7,8]

ACI is indicated for the treatment of medium to large, full-thickness, focal defects of articular cartilage. Ideally, the lesion is contained, thus providing a stable rim of intact cartilage to support the periosteal sutures. Defects that extend deeply into the subchondral bone (more than 6 to 8 mm) require staged or concomitant bone grafting. Lower extremity malalignment, ligamentous or patellar instability, and loss of motion should be evaluated preoperatively and addressed in a staged or concomitant fashion. History of active or recent infection, inflammatory arthritis, significant medical comorbidities, and inability to follow the complex postoperative rehabilitation contraindicate ACI.

Patients often present with knee pain and swelling, especially with impact activities. Frequently, they report a history of knee injury or prior surgical procedures such as meniscectomy or anterior cruciate ligament (ACL) reconstruction. Typical physical exam findings include activity-related soft tissue swelling and joint effusion, quadriceps atrophy, tenderness with palpation of the joint line and femoral condyle, and occasionally mild laxity due to loss of cartilage and/or meniscal substance; motion is generally preserved except in very advanced cases.

Radiographic work-up should include standard weightbearing anteroposterior views in extension, posteroanterior views in 45 degrees of flexion, and flexion lateral and axial sunrise views. Double-stance, weightbearing, long-leg radiographs are obtained to assess lower extremity alignment and to determine if corrective osteotomy is necessary. Magnetic resonance imaging (MRI) is useful for the evaluation of menisci and ligamentous structures, as well as to rule out or define associated pathology. However, high-resolution (1.5 Tesla or greater) MRI is necessary to accurately assess the articular cartilage.

Surgical Goals

The goal of ACI is to re-establish near-normal knee function by providing a high-quality repair tissue to fill large chondral defects. On careful examination, most chondral defects are associated with other abnormalities, including malalignment, patellar maltracking, ligamentous instability, and insufficiency of the menisci. It is imperative to address these comorbidities to maximize the potential for a successful outcome.

Malalignment shifts the load-bearing axis to one compartment, resulting in overload and accelerated degeneration of the articular surface. Ligamentous insufficiency, most commonly of the ACL, increases shear forces and thus contributes to chondral wear and graft failure. Meniscal insufficiency increases contact stresses by up to 300% in the respective compartment and is associated with the early onset of osteoarthritis. Patellar maltracking and instability lead to increased shear forces that are associated with a higher rate of transplant failure.

Operative Technique

Diagnostic Arthroscopy and Cartilage Biopsy

A diagnostic arthroscopy is performed to evaluate the defect and assess the joint for potential comorbidities. Ligamentous instability should be addressed either at this point or concomitantly with the re-implantation. Significant meniscal deficiency should be noted and treated with meniscal transplantation if deemed necessary. The number, size, and location of chondral defects is noted, and the opposing articular surfaces are thoroughly evaluated for kissing lesions.

The quality and thickness of the surrounding articular cartilage is assessed to determine whether the lesion is contained (having a rim of healthy cartilage) or uncontained, which will require suturing through adjacent synovium, small drill holes, or bone anchors. The posterior extent of the lesion is critical, as this can complicate access for periosteal suturing at the time of open arthrotomy.

If the defects are found to be amenable to ACI, a full-thickness cartilage biopsy is taken from the superior and lateral aspect of the intercondylar notch with a sharp gouge (Figure 7-1). A whittling, side-to-side twisting motion of the gouge will more accurately remove the tissue while protecting against unwanted slippage. We found it helpful to leave one end of the biopsy attached so that it may be more easily grasped. The biopsy should measure approximately 5 mm wide by 10 mm long and weigh 200 to 300 mg.

After removal from the joint, the biopsy is directly placed in sterile transport medium and shipped overnight for cell culturing (Figure 7-2). The cartilage matrix is enzymatically digested, and the approximately 200,000 to 300,000 cells contained within are expanded in an approximately 6-week process. This process can be interrupted after 2 weeks and the cells cryopreserved for up to 5 years, if needed.

Autologous Chondrocyte Implantation 85

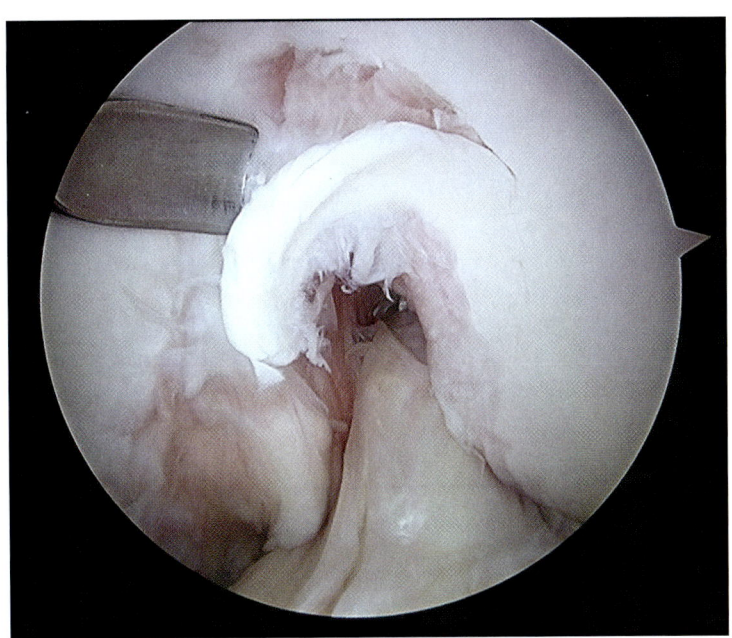

Figure 7-1. Cartilage biopsy being harvested from the intercondylar notch.

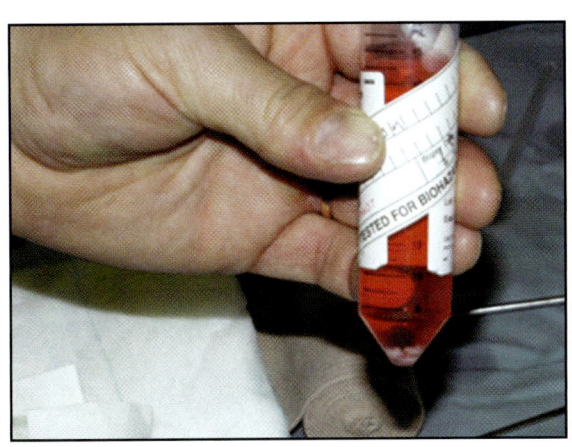

Figure 7-2. Cartilage biopsy in transport medium.

IMPLANTATION

Surgical steps for cell implantation include arthrotomy; defect preparation; periosteal patch harvest; patch fixation, integrity testing, and fibrin glue sealing; chondrocyte implantation; and wound closure.

Arthrotomy

* For single lesions of the femoral condyles, a limited medial or lateral parapatellar arthrotomy is performed.
* Adequate exposure is critical, and it may be necessary to mobilize the meniscus by incising the coronary ligament and taking down the intermeniscal ligament, with subsequent repair at the end of the procedure.
* Correct retractor placement is crucial, especially with limited exposures. We routinely place a bent Hohmann retractor into the notch, displacing the patella away from the defect. A

Figure 7-3. Chondral defect before preparation.

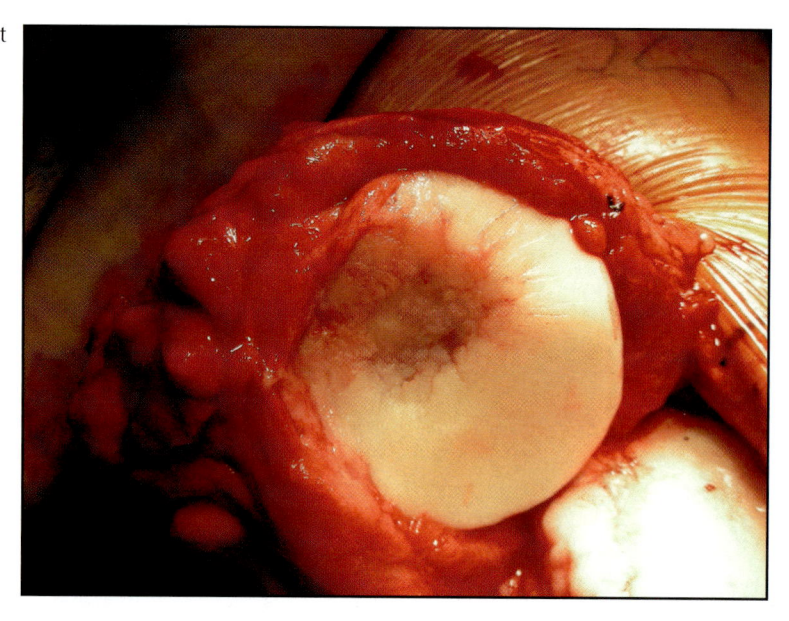

Z- or rake retractor is helpful to control the peripheral soft tissues. For large or multiple defects, a standard medial parapatellar arthrotomy is performed with lateral subluxation or dislocation of the patella (Figure 7-3).

Defect Preparation

* Careful defect preparation is crucial for graft attachment and, ultimately, success of the transplant. The defect bed must be cleaned of all degenerated tissue to achieve a stable rim with vertical shoulders. This is performed by first outlining the defect with a scalpel incision down to the subchondral bone. The degenerated cartilage is then débrided with small ring or conventional curettes, taking as much of the surrounding cartilage as needed to remove all unstable or undermined tissue (Figure 7-4).
* However, if this would result in an uncontained lesion, it is preferable to leave a small rim of degenerated cartilage to sew into, rather than using bone tunnels or suture anchors.
* During débridement, it is essential to not violate the subchondral plate because bleeding results in migration of a mixed mesenchymal cell population from the marrow cavity, resulting in a more fibrous repair tissue.
* Once a healthy defect bed is prepared, it is then measured in its length and width and templated with a sterile marking pen and tracing paper (glove packaging paper works well).
* The template should be oversized by approximately 2 mm in both dimensions because there is shrinkage of the periosteum as it is procured.

Periosteal Patch Harvest

* The most accessible site for procurement of the periosteal patch is the proximal medial tibia. The arthrotomy incision can be extended distally, or a second incision is made over the medial surface of the proximal tibia, starting 2 cm to 3 cm inferior to the pes anserinus insertion.
* The subcutaneous fat is incised superficially, and further dissection with Metzenbaum scissors will expose the tibial periosteum.

Autologous Chondrocyte Implantation 87

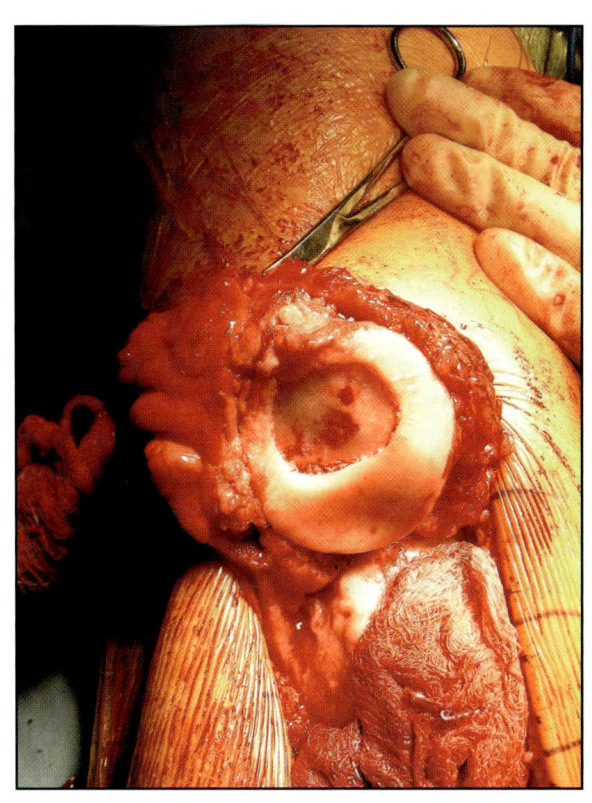

Figure 7-4. Chondral defect after preparation and before application of epinephrine-soaked sponges to address the minimal bleeding seen at the defect bed.

* A wet sponge can be used to gently sweep away loose tissue.
* The periosteal patch is now outlined with the template, and the orientation and superficial surface is marked.
* A fresh #15 blade is used to sharply divide the periosteum, which is then mobilized with a small sharp periosteal elevator. The patch should be very gently removed from its bony bed to avoid ripping; the periosteum is pulled upward with non-toothed micro forceps as it is gently mobilized with gentle push/pull and side-to-side motions of the periosteal elevator.
* After the patch has been harvested, it should be spread out on and covered by a moist sponge to avoid desiccation and shrinkage. If a tourniquet has been used, it can be deflated at this point for the remainder of the procedure.

Patch Fixation, Integrity Testing, and Fibrin Glue Sealing

* Minor punctate bleeding from the subchondral bone is not uncommon, especially after the tourniquet has been deflated and can usually be controlled with epinephrine or thrombin-soaked sponges or neuro-patties.
* Infrequently, a larger bone bleeder needs to be controlled with electrocautery or fibrin glue.
* Once the defect is completely dry, the periosteal patch is retrieved from the back table and placed over the defect, with the cambium layer facing toward the subchondral bone.
* The periosteum is gently unfolded and stretched with non-toothed forceps; an obviously oversized patch can be trimmed carefully at this time.

Figure 7-5. Suturing of the patch.

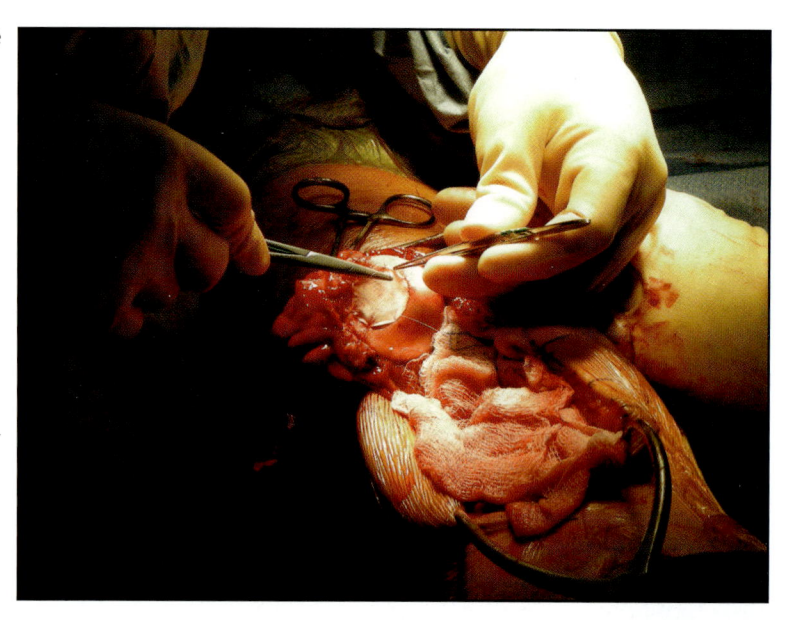

- Suturing is performed with 6-0 Vicryl on a P-1 cutting needle, which has been immersed in mineral oil or glycerin for better handling. The sutures are placed first through the periosteum and then the articular cartilage, exiting approximately 3 mm away from the defect edge, everting the periosteal edge slightly to provide a better seal against the defect wall (Figure 7-5).
- The knots are tied on the patch side, thus remaining below the level of the adjacent cartilage.
- Interrupted sutures are initially placed on each side of the patch (3, 6, 9, and 12 o'clock), adjusting the tension of the patch after each suture and trimming the periosteum as needed to obtain a patch that is neither too loose as to sag into the defect, nor so tight that it would cut out of the sutures.
- Thereafter, additional sutures are placed in between to circumferentially close the gaps.
- An opening wide enough to accept an angiocath is left in the most superior aspect of the periosteal patch to inject the chondrocytes.
- Water tightness of the suture line can now be tested by slowly injecting saline into the covered defect with a tuberculin syringe and plastic 18-gauge angiocath. Any leakage should be addressed with additional sutures or fibrin glue as needed.
- Lastly, the saline is re-aspirated to prepare the defect for chondrocyte implantation.

Chondrocyte Implantation

- The cells are now resuspended and steriley aspirated from the transport tubes with a tuberculin syringe through an 18-gauge or larger needle because smaller gauge needles can damage the cells.
- The needle is then removed and replaced with a flexible, plastic, 18-gauge, 2-inch angiocath.
- The angiocath is introduced into the defect through the residual opening of the periosteal patch. As the angiocath is slowly withdrawn, cells are injected until the defect is filled with fluid (Figure 7-6).

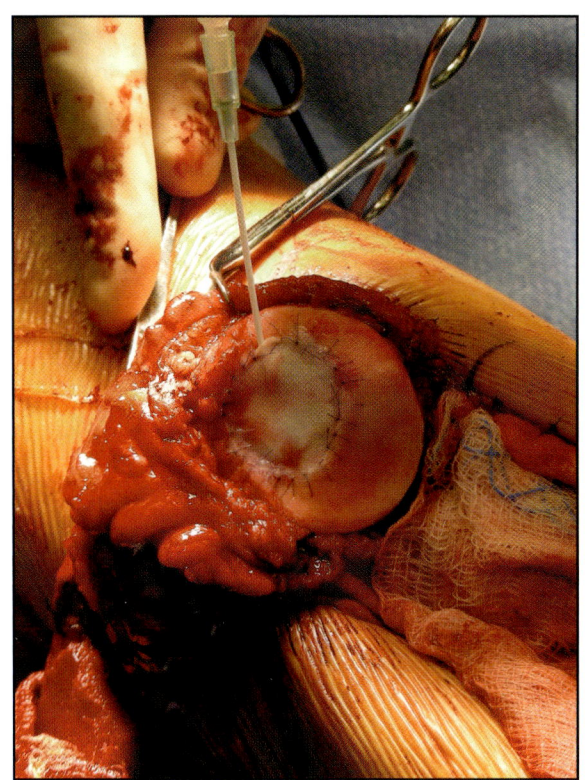

Figure 7-6. Cell injection from the 12 o'clock position.

* One or two additional sutures and fibrin glue are then used to close the injection site (Figure 7-7).

Wound Closure

* We minimize the use of intra-articular drains as to avoid damage to the periosteal patch. When drains are used, it should be without suction and with care to position the tubing away from the defect.
* The wound is closed in layers, and a soft dressing is applied to the knee. Prophylactic intravenous cephalosporin antibiotics are used for 24 hours after surgery.

Rehabilitation

A detailed rehab plan is critical to satisfy the dual, and occasionally conflicting, goals of addressing the risk of postoperative adhesions and protecting the periosteal patch and graft. Continuous passive motion (CPM) is started on postop day 1, generally at 0 to 40 degrees, for at least 6 hours a day. Patients with condylar lesions can increase their motion to 90 degrees as tolerated and are limited to touch-down weightbearing for 6 weeks, then transition to full weightbearing during the following 2 to 4 weeks. Trochlear and patellar lesions are limited to 40 degrees on the CPM because patellofemoral contact stresses increase at higher angles. To avoid stiffness, these patients should passively dangle the leg over the edge of the bed 3 times per day to achieve 90 degrees of flexion by 3 weeks. Patients remain touch-down weightbearing for 6 weeks if the defects were implanted in conjunction with a tibial tubercle osteotomy; otherwise, they are allowed to bear weight as tolerated in a knee immobilizer. Generally speaking, patients can

Figure 7-7. Final defect after closure of the injection site and application of fibrin glue.

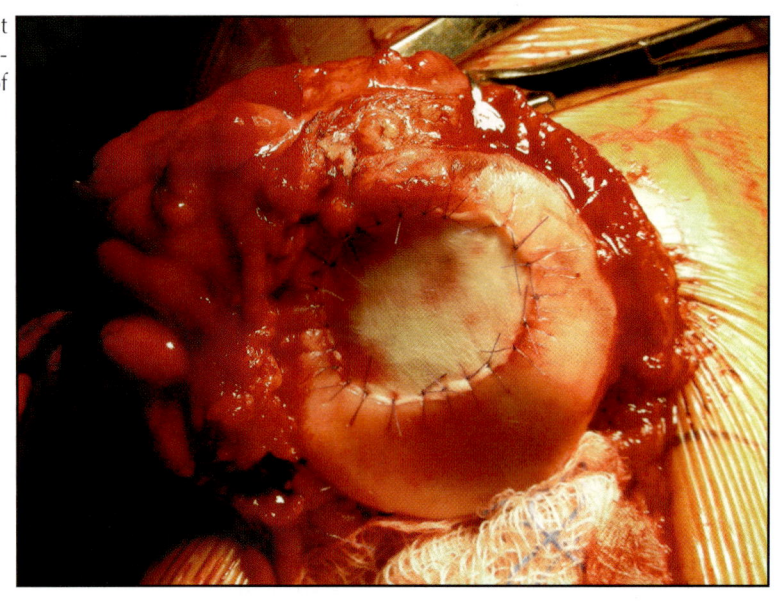

start non-impact activities such as stationary biking without resistance at 6 weeks, light-impact activities such as rollerblading at 6 months, and higher-impact or pivoting activities after 12 to 18 months.

TIPS AND PEARLS

- ✔ We have found the use of continuous epidural analgesia very helpful: the catheter is placed preoperatively and can be used to provide intraoperative analgesia, as well as postoperative pain control for the first 48 hours. This has allowed us to initiate full range of motion exercises and CPM immediately postoperatively.
- ✔ The patient is positioned supine on a standard operating table with a thigh tourniquet. For arthroscopy, we use either a lateral post or thigh-holder; no post is used during re-implantation. However, especially in posterior lesions of the femoral condyle, a leg positioning device is helpful to stabilize the knee in hyperflexion.
- ✔ Make sure to prep the lower leg into the field to just above the ankle to allow harvesting of the periosteal patch.
- ✔ Harvest the periosteum distal to the pes insertion because proximally fibers of the sartorius blend into the periosteum, which compromises the quality of the periosteal patch and complicates handling.
- ✔ Oversize the template by 1 to 2 mm to account for shrinkage of the periosteum.
- ✔ Intralesional osteophytes, which are commonly seen in previously microfractured or very chronic defects, can be removed with a high-speed burr.
- ✔ Micro instruments, such as used for vascular surgery, are very helpful for periosteal suturing. We routinely use fine, non-toothed microforceps, small needle holders, and iris scissors.
- ✔ Concomitant procedures such as high-tibial osteotomy or ACL reconstruction should be performed before periosteal suturing in order to not damage the fairly friable patch.

✔ The tourniquet is most helpful during the initial exposure and can be released as soon as the periosteal patch has been harvested to minimize ischemia time.

PITFALLS

✘ When possible, avoid harvesting periosteum from the intra-articular portion of the distal femur. In our experience, this increases the risk of arthrofibrosis and postoperative stiffness.

✘ If needed, position suction drain tubes away from the defect because they can become adherent and damage the patch upon removal.

✘ Be careful not to leave behind any degenerated or undermined cartilage surrounding the defect, even if this means making the defect substantially larger. Degenerated cartilage will continue to degrade, compromising the repair.

✘ Not correcting associated pathology such as ligamentous instability, meniscal deficiency, or malalignment will significantly increase the failure rate of cartilage repair.

REFERENCES

1. Brittberg M, Lindahl A, Nilsson A, Ohlsson C, Isaksson O, Peterson L. Treatment of deep cartilage defects in the knee with autologous chondrocyte transplantation. *N Engl J Med.* 1994;331(14):889-895.
2. Grande DA, Pitman MI, Peterson L, Menche D, Klein M. The repair of experimentally produced defects in rabbit articular cartilage by autologous chondrocyte transplantation. *J Orthop Res.* 1989;7(2):208-218.
3. Browne JE, Anderson AF, Arciero R, et al. Clinical outcome of autologous chondrocyte implantation at 5 years in US subjects. *Clin Orthop Relat Res.* 2005;436:237-245.
4. Micheli LJ, Browne JE, Erggelet C, et al. Autologous chondrocyte implantation of the knee: multicenter experience and minimum 3-year follow-up. *Clin J Sport Med.* 2001;11(4):223-228.
5. Minas T. Autologous chondrocyte implantation for focal chondral defects of the knee. *Clin Orthop Relat Res.* 2001;391(suppl):S349-S361.
6. Peterson L, Minas T, Brittberg M, Nilsson A, Sjogren-Jansson E, Lindahl A. Two- to 9-year outcome after autologous chondrocyte transplantation of the knee. *Clin Orthop Relat Res.* 2000;374:212-234.
7. Gomoll AH, Minas T, Farr J, Cole BJ. Treatment of chondral defects in the patellofemoral joint. *J Knee Surg.* 2006;19(4):285-295.
8. Minas T, Bryant T. The role of autologous chondrocyte implantation in the patellofemoral joint. *Clin Orthop Relat Res.* 2005;436:30-39.

Pediatric Osteochondral Injuries

Dennis E. Kramer, MD and Mininder S. Kocher, MD, MPH

Pediatric osteochondral knee injuries include both osteochondritis dissecans (OCD) lesions and traumatic osteochondral fractures. OCD lesions are stress fractures of subchondral bone that secondarily progress to involve the overlying cartilage.[1] They most commonly occur on the posterior aspect of the medial femoral condyle, but can also occur on the lateral femoral condyle, patella, and trochlea.[2-4] Numerous staging systems have been described based on radiographic, magnetic resonance imaging (MRI),[3,5] or arthroscopic[6] appearance. In general, OCD lesions are classified as stable (intact overlying cartilage) or unstable (overlying cartilage violated). Juvenile OCD lesions occur in children with open distal femoral physes and have a better prognosis with nonoperative management.[2,4]

Treatment recommendations are based on the stage of the OCD lesion and the status of the distal femoral physis. Stable lesions in children with open physes are generally treated conservatively with cessation of repetitive loading. Nonoperative management protocols often include an initial period of restricted weightbearing with knee bracing or immobilization followed by activity modification and physical therapy.[2] Factors associated with failure of nonoperative management include larger lesion size, skeletal maturity, and lesion instability.[1] The operative indications for juvenile OCD lesions include the following:

* All patients with detached or unstable lesions
* Symptomatic patients approaching physeal closure (within 6 to 12 months)
* Stable lesions that have not healed after 6 to 9 months of nonoperative management[2,4,7]

Symptomatic OCD lesions in skeletally mature children are generally treated operatively.[2]

Surgical treatment options for OCD lesions include transarticular drilling, internal fixation, and lesion excision with chondral resurfacing. Transarticular drilling is indicated for stable lesions with intact overlying cartilage that have failed conservative management.[4] Internal fixation is added for large stable lesions (>2 cm) and loose or unstable fragments with viable overlying cartilage. Fixation options include metal implants (Herbert screws or partially threaded cannulated screws), bioabsorbable pins or screws, and osteochondral plugs. OCD lesions in which the overlying cartilage is fragmented and unsalvageable or displaced with minimal subchondral bone are treated with fragment excision and a cartilage resurfacing technique, such as microfracture, mosaicplasty, or autologous chondrocyte implantation.[8,9]

Acute osteochondral fractures most commonly occur in the medial patellar facet or the lateral femoral condyle following a patellar dislocation. Adolescents are especially vulnerable to osteochondral fractures as the interface between the articular cartilage and subchondral bone is an area of potential weakness.[1] Fragment reduction and fixation are indicated for large fragments (>1 cm) with adequate subchondral bone where the donor site involves a weightbearing area. Fragment excision and donor site resurfacing are indicated for small loose fragments that have minimal subchondral bone attached, fragments from a non-weightbearing donor site, and fragments with a damaged and unsalvageable chondral surface.

Surgical Goals

The goal of transarticular drilling of an OCD lesion is to stimulate the underlying subchondral bone to repair itself and produce a stable construct of subchondral bone and overlying cartilage. This is thought to occur by creating channels for revascularization across the necrotic subchondral bone and into the marrow, which allows for osteogenic cells to enter the subchondral bone in the lesion.[4,10] Internal fixation is added to stabilize large or unstable lesions while the underlying subchondral bone heals itself to prevent further chondral damage and the formation of loose bodies. The goal of fragment excision is to remove unstable chondral fragments that can cause further injury to the knee. When the lesion has been débrided to stable edges, a chondral resurfacing technique is added either to stimulate the exposed subchondral bone to form fibrocartilage or to transplant articular cartilage into the defect. The goal of reduction and fixation of a loose osteochondral fracture is to repair the donor site with its native cartilage by stabilizing the loose fragment to its original site.

Operative Technique

Arthroscopic Transarticular Drilling of an Osteochondritis Dissecans Lesion

* The case is done as a same-day surgery. General anesthesia is employed.
* The patient is positioned supine, and a nonsterile tourniquet is applied to the upper thigh.
* Diagnostic knee arthroscopy is first performed through a standard anterolateral viewing portal and anteromedial working portal.
* The anterior fat pad is débrided over the lesion to improve arthroscopic visualization.
* Identify, localize, and inspect the lesion by palpating the cartilage with a probe, feeling for softening or indentation over the lesion, and assessing for lesion size and stability (Figure 8-1).
* Use a 0.045-inch smooth Kirschner wire for transarticular drilling.
* Using a freehand technique, percutaneously place the Kirschner wire through the skin beginning 1 to 2 cm below the corresponding arthroscopic portal and advance it to the softened area of cartilage at the center of the lesion.
* Flex and extend the knee as needed with various percutaneous starting points for Kirschner wire insertion to ensure that the Kirschner wire is as perpendicular as possible to the lesion. Make an accessory portal at the location that will provide the best access to the lesion.
* Using a power drill, advance the Kirschner wire retrograde across the lesion and into the underlying subchondral bone. Adequate penetration is confirmed by noting fat droplets or bleeding coming from the drill holes. The lesion is drilled both at its center as well as around its periphery, with drill holes placed several millimeters apart in order to maximize healing potential (Figure 8-2).

Pediatric Osteochondral Injuries | 95

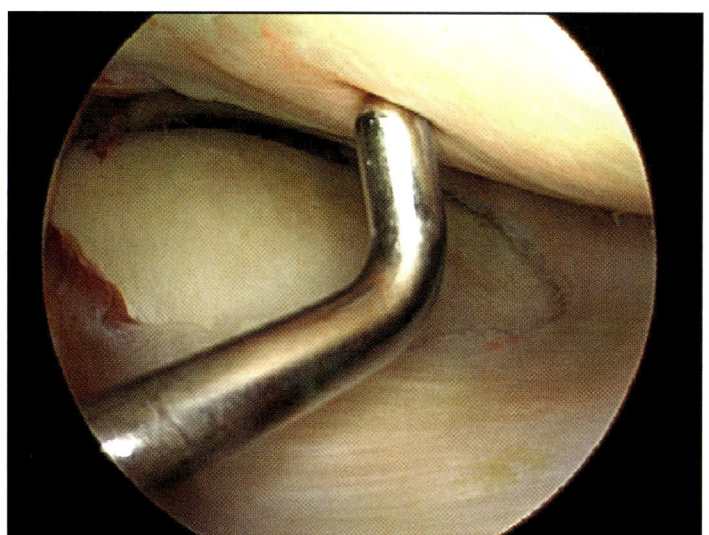

Figure 8-1. An arthroscopic probe is used to palpate the cartilage, feeling for softening over the lesion.

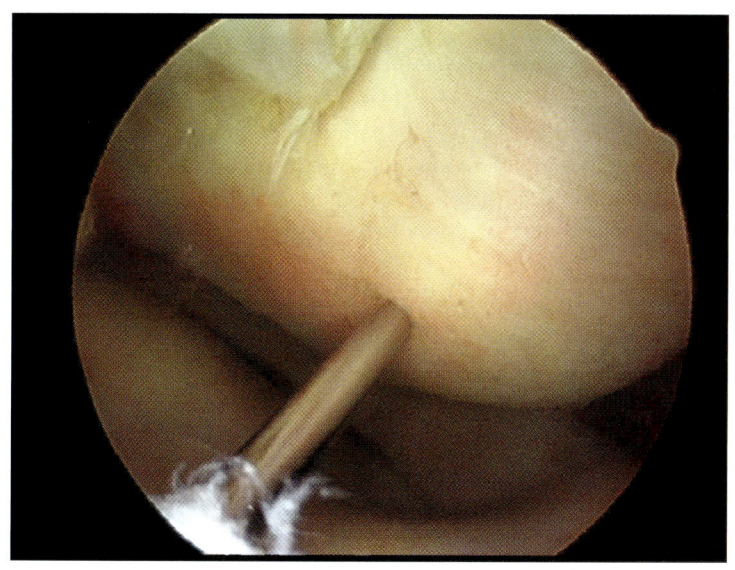

Figure 8-2. Arthroscopic image of retrograde transarticular drilling of a stable OCD lesion of the medial femoral condyle with an intact articular surface. The smooth Kirschner wire used is perpendicular to the articular surface.

* For lesions in the classic location at the posterior aspect of the medial femoral condyle, the arthroscope should be placed through the anterolateral portal, and Kirschner wire is placed percutaneously through the skin beginning just inferior to the anteromedial portal at the medial border of the patellar tendon. The knee is then hyperflexed beyond 90 degrees to expose the posterior border of the lesion.
* For lateral femoral condyle lesions, the arthroscope should be placed through the anteromedial portal, and the knee is either kept flexed or placed in the figure-of-4 position, whichever provides the best access to the lesion. The Kirschner wire is then placed percutaneously through the skin beginning just inferior to the anterolateral portal on the lateral border of the patellar tendon.
* Alternatively, the Kirschner wire can be placed through the patellar tendon, using a small vertical incision through the tendon to allow easier passage.

Figure 8-3. An open lateral release is used to assist with exposure and transarticular drilling of an OCD lesion on the patella.

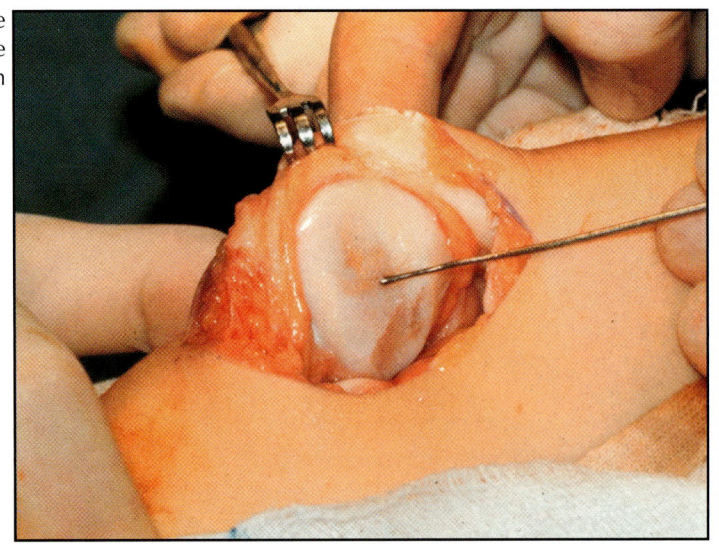

- For patellar and trochlear lesions, if a lateral release is planned, we perform an open lateral release and use the lateral arthrotomy to directly access the lesion (Figure 8-3).
- If no lateral release is planned, the patella must be manually tilted medially or laterally to expose the lesion for transarticular drilling. Arthroscopic visualization may be difficult in these cases. If visualization is inadequate, a mini-arthrotomy should be performed on the side of the patella corresponding to the location of the lesion.

FIXATION OF AN OSTEOCHONDRITIS DISSECANS LESION OR OSTEOCHONDRAL FRACTURE

- Cracks or fissuring in the articular cartilage over the lesion are indicative of an open and unstable lesion (Figure 8-4). In these lesions, fixation is added before or after transarticular drilling.
- If a partially unstable flap lesion is identified, fibrous tissue may exist between the osteochondral flap and underlying bone and should be débrided with curettes until bleeding bone is visualized while preserving the intact cartilaginous hinge.
- If significant subchondral bone loss exists, autologous bone graft should be packed into the crater before reduction and fixation.
- For loose OCD lesions or osteochondral fractures, anatomic reduction of the lesion prior to fixation is mandatory. Loose bodies often increase in size and may need to be trimmed prior to reduction and fixation back into the donor site.
- An arthrotomy is often necessary to achieve anatomic reduction of a loose fragment.
- Anatomically reduce the unstable or detached portion of the lesion, and temporarily fix the fragment with 2 Kirschner wires to control fragment rotation prior to fixation.
- Large posterior lesions may be difficult to access arthroscopically, and an arthrotomy may be necessary to allow complete access to the lesion for adequate fixation (Figure 8-5).
- Choice of fixation device depends on surgeon preference, lesion size, and stability. Partially threaded cannulated screws provide the most compression but leave an indentation on the articular surface. They may scuff the tibial surface and require later removal. Herbert

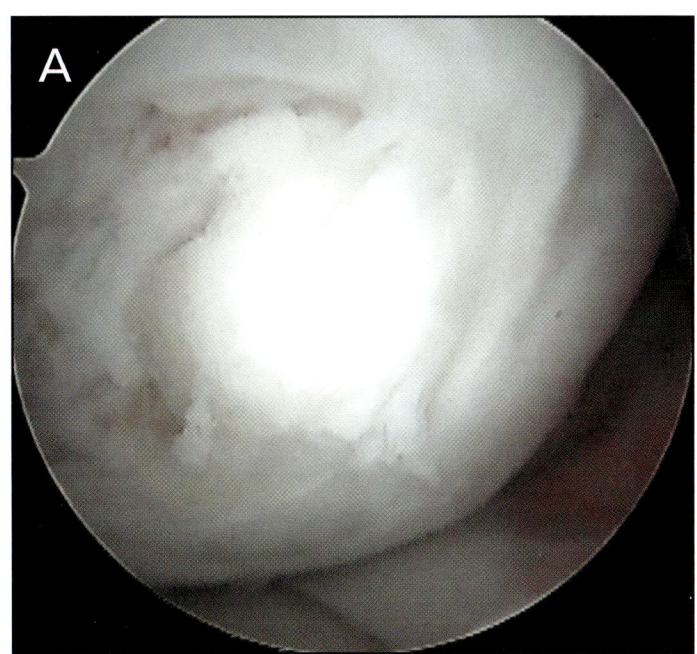

Figure 8-4. Arthroscopic images of unstable lesions. (A) Lesion in situ. (B) Hinged lesion. (Reprinted with permission from Ganley TJ, Gaugler RL, Kocher MS, Flynn JM, Jones KJ. Osteochondritis dissecans of the knee. *Op Tech Sports Med.* 2006;14:147-158. © Elsevier 2006.)

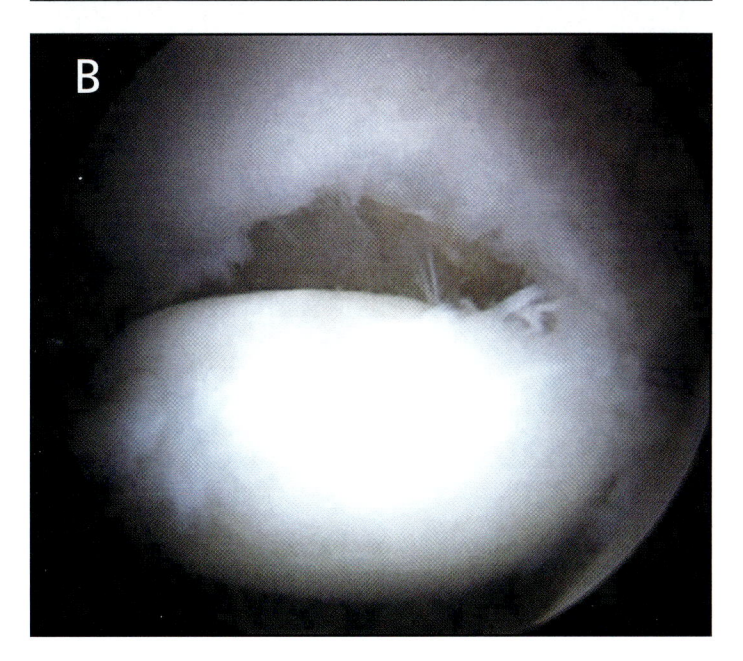

screws can be buried below the articular cartilage surface and provide some compression, but also require later screw removal. Bioabsorbable implants provide limited compression without the need for later screw removal.

* We prefer partially threaded cannulated screws or Herbert screws for larger lesions with sufficient subchondral bone in which lesion compression will stimulate healing (Figure 8-6). For smaller lesions, we use 1.5-mm bioabsorbable poly-lactic acid pins (Smart Nail, Bionix Implants, Tampere, Finland) or 2.7-mm Biocompression screws (Arthrex, Naples, FL) (Figure 8-7).

Figure 8-5. An arthrotomy is used to provide exposure for a large posterior lesion that required reduction and fixation.

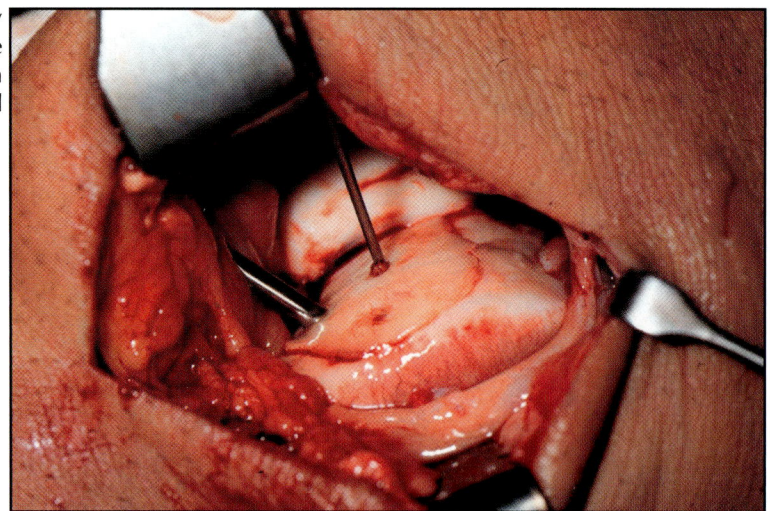

Figure 8-6. Fixation of juvenile OCD of the knee with Herbert screws.

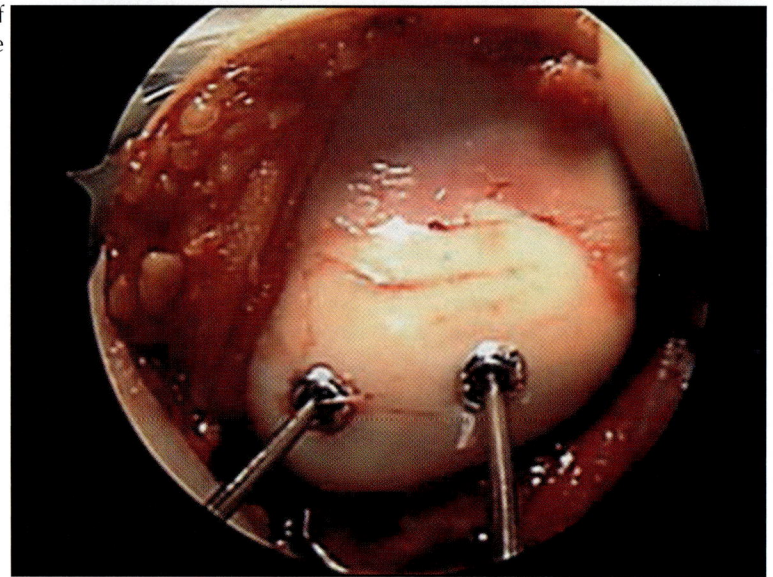

- Plan your placement of fixation devices. Use multiple fixation points for larger or more unstable lesions. If using a single point of fixation, go through the center of the fragment or through the area of the fragment with the most cancellous bone attached.
- Use a #11 blade knife to make an accessory portal in the area where the fixation device will be placed through. Clear a direct path to the lesion through this accessory portal to prevent the implant from getting caught in the fat pad.
- Make sure all fixation devices are seated 1 to 2 mm below the level of the articular cartilage.

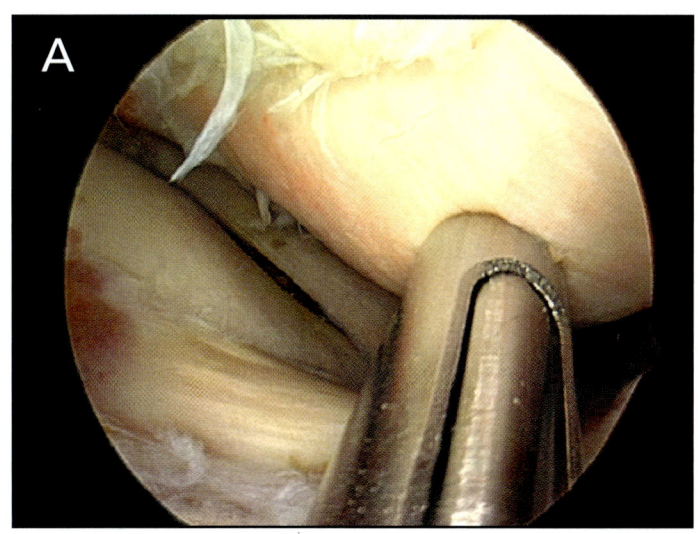

Figure 8-7. Bioabsorbable fixation of a juvenile OCD lesion. (A) the OCD lesion was drilled with a 1.5-mm step drill through a slotted drill guide. (B) A PLA copolymer tack (SmartNail, ConMed Linvatec, Utica, NY) was impacted in the drill hole. (C) The intraoperative arthroscopic photograph shows the lesion after SmartNail fixation.

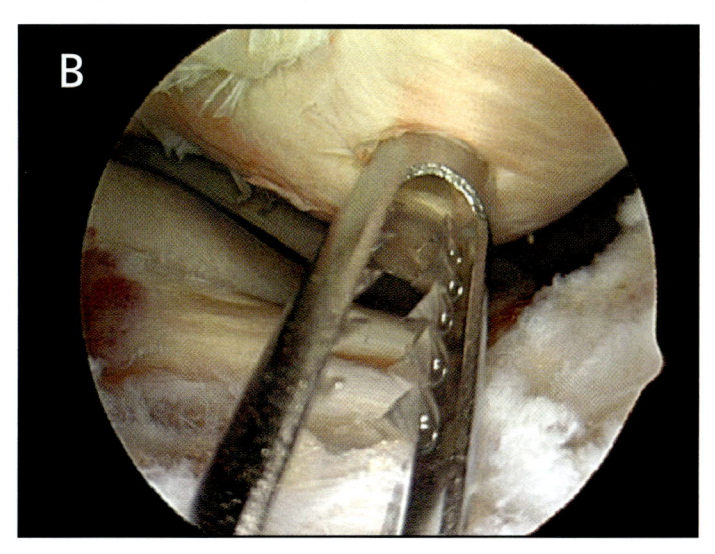

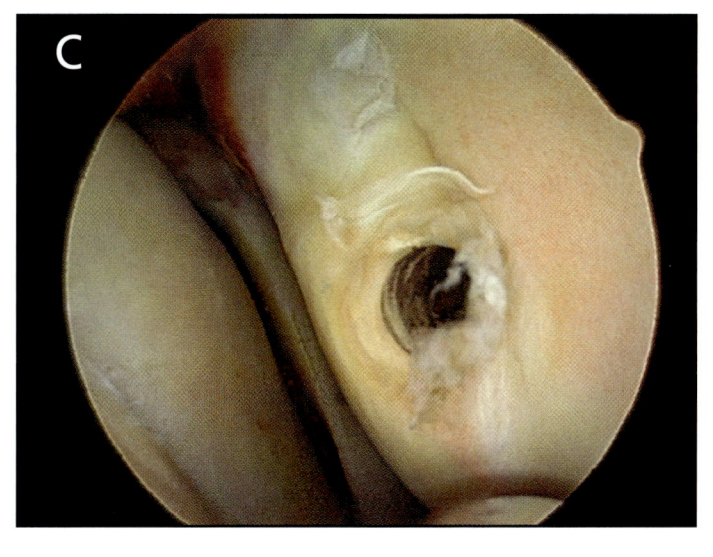

Fragment Excision and Chondral Resurfacing of an Osteochondritis Dissecans Lesion or Osteochondral Fracture

* Excise any loose and free-floating fragments.
* Débride the donor OCD lesion to stable edges with a hand-held curved curette and a full-radius resector. It is critical to make sure the lesion is "well shouldered" by removing any loose or marginally attached but unstable cartilage on the edges of the lesion.
* Our preference is to perform microfracture as the initial treatment of Grade IV chondral injuries. Other options include mosaicplasty, autologous chondrocyte implantation (ACI), and osteochondral allograft reconstruction.
* Standard microfracture techniques as described by Steadman and colleagues[11] remove the calcified cartilage layer with a hand-held curved curette looking for punctate bleeding from the underlying subchondral bone.
* Now use the 30- or 45-degree microfracture awls to create holes in the exposed subchondral bone 3- to 4-mm apart by placing the tip perpendicular to the subchondral bone (Figure 8-8).
* Hole depth should be about 2 to 4 mm to allow for access to the marrow elements.
* Begin at the periphery and proceed toward the center of the lesion.
* Patellar and trochlear lesions may be very difficult to access arthroscopically. Attempt to microfracture the lesion with the knee in extension using manual pressure on the 90-degree microfracture awl. If adequate exposure cannot be attained, make a mini-arthrotomy, and microfracture the lesion through this arthrotomy.
* Consider performing a chondral biopsy at the time of microfracture for large lesions (>3 cm) that may benefit from an ACI procedure in the future.

Tips and Pearls

✔ Carefully review the MRI preoperatively to predict lesion location and stability and to plan the operative approach. For femoral condyle lesions, note the posterior extent of the lesion with the knee flexed to determine the amount of knee flexion that will be necessary to arthroscopically localize the lesion (Figure 8-9).

✔ Always have available appropriate instruments for arthrotomy, various fixation devices, and a chondral biopsy kit.

✔ Intraoperatively, the exact margins of the OCD lesion may be difficult to localize. In these cases, fluoroscopy can be used to outline lesion position. Begin by placing a Kirschner wire at the suspected margin of the lesion before obtaining the fluoroscopic image.

✔ Often, the best location for transarticular drilling is through the inferior aspect of the patellar tendon. Make a vertical 1-cm incision through the skin and through the patellar tendon in this location to facilitate Kirschner wire passage.

✔ Grasp the Kirschner wire with the drill 3 cm from the skin edge before transarticular drilling of the lesion. Now, drill the Kirschner wire until the drill contacts the skin edge to confirm adequate drilling depth.

Pediatric Osteochondral Injuries | 101

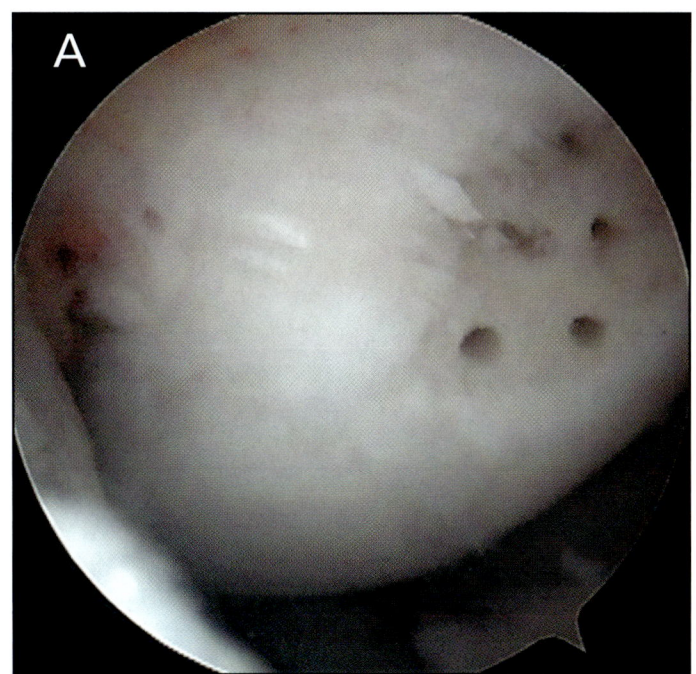

Figure 8-8. Arthroscopic images of a full-thickness OCD lesion treated with microfracture. (Reprinted with permission from Ganley TJ, Gaugler RL, Kocher MS, Flynn JM, Jones KJ. Osteochondritis dissecans of the knee. *Op Tech Sports Med.* 2006;14:147-158. © Elsevier 2006.)

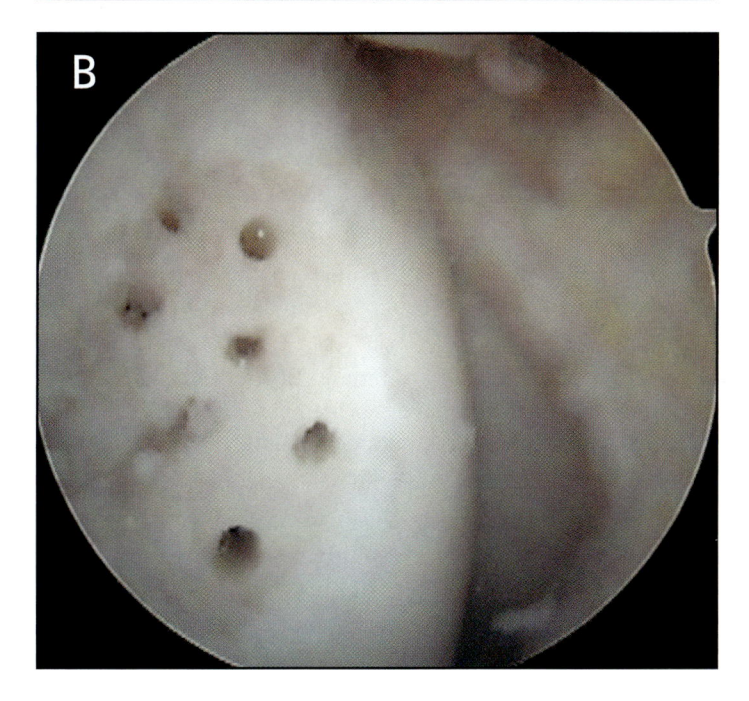

- ✔ Following arthroscopic transarticular drilling of the lesion, we routinely switch the arthroscope to the opposite portal to provide a different viewpoint and ensure the entire lesion has been addressed.
- ✔ For patellar lesions in patients with a tight lateral retinaculum, consider performing a mini-open or open lateral release. This allows the patella to be tilted laterally, and drilling can be done directly through this lateral arthrotomy incision.

Figure 8-9. Sagittal MRI shows the posterior extent of this juvenile OCD lesion on the medial femoral condyle.

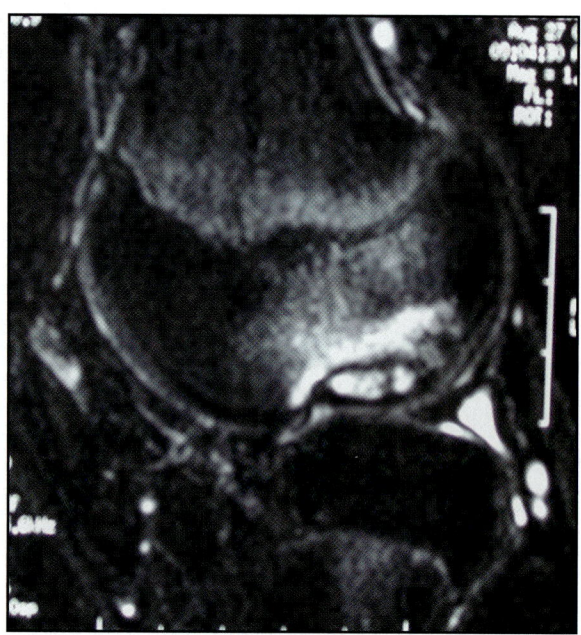

✔ If the patient has recurrent patellar instability with lateral patellar subluxation, consider adding an open medial plication or medial retinacular repair and accessing patellar chondral lesions through this open medial incision.

Pitfalls

✘ Inadequate fat pad débridement prior to drilling will result in obscured visualization during drilling as the Kirschner wire will likely get caught in the fat pad in front of the lesion.

✘ Adequate débridement of the crater base is necessary to remove fibrous tissue and maximize healing potential of the lesion, but avoid excessive débridement of the crater base to minimize loss of bone substance and subsequent fragment depression.

✘ If the tourniquet is inflated during drilling, you may not see bleeding from the drill holes.

✘ Often, the posterior border of the OCD lesion is the most difficult to access and is inadequately drilled.

✘ When placing a fixation screw arthroscopically, make sure that the path to the lesion has been débrided or the fixation device may get stuck in the fat pad before it is able to get to the lesion. This can be done by using a #11 blade knife and oscillating shaver to create an accessory portal with a direct path to the lesion for placement of the fixation device.

✘ Make sure that fixation devices are placed below the surface of the articular cartilage to prevent damage to weightbearing areas adjacent to the lesion.

REFERENCES

1. Ganley TJ, Flynn JM. Osteochondritis dissecans of the knee. In: Micheli LJ, Kocher MS, eds. *The Pediatric and Adolescent Knee*. Philadelphia, PA: Saunders; 2006:273-293.
2. Flynn JM, Kocher MS, Ganley TJ. Osteochondritis dissecans of the knee. *J Pediatr Orthop*. 2004;24(4):434-443.
3. Hefti F, Beguiristain J, Krauspe R, et al. Osteochondritis dissecans: a multicenter study of the European Pediatric Orthopedic Society. *J Pediatr Orthop B*. 1999;8(4):231-245.
4. Kocher MS, Tucker R, Ganley TJ, Flynn JM. Management of osteochondritis dissecans of the knee: current concepts review. *Am J Sports Med*. 2006;34(7):1181-1191.
5. De Smet AA, Ilahi OA, Graf BK. Untreated osteochondritis dissecans of the femoral condyles: prediction of patient outcome using radiographic and MR findings. *Skeletal Radiol*. 1997;26(8):463-467.
6. Guhl JF. Arthroscopic treatment of osteochondritis dissecans. *Clin Orthop Relat Res*. 1982;167:65-74.
7. Cahill BR. Osteochondritis dissecans of the knee: treatment of juvenile and adult forms. *J Am Acad Orthop Surg*. 1995;3(4):237-247.
8. Micheli L, Curtis C, Shervin N. Articular cartilage repair in the adolescent athlete: is autologous chondrocyte implantation the answer? *Clin J Sports Med*. 2006;16(6):465-470.
9. Peterson L, Minas T, Brittberg M, Lindahl A. Treatment of osteochondritis dissecans of the knee with autologous chondrocyte transplantation: results at two to ten years. *J Bone Joint Surg Am*. 2003;85(A Suppl 2):17-24.
10. Anderson AF, Richards DB, Pagnani MJ, Hovis WD. Antegrade drilling for osteochondritis dissecans of the knee. *Arthroscopy*. 1997;13(3):319-324.
11. Steadman JR, Miller BS, Karas SG, Schlegel TF, Briggs KK, Hawkins RJ. The microfracture technique in the treatment of full-thickness chondral lesions of the knee in National Football League players. *J Knee Surg*. 2003;16(2):83-86.

Single-Bundle ACL Reconstruction Using Patellar Tendon Grafts
Transtibial Endoscopic Hybrid Technique

Jerome J. Da Silva, MD; Champ L. Baker III, MD; and Bernard R. Bach Jr, MD

Bone-patellar tendon-bone disruption of the anterior cruciate ligament (ACL) is a potentially disabling injury. In the active individual, chronic ACL deficiency has been demonstrated to result in functional instability, meniscal injury, chondral damage, and the development of osteoarthritis.[1-3] Although the true natural history of the ACL-deficient knee has not yet been completely characterized, it is clear that not all patients with an ACL injury require reconstruction.[2] Few prospective studies exist comparing the outcomes of reconstruction versus non-operative treatment of the ACL-injured knee. Studies have demonstrated that early ACL reconstruction reduces the risk of subsequent meniscal injury when compared to late reconstruction; however, no rigid management guidelines presently exist.[2,4]

The decision to perform ACL reconstruction should be made after determination of the individual's activity level, occupation, expectations, and consideration of other surgical factors.[5] In the study by Daniel and colleagues, the 2 most important variables in predicting late meniscal surgery or ACL reconstruction were total pre-injury hours per year spent in participation of hard cutting, pivoting, and jumping sports (Category I sports) and KT-1000 arthrometer manual maximum side-to-side differences.[2] High-risk patients, including those active in hard cutting sports for more than 5 hours per week, and individuals with comparable physically demanding occupations or lifestyles should consider ACL reconstruction.[5,6] High skill level athletes or individuals at a lower level unwilling to modify activities are candidates for reconstruction. Patients with recurrent symptomatic instability despite modification of activities, appropriate rehabilitation, and bracing should consider reconstruction. Older age is not considered a contraindication to surgery if the individual is active in recreational sports and wants to maintain his or her activity level.[7,8] Patients with an acute ACL injury and an associated repairable meniscus tear should be considered for combined ACL reconstruction and meniscal repair due to the significantly increased healing rates for the meniscus versus isolated repair.[9,10] ACL tears associated with other severe knee ligamentous injuries also merit surgical intervention.[5,11]

SURGICAL GOALS

The goal of an ACL reconstruction is to restore knee stability, maintain normal motion, minimize donor site complications, and allow the patient to return to his or her desired level of functional activities. Associated ligament, meniscal, and chondral injuries are all addressed as necessary. The optimal graft choice has been a source of controversy. At our institution, the

Figure 9-1. Lachman exam under anesthesia.

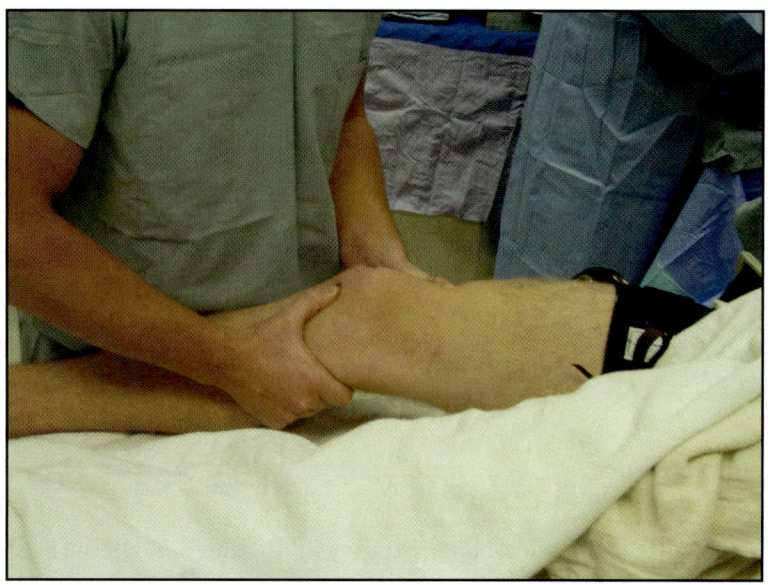

bone-patellar tendon-bone (BTB) autograft has been the preferred graft choice for more than 20 years.[12] We prefer the BTB autograft due to ease of harvest, excellent graft strength, and bone-to-bone healing. Additionally, we have observed a high rate of patient satisfaction, predictable clinical outcomes, and minimal patellar complications in short- and intermediate-term follow-up.[7,13-17] The use of allograft for ACL reconstruction has increased in the senior author's practice (BRB) from 2% of patients between 1986 and 1996 to almost 50% in 2008.[5,18] A study at our institution using BTB allograft demonstrated high rates of patient satisfaction, clinical outcomes, and arthrometric stability testing comparable to our institution's previously published results with patellar tendon autograft.[18] The option of allograft tissue is typically discussed or recommended with patients who are older than 40 years, have moderate patellofemoral crepitation or pain, have radiographic evidence of mild degenerative joint disease yet are clinically unstable, are of petite stature, have donor graft tissue of questionable quality, or have requested an allograft.[18] Allograft tissue is regularly used in patients with multi-ligament knee injuries requiring reconstruction and in 90% of our patients who present for revision ACL reconstruction.

TECHNIQUE

* The procedure begins with an exam under anesthesia. A Lachman exam and a pivot shift exam are performed on both the operative and contralateral extremity. The pivot shift phenomenon defines, in our opinion, functional ACL deficiency (Figures 9-1 and 9-2).
* The patient is positioned supine, with the waist of the bed slightly flexed and the foot of the bed flexed 90 degrees. A padded thigh tourniquet is placed around the operative thigh and then incorporated into an arthroscopic leg holder. This allows the leg to hang at 90 degrees. The contralateral leg is placed in a padded gynecological stirrup leg holder with the hip and knee flexed to protect the femoral and common peroneal nerve (Figures 9-3 and 9-4).
* BTB graft harvest is performed through an 8-cm longitudinal anterior skin incision positioned 1 cm medial to the tibial tubercle. This allows for both harvest of the graft and tibial tunnel drilling through the same incision. Next, 10-mm x 25-mm bone plugs are harvested from both the distal patella and tibial tubercle using a micro-sagittal saw and curved

Single-Bundle ACL Reconstruction Using Patellar Tendon Grafts 107

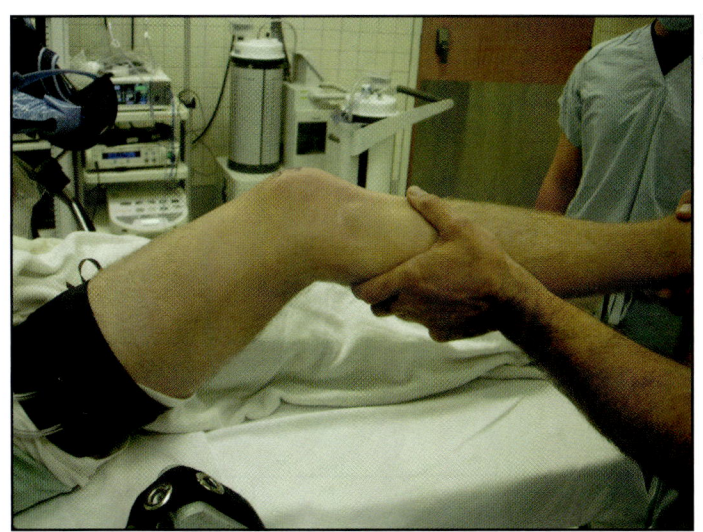

Figure 9-2. Pivot shift exam under anesthesia.

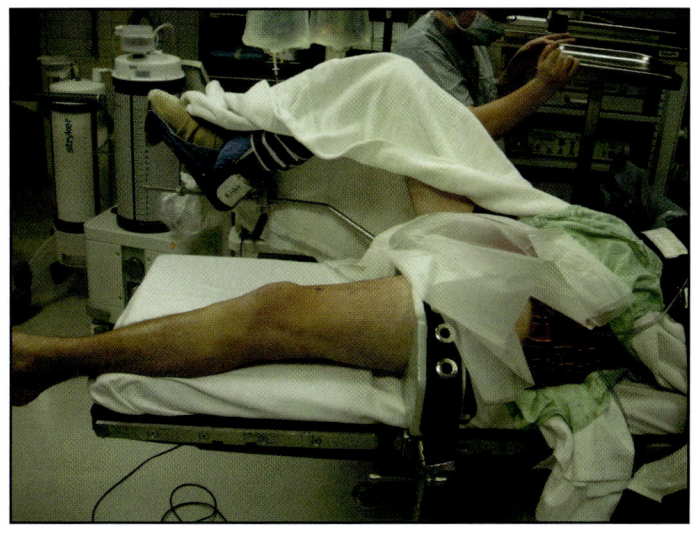

Figure 9-3. Patient positioned with arthroscopic leg holder and contralateral leg in stirrup.

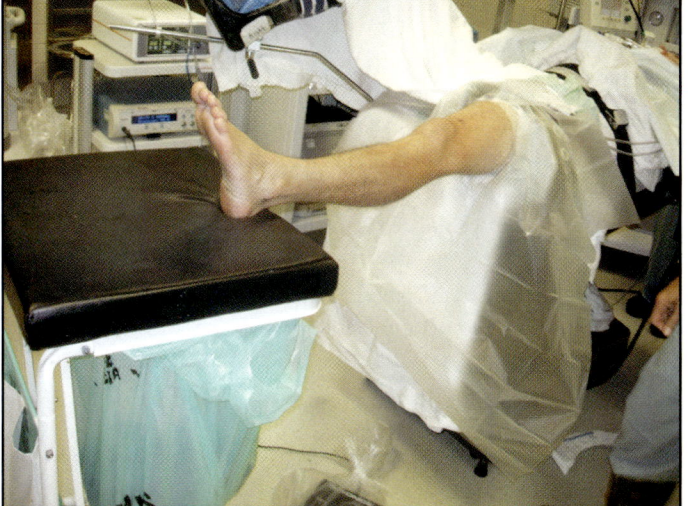

Figure 9-4. Operative extremity ready to be prepped with foot of table broken.

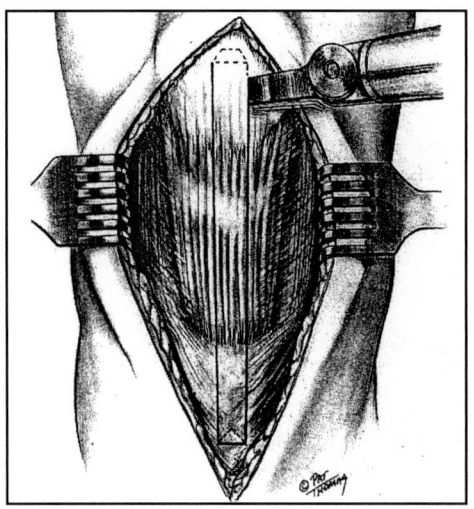

Figure 9-5. Harvest of BTB autograft using microsagittal saw. (Reprinted with permission from SLACK Incorporated from Hardin GT, Bach Jr. BR, Bush-Joseph CA, Farr J. Endoscopic single-incision anterior cruciate ligament reconstruction using patellar tendon autograft. *Am J Knee Surg.* 1992;5(3):144-155.)

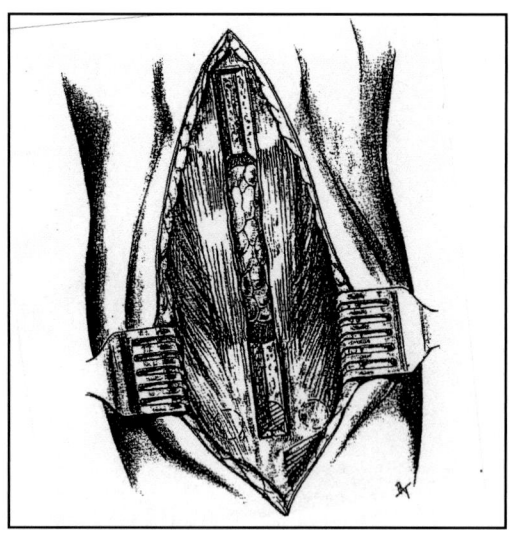

Figure 9-6. Patellar tendon following graft harvest with fat pad left in situ. (Reprinted with permission from SLACK Incorporated from Hardin GT, Bach Jr. BR, Bush-Joseph CA, Farr J. Endoscopic single-incision anterior cruciate ligament reconstruction using patellar tendon autograft. *Am J Knee Surg.* 1992;5(3):144-155.)

osteotomes. The saw cuts are carefully made at angles to create plugs of about 6- to 7-mm thickness. Osteotomes should never be used to lever the bone plugs as they may contribute to an intraoperative patellar fracture or bone plug fracture. The intervening tendon is carefully dissected away from the fat pad. This prevents extravasation of water during the procedure. A meticulously harvested graft makes the remainder of the procedure much easier (Figures 9-5 and 9-6).

* The graft is then prepared on the back table to allow passage of both bone plugs through a 10-mm graft passer (sizing tube). Two drill holes are made in the tibial bone plug using a 0.45-mm Steinman pin. These holes are drilled parallel to the cortex. This allows for passage of two #5 Ethibond sutures. The graft is then marked at the bone tendon junctions, as well as on the cortical surface of the tibial bone plug with a sterile marking pen (Figure 9-7).

* Diagnostic arthroscopy is then performed. We usually will harvest the graft prior to arthroscopy if an obvious pivot shift test is noted and the patient has normal radiographs. Anterolateral and anteromedial portals are established on either side of the patellar tendon at the level of the distal patellar pole. Separate skin incisions are unnecessary as these portals are placed within the longitudinal skin incision. A superomedial outflow portal is also established.

* Any additional meniscal or articular cartilage work is performed at this time. It is important to carefully document all meniscal and chondral pathology because, ultimately, these pathologies may impact the long-term result of an ACL reconstruction.

* Notch preparation and notchplasty is performed. Residual ACL tissue is débrided to provide visualization of the lateral wall and "over the top" region. This may be facilitated with arthroscopic scissors, electrocautery, and a motorized shaver. The goal of the notchplasty is

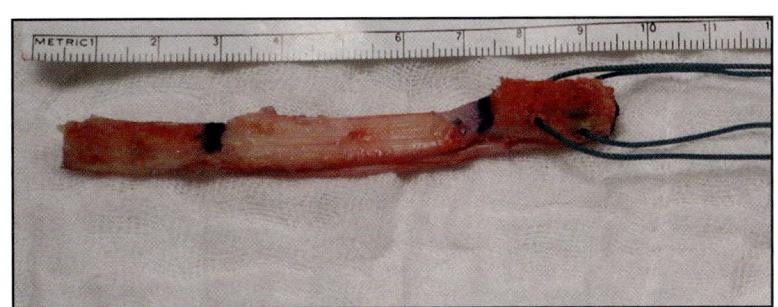

Figure 9-7. Prepared BTB autograft.

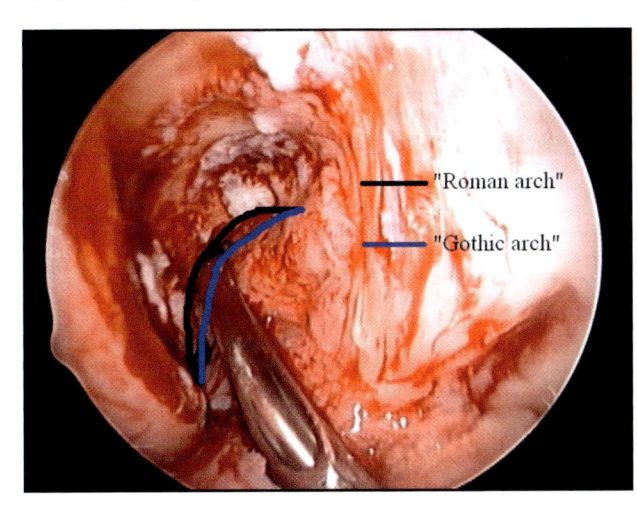

Figure 9-8. Following notchplasty, notch configuration should reveal a "Roman arch." (Reprinted with permission from Rue JPH, Lewis PB, Parameswaran AD, Bach Jr, BR. Single-bundle anterior cruciate ligament reconstruction: technique overview and comprehensive review of results. *J Bone Joint Surg.* 2008;90:67-74. Reprinted with permission from *The Journal of Bone and Joint Surgery Inc.*)

to create an opening of 10 mm between the lateral wall of the intercondylar notch and the lateral edge of the posterior cruciate ligament (PCL) to prevent impingement of the graft in the notch. We often will initiate the notchplasty with a curved 0.25-inch osteotome and mallet. Fragments are collected to graft the distal patellar defect if an autograft is used. The notchplasty is completed from anterior to posterior using a burr to expand the notch with superior and lateral expansion to prevent graft impingement in full extension. The final posterior over-the-top configuration should resemble a smooth "Roman arch" as opposed to a pointed "Gothic arch." This allows for easier placement of the femoral aiming guide at the 10:30 or 1:30 clock positions, depending on the side of the body, as the offset aimer may have a tendency to slide vertically (ie, toward the 11 o'clock or 1 o'clock position) with a more steeply oriented arch configuration (Figure 9-8).

* Once the notch has been adequately prepared, a tibial drill guide is used to intra-articularly position the guidepin. The guide is set based on the n + 10 rule, a modification of the n + 7 rule advocated by Miller,[19] by adding 10 to the tendinous graft length to set the guide in degrees (eg, 45 mm + 10 = 55 degrees). This assists in minimizing graft mismatch issues.[19,20] Generally, the tibial guide is set at a 55-degree angle and occasionally increased to 60 degrees for longer tendon graft lengths.

* Accurate tibial guidepin placement is performed by closely observing and adhering to 3 parameters: 1) the posterior aspect of the tibial ACL footprint; 2) 5 mm lateral to the medial tibial spine; and 3) 7 mm anterior to the PCL.[21-23] A simple general reference point for the pin to exit on the tibial articular surface is 3 to 4 mm posterior to the posterior edge of the anterior horn of the lateral meniscus (Figure 9-9).

Figure 9-9. Arthroscopic view of the tibial pin, showing appropriate position in relation to the PCL and the posterior aspect of the lateral meniscal anterior horn.

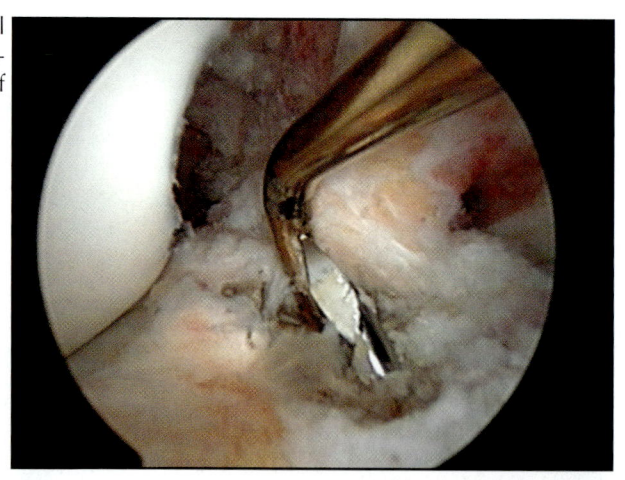

Figure 9-10. Tibial drill guide placed through the accessory inferomedial portal made through the graft harvest rent.

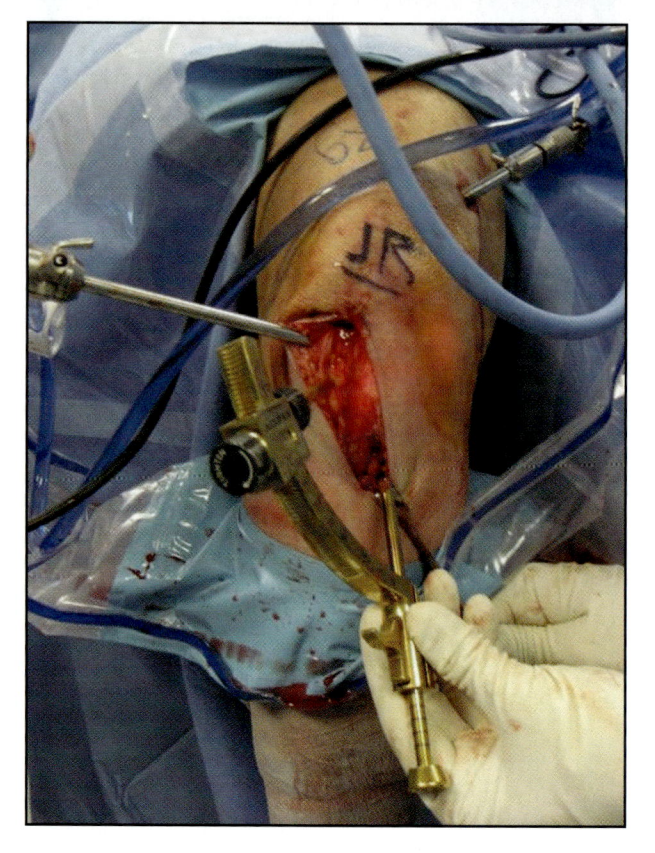

* The tibial drill guide is placed through an accessory inferomedial portal (Figure 9-10). This is important as it allows for a more appropriate medial to lateral (ie, oblique) orientation in the tibial tunnel so that accurate femoral tunnel placement can be achieved (Figure 9-11). This portal is made through the mid-patellar tendon rent when using BTB autograft or through the patellar tendon when using an allograft. This important "trick" allows more rotational flexibility in selecting the tibial orientation, which can impact the placement of the femoral tunnel when a transtibial technique is used. The tibial tunnel should be in the midline of the notch in the coronal plane, angled in such a way that the subsequent femoral

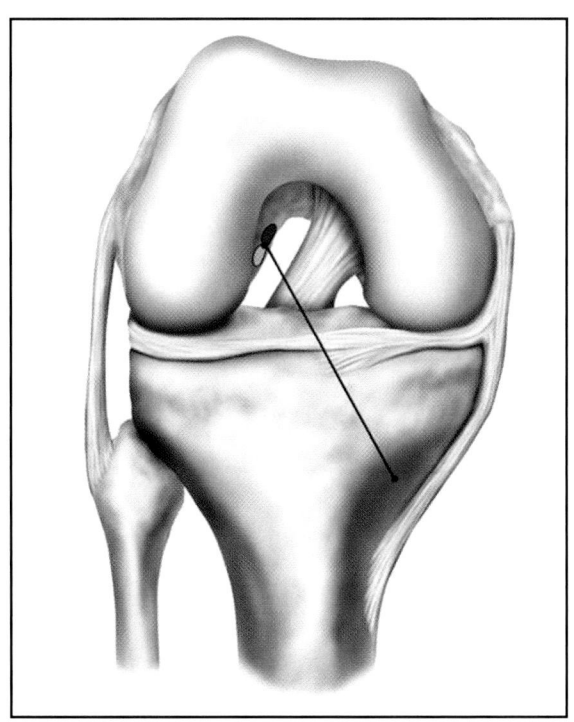

Figure 9-11. The tibial drill guide requires appropriate angulation to allow engagement of the femoral guide at the 10:30 position on the femoral condyle. (Reprinted with permission from Busam ML, Provencher MT, Bach Jr BR. Complications of anterior cruciate ligament reconstruction with bone-patellar tendon-bone constructs. *Am J Sports Med.* 2008;36:379-394.)

tunnel can easily be positioned at the 10:30 clock position on a right knee and the 1:30 clock position on a left knee. Failure to recognize the consequences of a malpositioned or malo-riented tibial tunnel will lead to vertical orientation of the femoral tunnel, which effectively will reconstruct preferentially more of the anteromedial bundle of the ACL. Clinically, this may eliminate the Lachman test but not provide rotational control. Currently, the goal is to place the femoral tunnel in a position that will fill portions of both of the posterolateral and anteromedial bundles. When properly achieved clinically, the Lachman and pivot shift tests are normalized. Alternatively, one could use an accessory portal to drill the tunnels with the knee hyperflexed as initially advocated by O'Donnell and Scerpella[24] and more recently repopularized by Harner et al.[25]

* Once the pin is drilled intra-articularly, we extend the knee to make certain that the pin is posterior to the apex of the intracondylar notch in knee extension. The pin is then tapped up into the femoral roof with a mallet to stabilize it while it is over-reamed. This will reduce the amount of posterior lip that may occur when the reamer enters the joint. The guidepin is then over-drilled with a cannulated reamer 1 mm larger than the tibial bone block (typically 11 mm). We usually will over-ream by 1 mm to make graft passage easier through the tibial tunnel; this reduces the likelihood of delaminating the graft during graft passage.

* The tunnel is plugged with a rubber stopper, and a shaver is used to remove osteochondral fragments from the intra-articular opening of the tibial tunnel. A chamfer reamer and curved hand rasp are used successively to smooth the posterior edge of the tunnel's proximal opening (Figures 9-12, 9-13, and 9-14). This is an important step, as this posterior lip may push the femoral offset aimer anteriorly when one attempts to position the femoral aimer. To position the aimer appropriately, one might have to extend the knee to allow the aimer to hook over the posterior cortical ridge. In doing so, the knee may be extended, and one can ream out through the posterior wall despite entering in what appears to be an appropriate location.

Figure 9-12. After drilling the tibial tunnel, a chamfer reamer and curved hand rasp are used to produce a smoother posterior surface for the graft to lie against. (Reprinted with permission from Ferrari JD, Bush-Joseph CA, Bach Jr BR. Arthroscopic-assisted anterior cruciate ligament reconstruction using patellar tendon autograft substitution—two-incision technique. *Techniques in Orthopaedics.* 1998;13(3):242-252.)

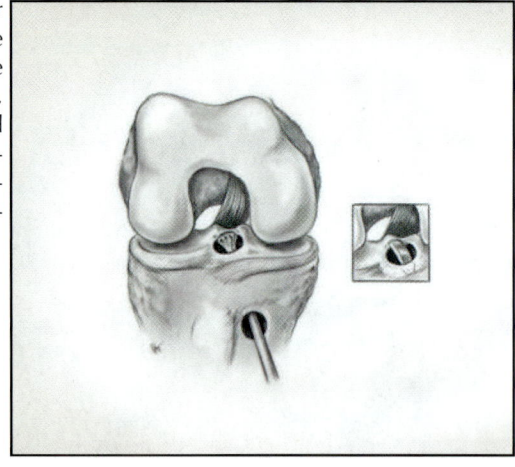

Figure 9-13. Arthroscopic view of chamfer reamer.

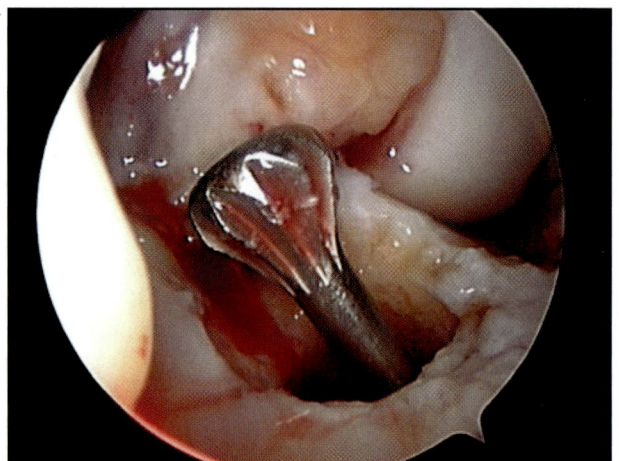

Figure 9-14. Arthroscopic view of curved hand rasp.

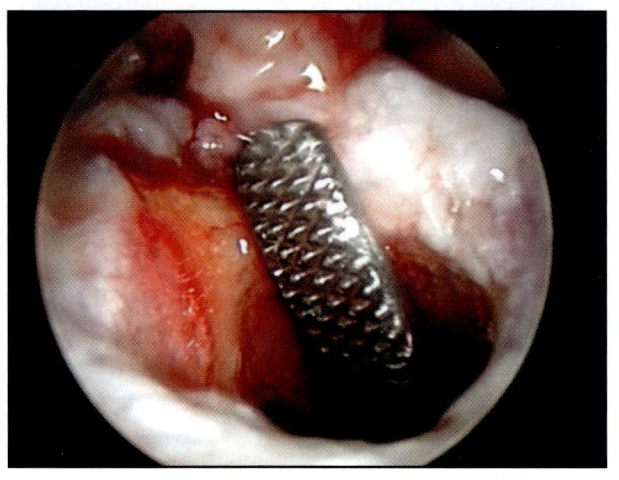

* A 7-mm femoral offset guide is inserted through the tibial tunnel, passed through the joint, and hooked at the "over-the-top" position (Figure 9-15). The surgeon should be able to perform this with the knee flexed between 75 and 90 degrees of knee flexion. The guide is then

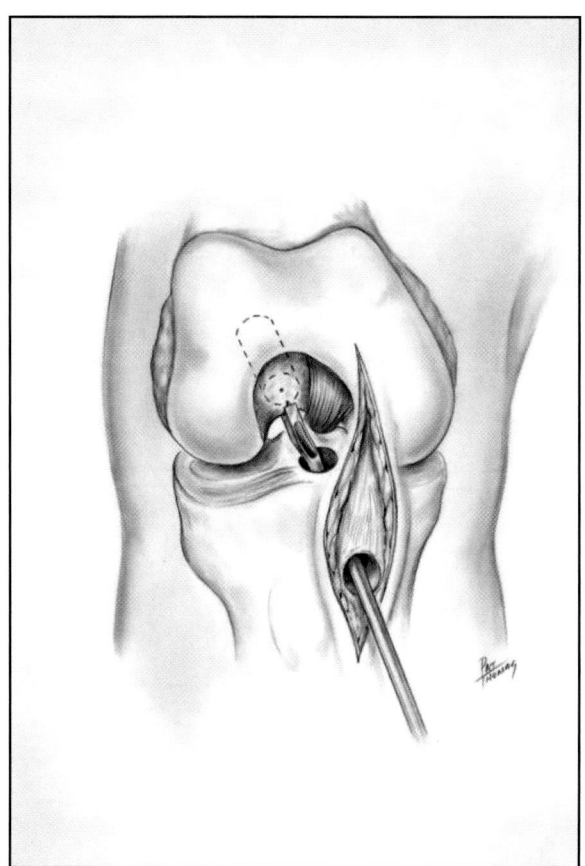

Figure 9-15. Transtibial tunnel placement of the femoral offset guide. (Reprinted with permission from Ferrari JD, Bush-Joseph CA, Bach Jr BR. Endoscopic anterior cruciate ligament reconstruction with patellar tendon autograft: surgical technique. *Techniques in Orthopaedics*. 1998;13(3):262-274.)

positioned and rotated laterally to achieve the proper orientation obliquely on the femur, corresponding to a position roughly between the anteromedial and posterolateral bundle origins.[26] This is approximately at the 10:30 clock position in a right knee or the 1:30 clock position in a left knee (Figures 9-16 and 9-17).

* Once the guide is properly anchored, the guidepin is drilled approximately 35 mm, or until it engages the far cortex (Figure 9-18).

* To ensure the integrity of the posterior cortical wall, a femoral tunnel "footprint" is reamed 10 mm into the femur before fully reaming the tunnel. This footprint is then probed to confirm cortical integrity and appropriate posterior bone thickness of 1 to 2 mm prior to reaming the tunnel to a depth of 35 mm (Figure 9-19). This step allows the surgeon to make certain that the posterior cortex will not be violated. Integrity of the femoral tunnel can be confirmed after reaming by inserting the arthroscope through the tibial tunnel in a retrograde fashion and examining the femoral socket under direct visualization (Figure 9-20).

* The graft can now be passed using a "push-in" technique. This requires the graft to be pushed through the tibial tunnel into the notch using a 2-prong graft pusher (Figure 9-21). With the bone plug in the notch, a curved hemostat is placed through the inferomedial portal to grasp the bone plug and guide it into the femoral tunnel (Figure 9-22). On the femoral side, the graft is positioned with the cancellous portion of the bone plug anterior and the cortical side posterior. This allows a more posterior placement of the tendon fibers and reduces the possibility of graft laceration during screw placement. Fixation is achieved using a metallic interference screw (7 mm x 25 mm) (Figure 9-23). The knee is further

Figure 9-16. The "clock face" orientation of the femoral notch. (Reprinted with permission from Rue JPH, Busam ML, Bach Jr BR. Hybrid single-bundle anterior cruciate ligament reconstruction technique using a transtibial drilled femoral tunnel. *Tech Knee Surg.* 2008;7:107-114.)

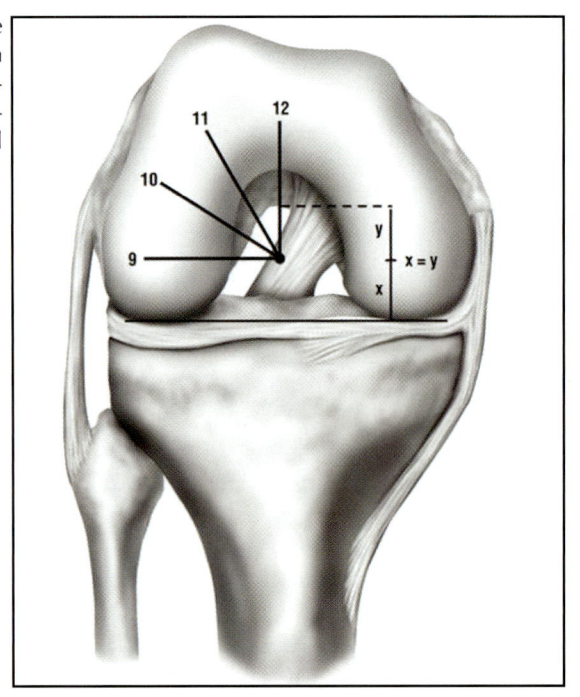

Figure 9-17. Placement of the femoral offset guide in the 10:30 position. (Reprinted with permission from Rue JPH, Lewis PB, Parameswaran AD, Bach Jr BR. Single-bundle anterior cruciate ligament reconstruction: technique overview and comprehensive review of results. *J Bone Joint Surg.* 2008;90:67-74. Reprinted with permission from *The Journal of Bone and Joint Surgery Inc.*)

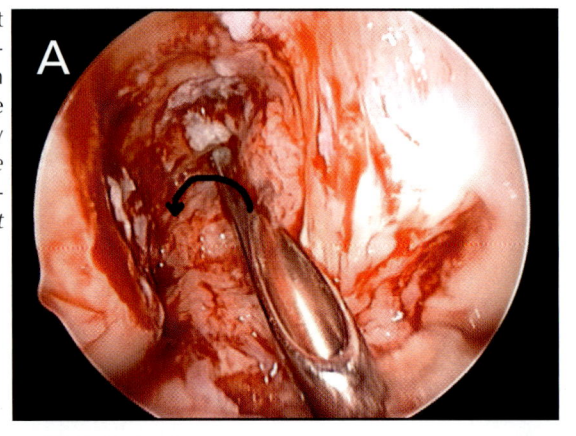

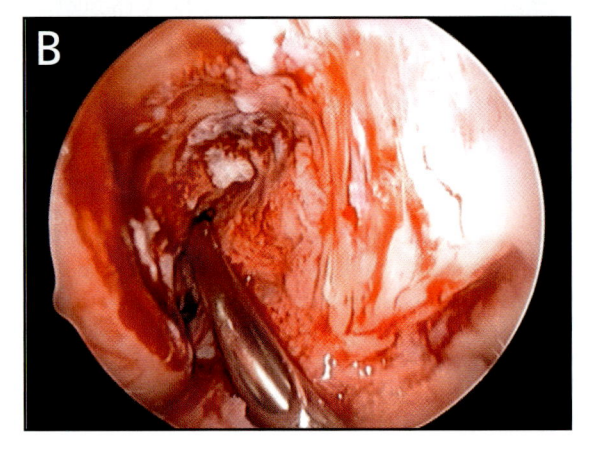

Single-Bundle ACL Reconstruction Using Patellar Tendon Grafts | 115

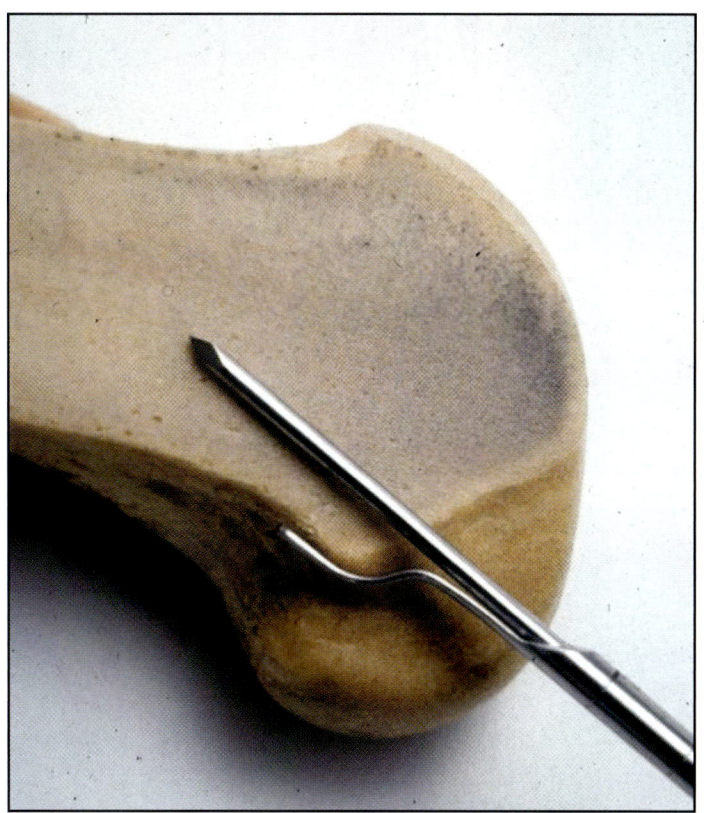

Figure 9-18. Guidepin placement using the 7-mm offset guide will leave a 2 mm posterior wall. (Reprinted with permission from SLACK Incorporated from Hardin GT, Bach Jr. BR, Bush-Joseph CA, Farr J. Endoscopic single-incision anterior cruciate ligament reconstruction using patellar tendon autograft: surgical technique. *Am J Knee Surg.* 1992;5(3):144-155.)

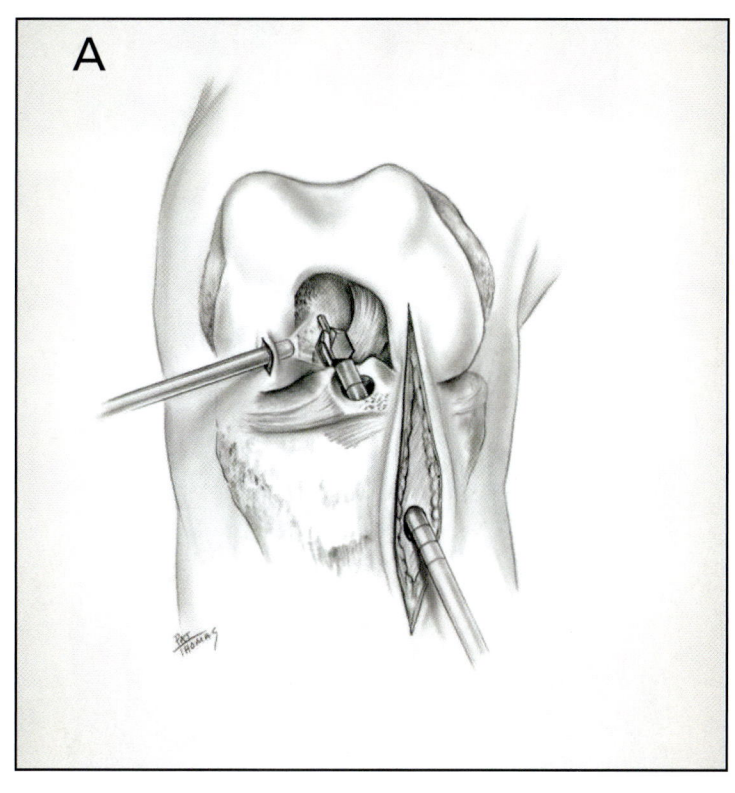

Figure 9-19A. Femoral tunnel reaming using a 10-mm reamer. (Reprinted with permission from SLACK Incorporated from Hardin GT, Bach Jr. BR, Bush-Joseph CA, Farr J. Endoscopic single-incision anterior cruciate ligament reconstruction using patellar tendon autograft: surgical technique. *Am J Knee Surg. 1992;*5(3):144-155.)

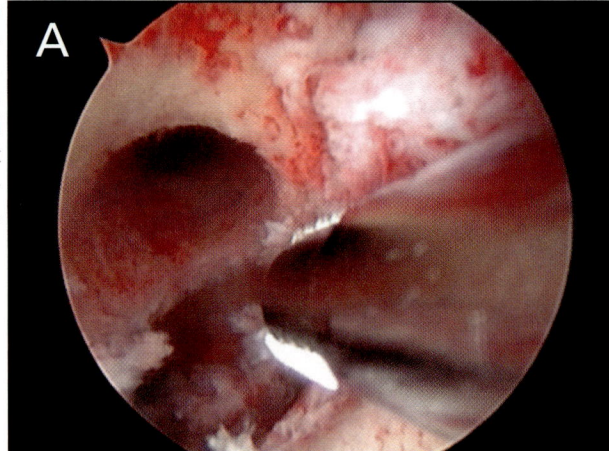

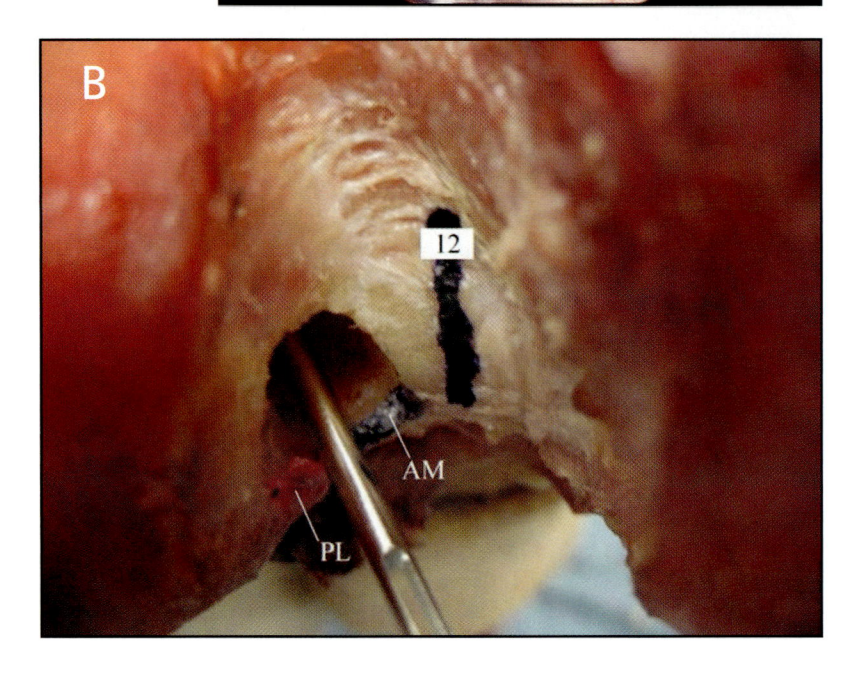

Figure 9-19B. Femoral tunnel reaming using a 10-mm reamer. (Reprinted with permission from SLACK Incorporated from Hardin GT, Bach Jr. BR, Bush-Joseph CA, Farr J. Endoscopic single-incision anterior cruciate ligament reconstruction using patellar tendon autograft: surgical technique. *Am J Knee Surg.* 1992;5(3):144-155.)

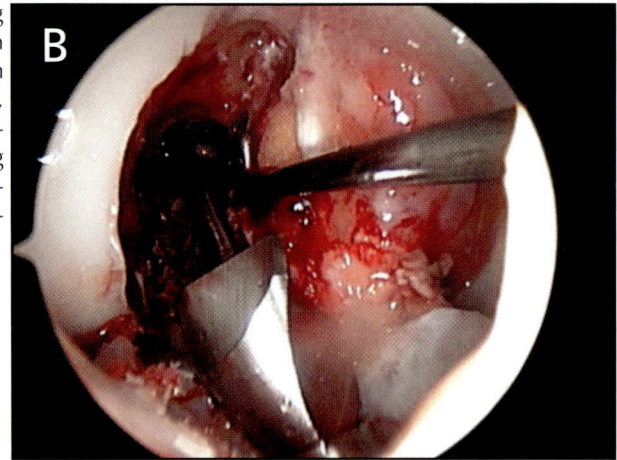

Figure 9-20. Femoral tunnel placement in the 10:30 position, bisecting the posterolateral and anteromedial bundle insertions. (Figure B reprinted with permission from Rue JPH, Busam ML, Bach Jr BR. Hybrid single-bundle anterior cruciate ligament reconstruction technique using a transtibial drilled femoral tunnel. *Tech Knee Surg.* 2008;7:107-114.)

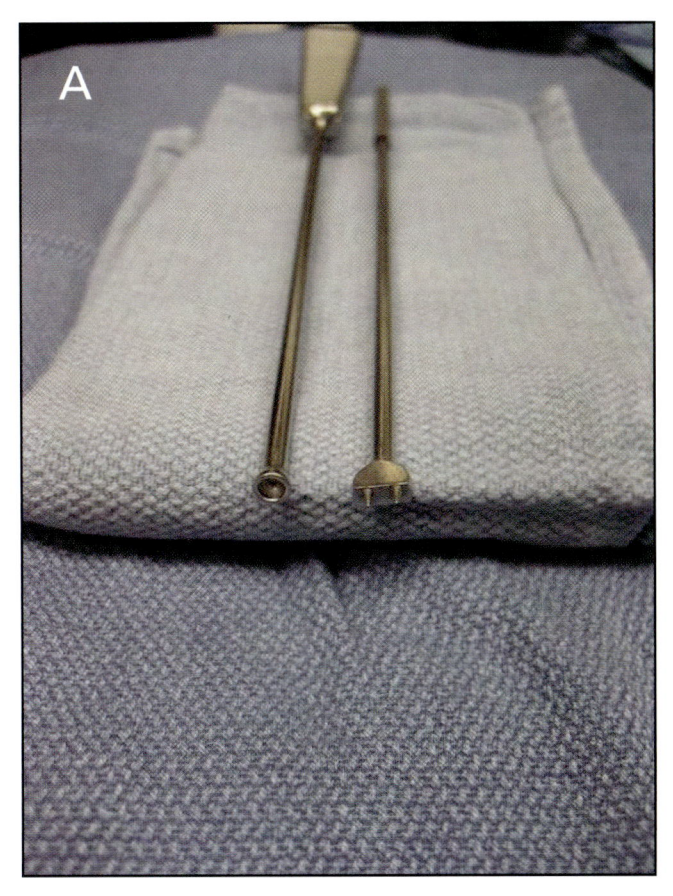

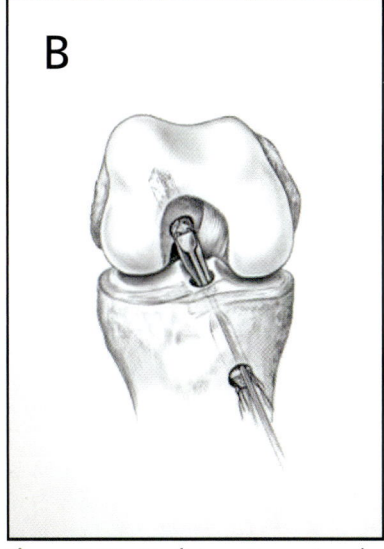

Figure 9-21. Graft insertion using the 2-pronged graft pusher. (Figure B reprinted with permission from SLACK Incorporated from Hardin GT, Bach Jr. BR, Bush-Joseph CA, Farr J. Endoscopic single-incision anterior cruciate ligament reconstruction using patellar tendon autograft: surgical technique. *Am J Knee Surg.* 1992;5(3):144-155.)

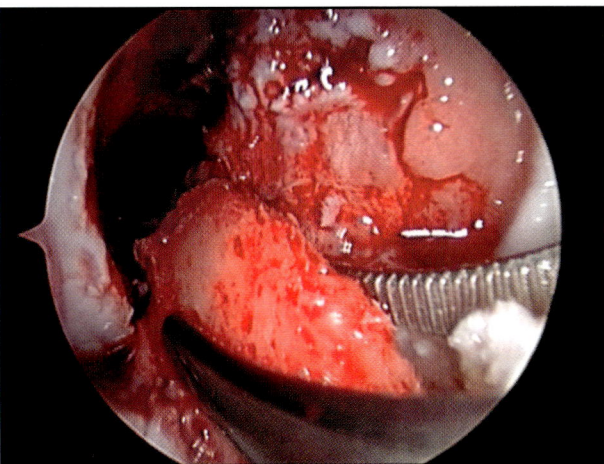

Figure 9-22. Guiding the graft into the femoral tunnel using a curved hemostat.

flexed during screw placement to account for the angle difference between the tibial tunnel and the inferomedial portal used for screw placement. This will enhance the potential for parallel screw placement and reduce the possibility of graft laceration. During screw placement, observe for tissue rotation as the screw is inserted. If this occurs, stop and carefully reassess to avoid lacerating the graft. Once the graft is securely fixed in the femoral tunnel, the graft is rotated laterally (toward the lateral wall) 180 degrees. This better replicates the

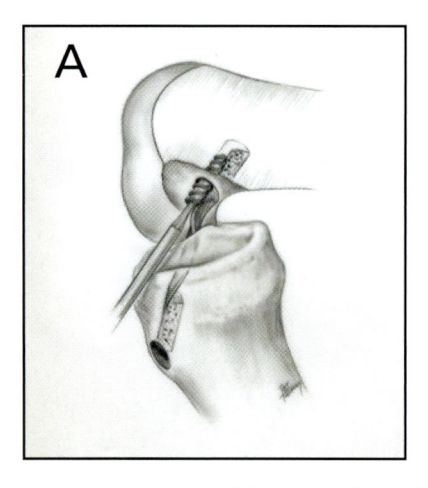

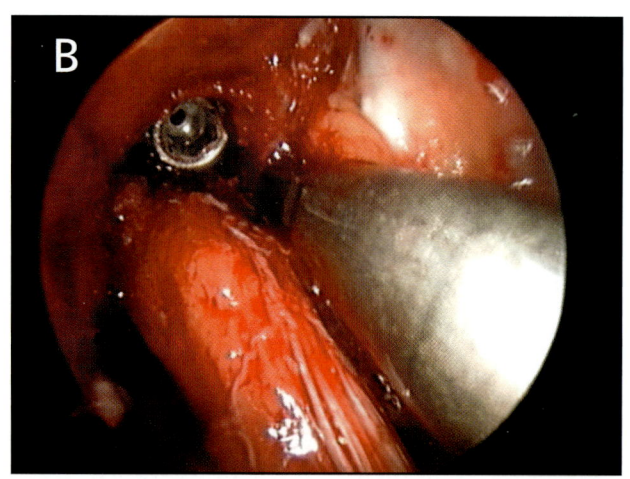

Figure 9-23. Femoral fixation achieved using an interference screw placed through the anteromedial portal. (Figure A reprinted with permission from SLACK Incorporated from Hardin GT, Bach Jr. BR, Bush-Joseph CA, Farr J. Endoscopic single-incision anterior cruciate ligament reconstruction using patellar tendon autograft: surgical technique. *Am J Knee Surg.* 1992;5(3):144-155.)

anatomic fiber orientation of the native ACL. Tibial screw fixation is achieved with the knee in extension or hyperextension. The knee is axially loaded by having the patient's foot fixed firmly on the surgeon's abdomen while the graft is tensioned. A metallic interference screw (usually 9 mm x 20 mm) is placed on the anterior aspect of the bone plug on the cortical surface. The screw is placed anteriorly on the cortical surface of the plug for several reasons: 1) the screw is less likely to wander and become divergent, 2) cancellous-to-cancellous fixation in the tibia is superior to cancellous-to-cortical fixation biomechanically, 3) one can place the screw beyond the tendo-osseous junction in graft construct mismatch situations and reduce the possibility of graft soft tissue injury, and 4) the screw will further position the graft posteriorly (Figure 9-24).

TIPS AND PEARLS

✔ Ensure that the final posterior intercondylar notch configuration resembles a smooth "Roman arch" as opposed to a pointed "Gothic arch." This allows for easier placement of the aiming guide at the 10:30 or 1:30 clock positions, as the offset aimer may have a tendency to slide vertically (ie, toward the 11 o'clock or 1 o'clock position) with a more steeply oriented arch configuration.

✔ The accessory inferomedial portal (transpatellar rent or tendon) allows improved mobility of the tibial guide device and allows for easier medial to lateral (ie, oblique) orientation of the guide than when it is placed through the standard medial portal.

✔ Position the 7-mm femoral offset guide at the most lateral (ie, oblique) position possible. Hook the "over-the-top" position, and then rotate the guide laterally to achieve the 10:30 or 1:30 clock position.

✔ If a graft construct mismatch exists, one can recess the graft on the femur, perform a "free bone block" form of fixation,[27] hyper-rotate the graft (up to 540 degrees can shorten the graft 8 mm), or rely on extra tunnel fixation (staple fixation).[28]

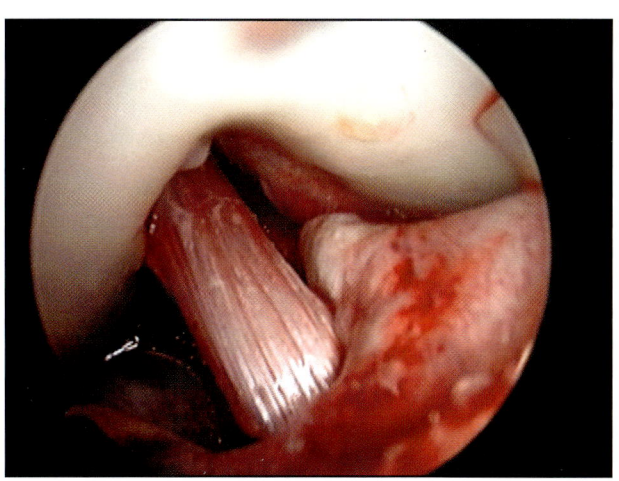

Figure 9-24. Final view of ACL graft.

PITFALLS

✘ Avoid removing the retropatellar fat pad during tendon harvest, as this can lead to excessive fluid extravasation. Do not lever the graft with an osteotome. Do not pass the graft away from the operative field; personally walk the graft to the preparation table to reduce the likelihood of dropping the graft. Inform everyone in the room where the graft is placed after preparation to avoid inadvertently passing the graft off the operative field.

✘ During notch preparation, avoid tapering the notchplasty as you progress posteriorly. Use the burr to remove equal amounts of bone from the notch at both the anterior aspect and the posterior aspect.

✘ Avoid placing the tibial tunnel without adequate medial-to-lateral obliquity. Without appropriate obliquity, it will be very difficult to use the transtibial technique to get to the 10:30 or 2:30 clock position for the femoral tunnel. The accessory inferior portal will also allow a more distal entrance site on the tibia and reduce the possibility of a graft construct mismatch.

✘ Always ream the first 10 mm of the femoral tunnel, and then stop and check to ensure that there is appropriate posterior bone. This will help prevent "blow-outs" of the femoral tunnel.

REFERENCES

1. Barrack RL, Bruckner JD, Kneisl J, et al. The outcome of non-operatively treated complete tears of the anterior cruciate ligament in active young adults. *Clin Orthop Relat Res.* 1990;259:192-199.
2. Daniel DM, Stone ML, Dobson BE, et al. Fate of the ACL-injured patient: a prospective outcome study. *Am J Sports Med.* 1994;22:632-644.
3. Noyes FR, Mooar PA, Matthews DS, et al. The symptomatic anterior cruciate deficient knee: part I. the long term functional disability on athletically active individuals. *J Bone Joint Surg Am.* 1983;65:154-162.
4. Fithian DC, Paxton EW, Stone ML, et al. Prospective trial of a treatment algorithm for the management of the anterior cruciate ligament-injured knee. *Am J Sports Med.* 2005;33:335-346.
5. Busam ML, Rue JP, Bach BR Jr. Fresh-frozen allograft anterior cruciate ligament reconstruction. *Clin Sports Med.* 2007;26:607-623.
6. Bach BR Jr, Nho SJ. Anterior cruciate ligament: diagnosis and decision making. In: Miller MD, Cole BJ, eds. *Textbook of Arthroscopy.* Philadelphia, PA: Elsevier; 2004:633-643.

7. Novak PJ, Bach BR Jr, Hager CA. Clinical and functional outcome of anterior cruciate ligament reconstruction in the recreational athlete over the age of 35. *Am J Knee Surg.* 1996;9:111-116.
8. Plancher KD, Steadman JR, Briggs KK, et al. Reconstruction of the anterior cruciate ligament in patients who are at least forty years old: a long term follow-up and outcome study. *J Bone Joint Surg Am.* 1998;80:184-197.
9. Cannon WD Jr, Vittori JM. The incidence of healing in arthroscopic meniscal repairs in anterior cruciate ligament-reconstructed knees versus stable knees. *Am J Sports Med.* 1992;20:176-181.
10. Tuneta JJ, Arciero RA. Arthroscopic evaluation of meniscal repairs: factors that affect healing. *Am J Sports Med.* 1994;22:797-802.
11. Beynnon BD, Johnson RJ, Abate JA, et al. Treatment of anterior cruciate ligament injuries, part 1. *Am J Sports Med.* 2005;33:1579-1602.
12. Glenn RE Jr, Bach BR Jr, Bush-Joseph CA. Anterior cruciate ligament reconstruction: the Rush experience. *Techniques in Orthopaedics.* 2005;20:396-404.
13. Bach BR Jr, Jones GT, Sweet FA, et al. Arthroscopic assisted ACL reconstruction using patellar tendon substitution: two year follow up study. *Am J Sports Med.* 1994;22:758-767.
14. Bach BR Jr, Levy ME, Bojchuk J, et al. Single-incision endoscopic anterior cruciate ligament reconstruction using patellar tendon autograft: minimum two year follow-up evaluation. *Am J Sports Med.* 1998;26:30-40.
15. Bach BR Jr, Tradonsky S, Bojchuk J, et al. Arthroscopically assisted anterior cruciate ligament reconstruction using patellar tendon autograft: five to nine year follow-up evaluation. *Am J Sports Med.* 1998;26:20-29.
16. Ferrari JD, Bach BR Jr, Bush-Joseph CA, et al. Anterior cruciate ligament reconstruction in men and women: an outcome analysis comparing gender. *Arthroscopy.* 2001;17:588-596.
17. Wexler G, Bach BR Jr, Bush-Joseph CA, et al. Outcomes of anterior cruciate ligament reconstruction in patients with Workers' Compensation claims. *Arthroscopy.* 2000;16:49-58.
18. Bach BR Jr, Aadalen KJ, Dennis MG, et al. Primary anterior cruciate ligament reconstruction using fresh-frozen, nonirradiated patellar tendon allograft: minimum 2-year follow-up. *Am J Sports Med.* 2005;33:284-292.
19. Miller MD, Hinkin DT. The "N + 7 rule" for tibial tunnel placement in endoscopic anterior cruciate ligament reconstruction. *Arthroscopy.* 1996;12:124-126.
20. Olszewski AD, Miller MD, Ritchie JR. Ideal tibial tunnel length for endoscopic anterior cruciate ligament reconstruction. *Arthroscopy.* 1998;14:9-14.
21. Howell SM, Clark JA. Tibial tunnel placement in anterior cruciate ligament reconstructions and graft impingement. *Clin Orthop Relat Res.* 1992;283:187-195.
22. Jackson DW, Gasser SI. Tibial tunnel placement in ACL reconstruction. *Arthroscopy.* 1994;10:124-131.
23. Morgan CD, Kalman VR, Grawl DM. Definitive landmarks for reproducible tibial tunnel placement in anterior cruciate ligament reconstruction. *Arthroscopy.* 1995;11:275-288.
24. O'Donnell JB, Scerpella TA. Endoscopic anterior cruciate ligament reconstruction: modified technique and radiographic review. *Arthroscopy.* 1995;11:577-584.
25. Harner CD, Honkamp NJ, Ranawat AS. Anteromedial portal technique for creating the anterior cruciate ligament femoral tunnel. *Arthroscopy.* 2008;24:113-115.
26. Rue JP, Ghodadra N, Bach BR Jr. Femoral tunnel placement in single-bundle anterior cruciate ligament reconstruction: a cadaveric study relating transtibial lateralized femoral tunnel position to the anteromedial and posterolateral bundle femoral origins of the anterior cruciate ligament. *Am J Sports Med.* 2008;36:73-79.
27. Novak PJ, Wexler GM, Williams JS Jr, et al. Comparison of screw post fixation and free bone block interference fixation for anterior cruciate ligament soft tissue grafts: biomechanical considerations. *Arthroscopy.* 1996;12:470-473.
28. Busam ML, Provencher MT, Bach BR Jr. Complications of anterior cruciate ligament reconstruction with bone-patellar tendon-bone constructs: care and prevention. *Am J Sports Med.* 2008;36:379-394.

10

Anatomic Double-Bundle ACL Reconstruction

Susan S. Jordan, MD; Wei Shen, MD, PhD; and Freddie H. Fu, MD, DSc

Double-bundle anterior cruciate ligament (DB ACL) reconstruction is our preferred surgical option for ACL-deficient patients with symptomatic instability. There are contraindications to DB ACL reconstruction, however, that include skeletal immaturity, multiple ligament injury, and significant chondral abnormalities. We make the final decision to perform DB ACL reconstruction intraoperatively. At the time of arthroscopy, we measure the dimensions of the anteromedial (AM) and posterolateral (PL) attachment sites on the femur and tibia. To perform a DB ACL reconstruction, the attachment sites must be of adequate size to accommodate 2 grafts. We consider each knee individually and tailor the ACL reconstruction to fit the individual anatomy of the knee. In knees with attachment sites that measure less than 12 mm from anterior to posterior, we perform single-bundle reconstructions, whereas in those with tibial attachment sites greater than 12 mm in length, we perform DB ACL reconstruction.

We routinely use tibialis anterior allografts for both the AM and PL bundles in DB ACL reconstruction. We measure the size of the tibial and femoral footprints of the AM and PL bundles and fashion individual allografts to match the native size of each bundle (commonly, 7-mm diameter for the PL and 8 mm for the AM). Hamstring autograft can also be used, but we prefer allograft because its consistent size allows the surgeon to match the graft to the size of the AM and PL bundles. Hamstring autograft is often too small to cover the entire footprint of each bundle and, therefore, could lead to a non-anatomic reconstruction.

SURGICAL GOALS

The primary goals of DB ACL reconstruction are restoration of the anatomy of the native ACL and restoration of the stability of the native ACL. Anatomic studies have shown that the native ACL consists of 2 bundles: the AM and PL bundles[1,2] (Figures 10-1 and 10-2). The bundles exhibit different tensioning patterns throughout the knee range of motion and contribute differently to knee stability. The AM bundle appears to have a significant role in knee stability in the anteroposterior (AP) plane, while the PL bundle controls both AP and rotational stability.[3-5] Studies have shown that single-bundle (SB) ACL reconstruction fails to restore normal knee kinematics and stability.[6] DB ACL reconstruction appears to improve rotational stability and more closely restore normal knee kinematics.[7,8]

Our DB technique involves creation of 2 femoral and 2 tibial tunnels to recreate the AM and PL bundles. With an anatomically based ACL reconstruction, our goal is to return patients to their pre-injury level of activity with a pain-free, stable knee.

Figure 10-1. Arthroscopic picture of a left knee shows the 2 functional bundles of the ACL (the AM bundle and the PL bundle) attaching to the lateral femoral condyle. When the knee is flexed, the femoral PL attachment lies anterior to the AM attachment.

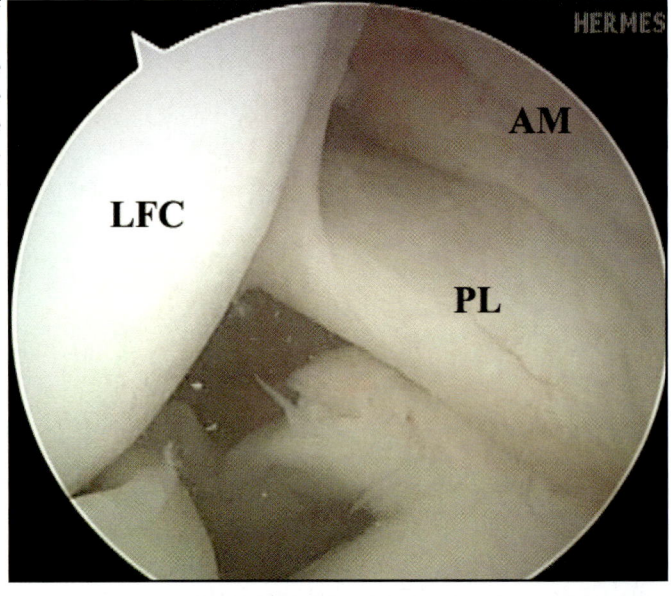

Figure 10-2. The AM and PL bundles of the normal ACL are clearly visible on this sagittal MRI image as 2 distinct structures.

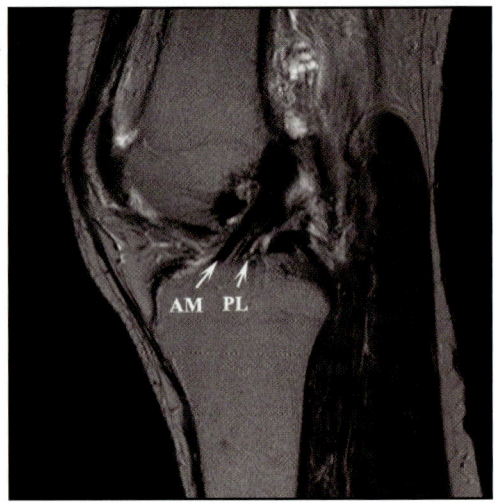

OPERATIVE STEPS

* A complete exam under anesthesia is performed to document Lachman, pivot shift, and range of motion.
* A tourniquet is applied to the operative limb, and the thigh is placed in a thigh holder, with the distal part of the bed flexed. The nonoperative leg is placed in a well-padded leg holder in the abducted position (Figure 10-3). The operative lower extremity is prepped with alcohol and Betadine (Alcon, Fort Worth, TX) and draped.
* Arthroscopy is performed using 3 portals (Figure 10-4). The anterolateral (AL) portal is established just at the lateral edge of the patellar tendon at the level of the inferior pole of the patella. We establish this portal with the knee at 45 degrees of flexion to avoid injuring the patella. We also use an AM portal and an accessory anteromedial (AAM) portal. The AM portal is placed inferior to the AL portal, along the medial border of the patellar tendon. To

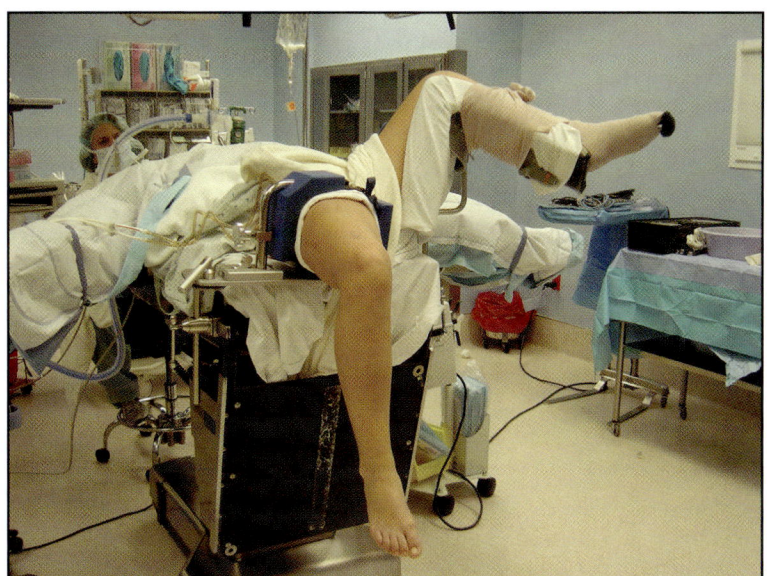

Figure 10-3. Positioning of the patient for a right DB ACL reconstruction is shown. This set-up allows knee range of motion from full extension to hyperflexion past 120 degrees.

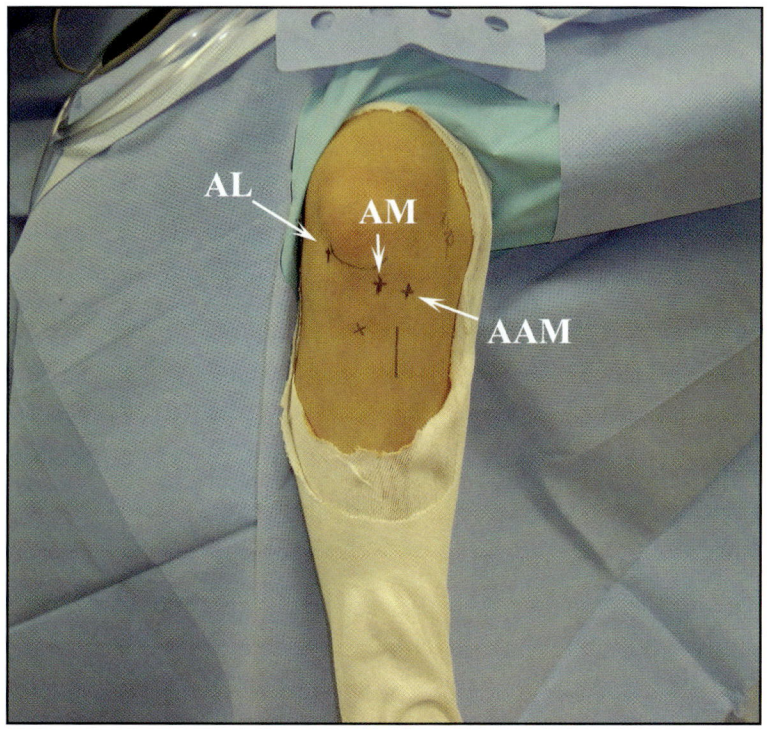

Figure 10-4. The locations of the 3 arthroscopic portals are shown: the AL portal, the AM portal, and the AAM portal.

create the AAM portal, we place the arthroscope in the AM portal and insert an 18-gauge spinal needle just above the medial meniscus, medial and distal to the AM portal. The trajectory of the needle should reach the center of the femoral footprint of the PL bundle. When establishing the AAM portal, the surgeon must ensure that the spinal needle does not damage the medial meniscus or the medial femoral condyle.

* Viewing through the AL portal, the fat pad is resected to permit visualization of the ACL bundle insertion sites. Associated meniscal injuries are addressed before beginning the ACL reconstruction.

Figure 10-5. The injury pattern of the 2 bundles is identified by careful dissection of the intact fibers. In this case, the PL bundle is stretched on the femoral side, and the AM bundle is torn off the femoral side.

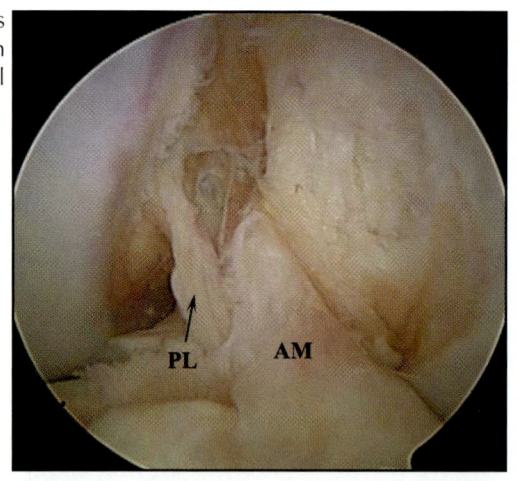

Figure 10-6. The femoral insertion sites of the AM and PL bundles have been identified and marked with the thermal device. We have identified 2 bony landmarks that can guide placement of femoral AM and PL tunnels. When in 90 degrees of knee flexion, the lateral intercondylar ridge (arrow heads) defines the upper border of both AM and PL insertion sites, while the lateral bifurcate ridge (arrows) divides them. Placing the arthroscope in the AM portal allows excellent visualization of the femoral insertions of the AM and PL bundles and makes notchplasty unnecessary.

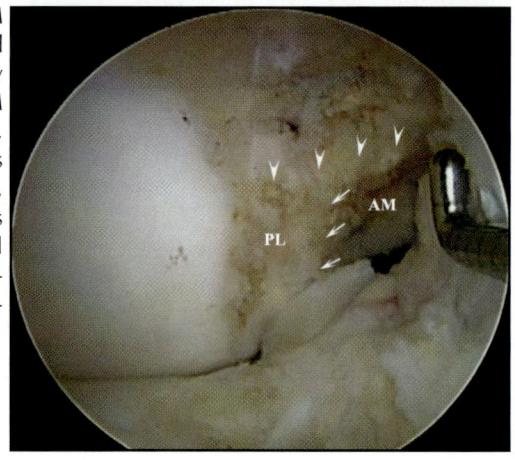

* Using a thermal device (Arthrocare Corporation, Sunnyvale, CA), we perform a gentle dissection of the ACL bundles, taking particular care to preserve the soft tissue remnants at the tibial and femoral attachments. We assess the rupture pattern (whether one or both bundles are torn, and from which attachment—femoral or tibial) (Figure 10-5). When one of the bundles is found to be intact, we preserve that bundle and augment it with a reconstruction of the injured bundle only.

* We identify 2 bony ridges along the lateral intercondylar wall: the lateral intercondylar ridge and the lateral bifurcate ridge (Figure 10-6). With the knee at 90 degrees of flexion, the lateral intercondylar ridge (also known as the "resident's ridge") defines the superior border of the AM and PL bundles. The lateral bifurcate ridge separates the AM and PL insertions. These ridges help guide identification of bundle attachment sites and tunnel placement.[9]

* The femoral and tibial footprints of both AM and PL bundles are marked with the thermal device. The lengths of the footprints are measured, and the graft size for each bundle is determined based on these measurements (Figure 10-7).

* A curved Steadman awl is used to create a small hole in the center of the femoral AM and PL footprints for subsequent guidewire placement.

* On the back table, an assistant begins graft preparation of 2 tibialis anterior grafts, which are thawed and rinsed in antibiotic solution. These allografts are usually between

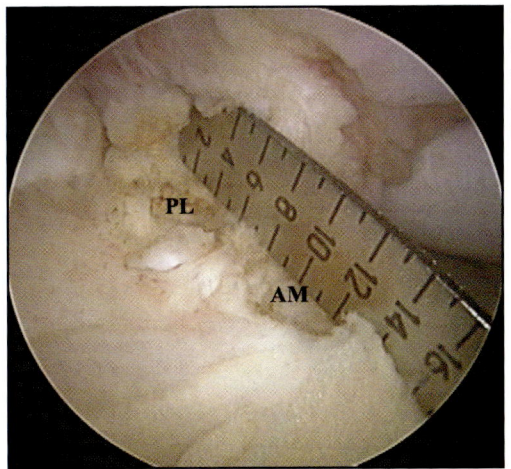

Anatomic Double-Bundle ACL Reconstruction 127

Figure 10-7. After gentle dissection, the tibial AM and PL insertion sites are marked with the thermal device. The length and width of the insertion sites are measured to tailor the tunnel and graft size for each individual knee.

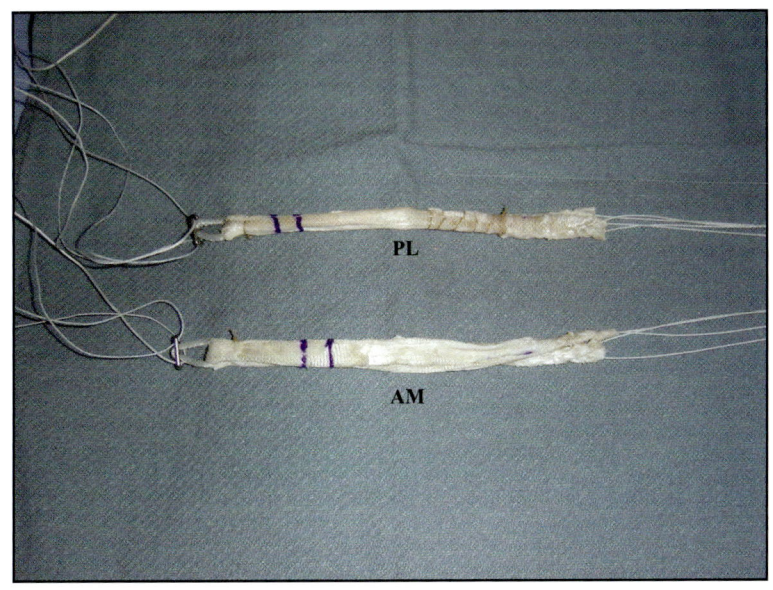

Figure 10-8. Doubled-over tibialis anterior allograft is commonly used for both AM and PL bundles. EndoButton fixation is often used on the femoral side for both grafts as shown here.

24 and 30 cm in length. Once trimmed to the appropriate diameter, the ends of the grafts are sutured using a baseball stitch with #2 Ticron sutures for a length of 2.5 cm. An EndoButton CL (Smith & Nephew, Inc, London, United Kingdom) is placed on each graft, resulting in a double-stranded graft of approximately 12 to 15 cm in length (Figure 10-8). We most commonly use a 15-mm length loop with the EndoButton, but the EndoButton Direct can also be used if tunnel lengths are short.

* The first tunnel we prepare is the PL femoral tunnel. Viewing through the AM portal, we place a 3.2-mm guidewire through the AAM portal at the center of the femoral footprint of the PL bundle. The location for PL femoral tunnel pin placement is usually 5 to 7 mm from the anterior lateral femoral condyle (LFC) cartilage and 3 mm from the inferior edge of the LFC cartilage. It is critical to flex the knee to at least 110 degrees during PL femoral tunnel preparation to protect the peroneal nerve and to ensure adequate tunnel length. A small (usually 6 mm) cannulated acorn reamer is placed over the guidewire, and the tunnel is reamed to a depth of 25 to 30 mm. The far cortex is breached with a 4.5-mm EndoButton

Figure 10-9. Guidewires for the AM and PL tibial tunnels are placed, centered in the insertions of the AM and PL bundles.

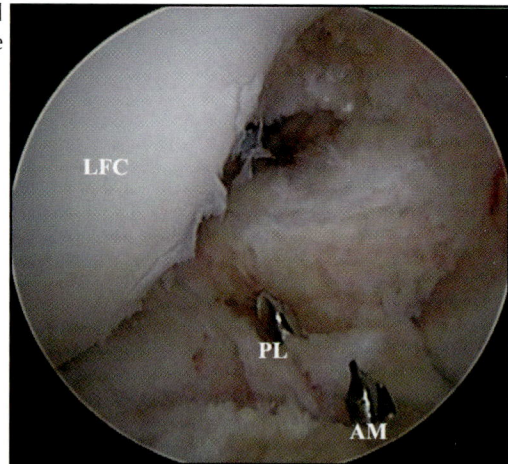

Figure 10-10. The AM and PL tunnels are usually dilated to 8 mm and 7 mm, respectively. However, the size of the tunnels is dictated by our measurement of native ACL insertion site size.

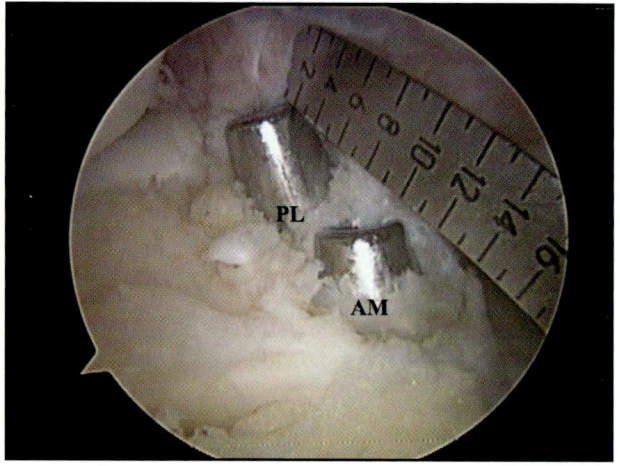

drill (Smith & Nephew, Inc), and the tunnel length is measured. The tunnel is reamed to the appropriate depth with the appropriate-sized acorn reamer on hand.

* The PL tibial tunnel is drilled next, after a 3- to 4-cm skin incision is made over the AM proximal tibia. The elbow ACL tibial drill guide is set at 45 degrees, and the tip of the drill guide is placed on the tibial footprint of the PL bundle through the AAM portal, while viewing through the AL portal. The tunnel begins just anterior to the superficial medial collateral ligament fibers.

* The AM tibial tunnel is drilled with the elbow ACL tibial drill guide set at 45 degrees and inserted through the AM portal (Figure 10-9). The location for the starting point for the AM bundle is halfway between the PL tibial tunnel and the tibial tuberosity. The surgeon must verify that the distance between these 2 pins will allow enough of a bony bridge between the tunnels. The AM and PL tibial tunnels are then over-drilled using a cannulated drill, and then dilators are used to dilate up to the ultimate tunnel diameter (Figure 10-10).

* The femoral AM tunnel is the last tunnel to be drilled, while viewing through the AM portal. First, we place the guidewire transtibially through the AM tibial tunnel (Figure 10-11A). If this places the guidewire too high and too far anterior on the medial wall of the LFC (outside of the anatomical footprint), then the wire is placed transtibially through the PL tibial tunnel (Figure 10-11B). When the trajectory of the guidewire is still too high and outside of

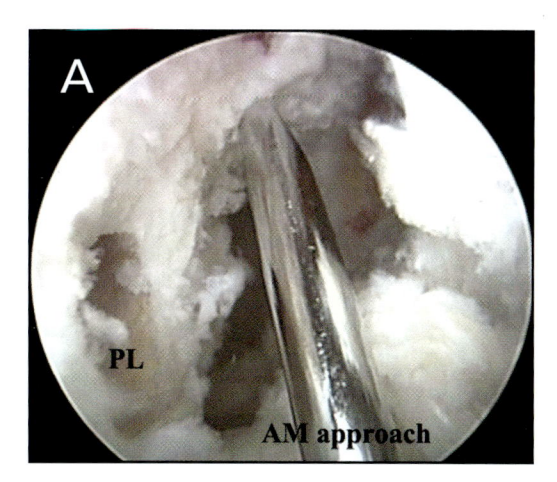

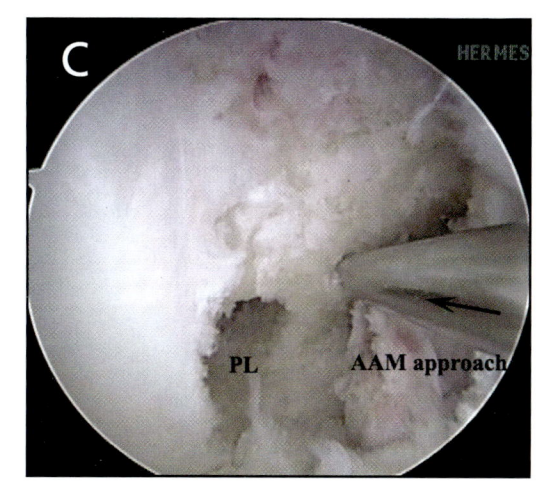

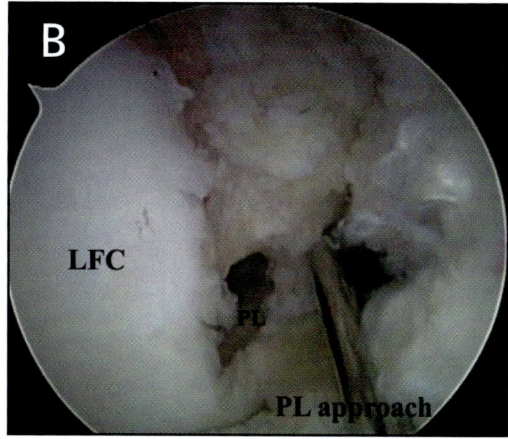

Figure 10-11. The guidewire can be inserted in 1 of 3 ways to reach the AM femoral attachment site for AM femoral tunnel preparation: transtibially through the (A) AM tibial tunnel, (B) transtibially through the PL tibial tunnel, or (C) through the AAM portal. In the case of (A), the trajectory of the wire is not anatomic—the wire aims above the AM femoral attachment.

the AM femoral footprint, we place the guidewire through the AAM portal, with the knee hyperflexed to position the pin appropriately in the center of the AM bundle attachment (Figures 10-11C and 10-12). A cannulated acorn reamer is inserted over the guidewire, drilling to a depth of 20 to 30 mm. We drill a shorter distance when drilling through the AAM portal than if we are drilling transtibially, because the distance to the femoral cortex is shorter. The 4.5-mm EndoButton drill is used to perforate the femoral cortex, and the tunnel length is measured. The tunnel is then reamed by hand to the appropriate depth using the acorn reamer (Figure 10-13).

* Finally, we pass the grafts. A beath pin with a looped suture is passed through the AAM portal and out through the PL femoral tunnel. The looped suture is retrieved using an arthroscopic suture grasper placed through the PL tibial tunnel. Similarly, a beath pin is passed into the AM femoral tunnel, passing the pin through the tunnel or portal that was used to drill the AM femoral tunnel and then retrieving it through the AM tibial tunnel. Both beath pins should be passed before actually passing either graft to prevent the grafts from injury from the pins.

* The PL graft is passed first, and the EndoButton is then flipped for this graft (Figure 10-14). The AM graft is then passed in similar fashion (Figure 10-15). Preconditioning of the grafts is performed by flexing and extending the knee through a range of motion from 0 to 120 degrees approximately 20 to 30 times.

Figure 10-12. The guidepin is placed in the AAM portal for preparation of the AM femoral tunnel. The dilators are shown exiting the AM and PL tibial tunnels.

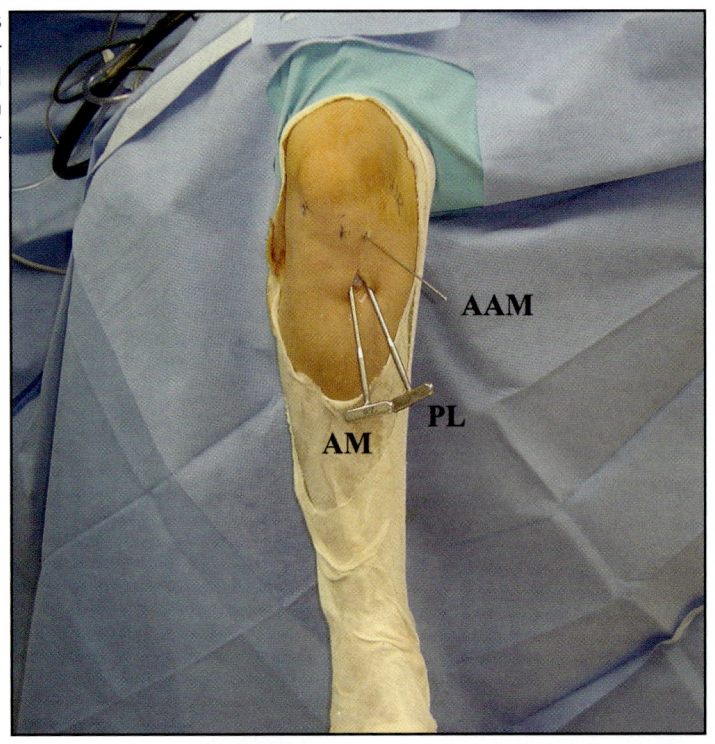

Figure 10-13. The final appearance of the femoral tunnels prior to graft passage, with dilators protruding from the AM and PL tibial tunnels.

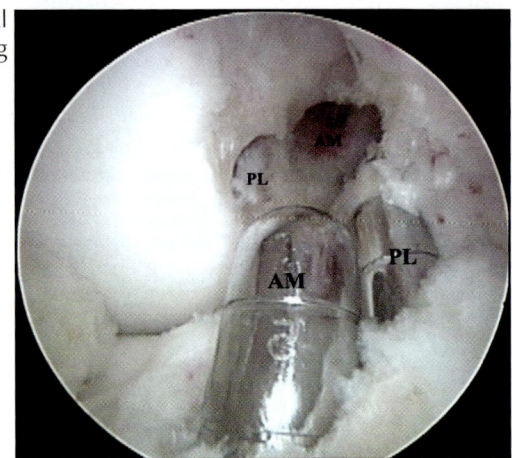

* Tibial fixation is performed with bioabsorbable screws. The grafts are tensioned manually by the surgeon during fixation. The PL graft is fixed with the knee in extension (Figure 10-16), while the AM graft is fixed at 60 degrees of flexion.
* After tibial fixation, a final arthroscopic inspection is performed to confirm the correct position and tension of the grafts. We have never seen impingement on the PCL using our anatomic DB technique (Figure 10-17).

Anatomic Double-Bundle ACL Reconstruction | **131**

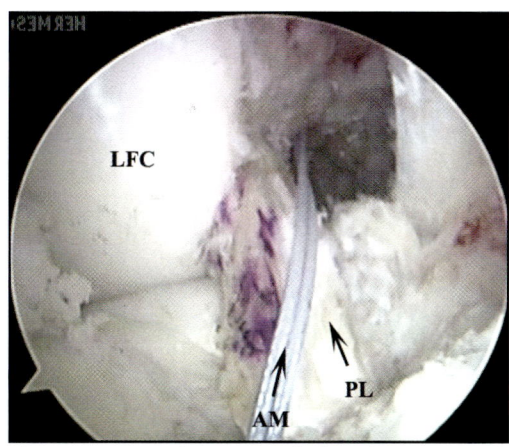

Figure 10-14. The PL graft has been passed. The suture loop of the AM graft is shown. The 2 bundles cross over each other at 90 degrees of knee flexion, as shown in this image.

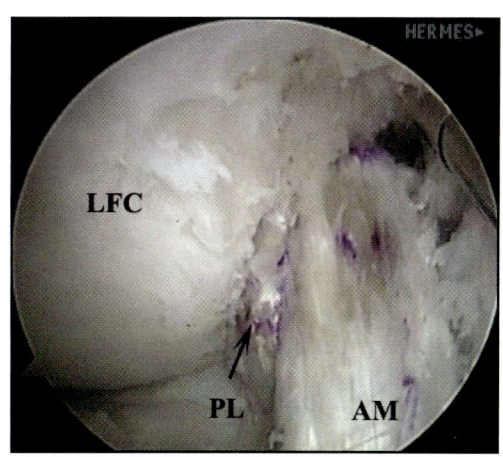

Figure 10-15. The final appearance after AM and PL graft passage shows a crossing pattern when in flexion. Also, note that the PL bundle is mostly covered up by the AM bundle.

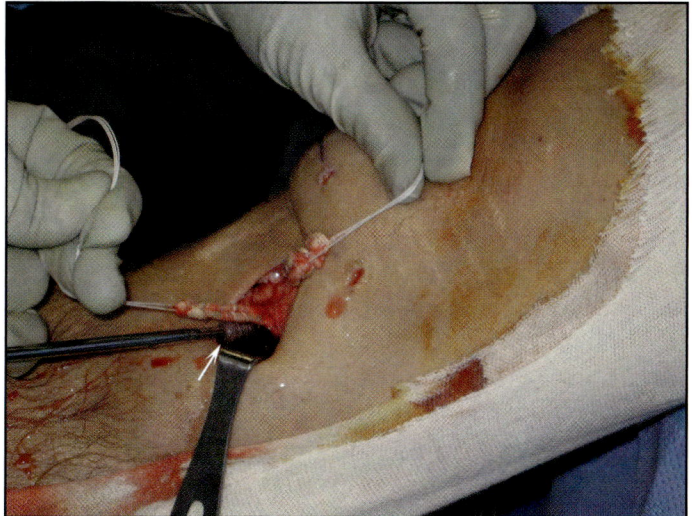

Figure 10-16. PL graft is fixed by a bioabsorbable screw (arrow) at 0 to 10 degrees of flexion as shown in this figure, while the AM graft is fixed by a bioabsorbable screw at 45 to 60 degrees of flexion, in order to restore the native tension pattern of the 2 bundles.

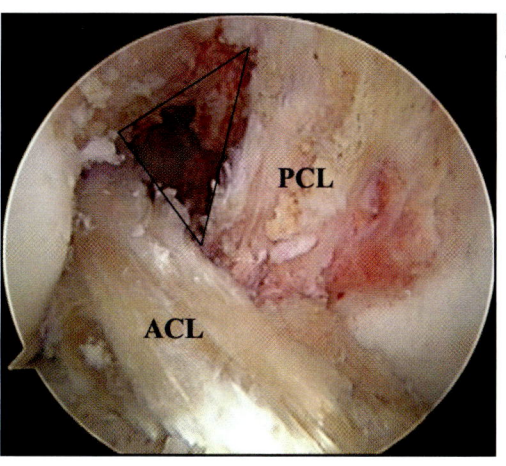

Figure 10-17. The ACL-PCL triangle is shown here after DB ACL reconstruction. There is no graft impingement if the tunnels are anatomically placed.

Tips and Pearls

✔ Portal location is critical for the DB ACL reconstruction. In particular, the AAM portal must be placed accurately in order to obtain the correct trajectory for the PL femoral tunnel. Using a spinal needle to identify the correct location and trajectory will avoid errant portal placement. The surgeon must ensure that the needle does not violate the medial meniscus or the medial femoral condyle, because reamers will pass through this portal during femoral tunnel drilling.

✔ Preservation of the soft tissue attachments of the AM and PL bundles on the femur and tibia allows accurate identification of the anatomic locations for tunnel placement. We perform gentle dissection of these attachments using a thermal device, taking care to leave as much soft tissue as possible.

✔ Identifying 2 bony ridges along the lateral femoral wall (the lateral intercondylar ridge and the lateral bifurcate ridge) helps with identification of native AM and PL attachment sites on the femoral side. In chronic situations where soft tissue attachment sites are not intact, these ridges are important guides to native ACL anatomy.

✔ Viewing through the AM portal (instead of the AL portal, as is traditionally done) allows improved visualization of the femoral footprints of the AM and PL bundles. We find that viewing through the AM portal makes notchplasty unnecessary in almost every case because of the excellent view obtained through this portal. Furthermore, notchplasty destroys the important bony ridges that help guide femoral tunnel placement and, therefore, should be avoided.

✔ Knowledge of the anatomy of the individual bundle attachments allows creation of anatomically accurate tunnels. For example, the PL tibial attachment is adjacent to the posterior root of the lateral meniscus, anterior and medial to it. The PL tibial attachment is lateral and anterior to the PCL and PL to the AM bundle insertion site. The AM bundle, PCL, and posterior root of the lateral meniscus form a triangle around the PL tibial insertion site.

✔ It is important to understand that insertion site alignment changes from vertical to horizontal when the knee joint is moved from full extension to 90 degrees of flexion.

✔ When establishing the AM femoral tunnel, the guidewire may be placed in 1 of 3 ways: transtibially through the AM tunnel, transtibially through the PL tunnel, or through the AAM portal. The method that places the wire in the center of the anatomic footprint is preferred. Transtibial approaches are attempted first because they achieve long and divergent tunnels. However, accurate insertion site position is the most important goal.

✔ The size of the ACL insertion varies from patient to patient. We measure the femoral and tibial footprints and tailor our reconstruction so that the individual AM and PL grafts match the bundle sizes for that particular knee.

Pitfalls

✘ During tibial tunnel preparation, the surgeon must confirm that there is adequate distance between the guidepins for the AM and PL tunnels to ensure sufficient bony bridge between the tunnels and avoid tunnel convergence.

✘ During preparation of the PL femoral tunnel, the knee should be hyperflexed to 110 degrees to protect the peroneal nerve and to ensure adequate PL femoral tunnel length. The knee must also be hyperflexed during PL graft passage, or the graft will not pass easily.

✘ When preparing the AM femoral tunnel through the AAM portal, the tunnel tends to be shorter than if prepared through a transtibial method. If the tunnel is short, traditional EndoButton fixation will not permit adequate graft material in the tunnel. In this case, fixation options such as the EndoButton Direct or an Endoloop with a post should be used to maximize the amount of graft in the tunnel.

References

1. Chhabra A, Starman JS, Ferretti M, Vidal AF, Zantop T, Fu FH. Anatomic, radiographic, biomechanical, and kinematic evaluation of the anterior cruciate ligament and its two functional bundles. *J Bone Joint Surg Am.* 2006;88(suppl 4):2-10.
2. Ferretti M, Levicoff EA, Macpherson TA, Moreland MS, Cohen M, Fu FH. The fetal anterior cruciate ligament: an anatomic and histologic study. *Arthroscopy.* 2007;23(3):278-283.
3. Buoncristiani AM, Tjoumakaris FP, Starman JS, Ferretti M, Fu FH. Anatomic double-bundle anterior cruciate ligament reconstruction. *Arthroscopy.* 2006;22(9):1000-1006.
4. Gabriel MT, Wong EK, Woo SL, Yagi M, Debski RE. Distribution of in situ forces in the anterior cruciate ligament in response to rotatory loads. *J Orthop Res.* 2004;22(1):85-89.
5. Sakane M, Fox RJ, Woo SL, Livesay GA, Li G, Fu FH. In situ forces in the anterior cruciate ligament and its bundles in response to anterior tibial loads. *J Orthop Res.* 1997;15(2):285-293.
6. Tashman S, Collon D, Anderson K, Kolowich P, Anderst W. Abnormal rotational knee motion during running after anterior cruciate ligament reconstruction. *Am J Sports Med.* 2004;32(4):975-983.
7. Yagi M, Kuroda R, Nagamune K, Yoshiya S, Kurosaka M. Double-bundle ACL reconstruction can improve rotational stability. *Clin Orthop Relat Res.* 2007;454:100-107.
8. Yagi M, Wong EK, Kanamori A, Debski RE, Fu FH, Woo SL. Biomechanical analysis of an anatomic anterior cruciate ligament reconstruction. *Am J Sports Med.* 2002;30(5):660-666.
9. Ferretti M, Ekdahl M, Shen W, Fu FH. Osseous landmarks of the femoral attachment of the anterior cruciate ligament: an anatomic study. *Arthroscopy.* 2007;23(11):1218-1225.

ACL—Arthroscopically Assisted Internal Fixation of Tibial Spine Avulsion Fractures

Bojan Zoric, MD and William Sterett, MD

Avulsion fractures of the tibial spine represent a variant of anterior cruciate ligament (ACL) disruption in which the bony insertion point of the ligament is avulsed. Noyes and colleagues have shown that as the ACL pulls off of the subchondral bone, a stretch injury or elongation of the ACL may occur.[1] These injuries frequently occur in children between the ages of 8 and 13 years and are often due to a sports-related incident.[2] Meyers and Mckeever reported that the most common mechanism of injury in their series was a fall from a bicycle.[2] There is increasing incidence of tibial spine fractures in children due to early participation in sports. Approximately 20% of children's injuries in sports require internal fixation.[3] Although tibial avulsion fractures are generally associated with children and adolescents, these injuries still do occur after skeletal maturity, but are usually associated with higher energy mechanisms and have associated injuries.[1,4,5] And, in general populations, as the skeletally immature transition into skeletally mature individuals, tibial avulsion fractures become less frequent, and ACL tears become more prevalent.[6] Tibial eminence fractures were once thought to be the pediatric equivalent of ACL tears in adults[4,7]; however, in our patient population of skiing injuries, adults with tibial eminence fractures have outweighed adolescents by an estimated 10 to 1.

After injury, pain and effusion from a hemarthrosis are the typical presenting symptoms.[2] Reluctance to bear weight and decreased range of motion may also be present. Physical examination should include a thorough evaluation of ligamentous stability and possible physeal injury in skeletally immature patients. Radiographic examination should include anteroposterior and lateral radiographs (Figure 11-1). Magnetic resonance imaging (MRI), as well as a computed tomography (CT) scan, may be of value to determine associated injuries.[8] In our population, we often get an MRI to evaluate associated ligamentous injuries, as well as a CT to better evaluate bony injury (Figure 11-2).

Meyers and Mckeever proposed a classification of tibial spine fractures based on the degree of displacement (Table 11-1).[2] Zaricznyj also proposed a modification of the initial classification by Meyers and Mckeever to include comminuted fracture of the tibial eminence (see Table 11-1).[9]

INDICATIONS

Treatment is based on degree of displacement and classification of avulsion fracture. Type I fractures with little or no displacement can be treated nonoperatively in a long leg cast in full extension or slight (20 degrees) flexion for 6 weeks. This is followed by rehabilitation, including motion, followed by strengthening. In our practice, we rarely treat by use of a long leg cast.

Figure 11-1. Preoperative lateral radiograph of a tibial spine avulsion fracture.

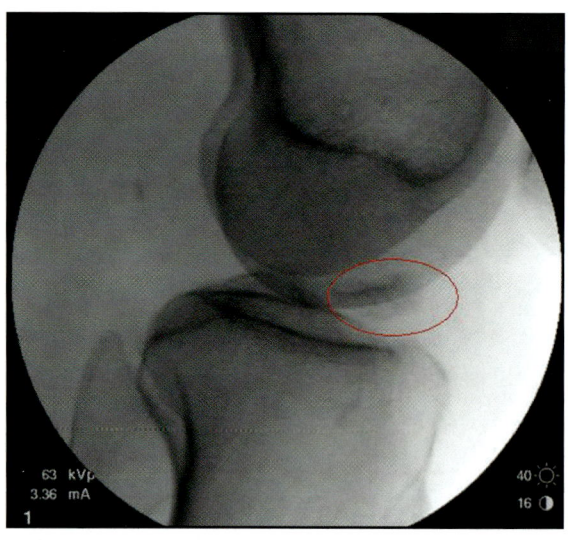

Table 11-1

CLASSIFICATION OF TIBIAL SPINE FRACTURES BASED ON DEGREE OF DISPLACEMENT

Type I	Minimal displacement of avulsed fragment from the proximal tibial physis.[2]
Type II	Displacement of the anterior one third to one half of the fragment superiorly with an intact posterior hinge that remains in contact with the proximal tibia.[2]
Type III	Displacement of the entire fragment with complete separation from the proximal tibial physis, associated with upward displacement and rotation.[2]
Type IV	Marked displacement of the fragments close to the medial plateau of the tibia or comminuted.

Adapted from Zaricznyj B. Avulsion fracture of the tibial eminence: treatment by open reduction and pinning. *J Bone Joint Surg Am.* 1977;59:1111-1114.

Figure 11-2. Computed tomography scan of a tibial spine avulsion fracture.

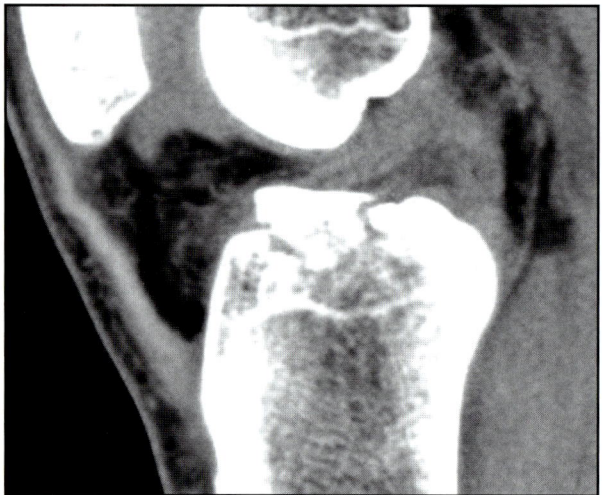

Although we rarely see type I fractures, we would instead treat these fractures through immobilization and do very limited and controlled passive range of motion exercises. If there is concern about the amount of displacement seen on plain radiographs, a CT scan would then be obtained to further evaluate the injury.

Type II fractures have historically been treated with closed reduction in extension and casting. We have found this protocol leads to unpredictable results. Although good results are possible, the ligament may have intrasubstance damage, leading to residual laxity, or the trauma and immobilization may lead to residual stiffness. In any case, this treatment should never be used unless anatomic reduction can be obtained in extension.

Type II and III fractures are typically not reducible in a closed fashion, secondary to displacement and blockage by the intermeniscal ligament. This transverse structure is typically interposed between the fracture fragment and its bed. If the ligament has minimal damage, we will reduce the bony fragment below the intermeniscal ligament and then stabilize it with either suture or screw fixation, depending on the age of the patient. These fractures require open reduction, correct tensioning, internal fixation, and proper rehabilitation.[10] We find that the benefits of early mobilization with stable fixation outweigh the surgical risks.

Typically, type II, III, and IV fractures are treated operatively in our practice. Treatment algorithms are based on age of the patient, quality of the ligament, and the comminution of the bony fragment.

Surgical Goals

Arthroscopic fixation of tibial eminence fractures involves several points. The main goal of the surgery is to obtain anatomic reduction and stable fixation of the avulsed fragment in order to have early mobility and a functional ACL.[11] With proper treatment of tibial eminence fractures, knee stability can be regained.[12,13]

Equally important is the evaluation of the entire joint. There are often associated injuries to meniscus and articular surfaces. Monto and colleagues found that 100% of these fractures had other associated chondral or meniscal injuries.[8] In another study, Kocher and colleagues found that meniscal entrapment was common in young patients with type II and III tibial eminence fractures.[7] Evaluating the avulsed fragment for comminution and size is essential for operative fixation. Removing any block to reduction, such as a clot, loose bony fragments, or interposed intermeniscal ligament/meniscus, is also a necessary portion of the procedure in order to restore anatomic reduction.[14]

When mild to moderate comminution is present, a washer may be added to the cannulated screw for fixation. In cases where there is excessive comminution or the ligament has significant damage, the entire ACL fracture construct should be excised. A primary ACL reconstruction can then be performed. Despite the "countersinking" of the new ligament being required, we have had good success with this.

If the tibial spine is allowed to heal in an elevated position, one of two outcomes may occur: the elevated fragment may block extension and limit terminal motion or it may lead to pathological laxity and decreased function.

Figure 11-3. Arthroscopic view of a tibial spine avulsion.

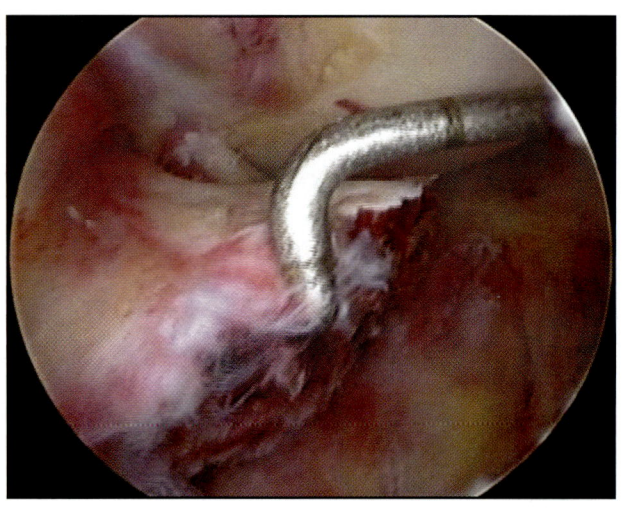

Arthroscopic Reduction and Internal Fixation of Tibial Spine Fractures Using Cannulated Screws

A treatment option for tibial eminence fractures includes the use of cannulated screws via arthroscopic reduction and internal fixation.[15]

* General or regional anesthesia is performed. A nonsterile tourniquet is applied on the upper thigh of the affected leg. The patient is placed supine with the affected leg in a leg holder. Standard arthroscopic instrumentation and set-up are used, and preoperative antibiotics are administered. The leg is exsanguinated with an Esmarch bandage. Arthroscopy is performed through the standard anterolateral viewing portal and the anteromedial portal for instrumentation.

* The fracture hematoma is evacuated for visualization, and the fat pad is removed as necessary. A diagnostic arthroscopy is subsequently performed to evaluate any associated pathology. Any block to reduction, such as meniscal interposition or bony fragments, is corrected (Figure 11-3).

* Débridement of the area under the avulsed tibial spine is done using an arthroscopic shaver and small curettes so that the fracture line can be identified.

* Reduction of the avulsed fragment should be performed. Often, it helps to translate the tibia posteriorly and keep the knee at approximately 40 degrees of flexion to decrease tension on the ACL (Figure 11-4).

* If the meniscus is blocking reduction, an outside-in suture can be placed around the meniscus to create traction while the fragment is reduced. Once reduction has been obtained, the knee is retained in flexion for both arthroscopic and fluoroscopic visualization.

* An additional high parapatellar portal on the medial side, at the level of the superior third of the patella, is created.

* A guidepin from the 4.5-mm cannulated set is passed through this portal under the medial facet of the patella, down into the medial half of the tibial eminence (Figure 11-5).

* Using the 4.5- or 4.0-mm cannulated screw system, the guidepin is then passed into the knee to the reduced fragment using the medial high accessory portal under both arthroscopic and fluoroscopic visualization.

ACL—Arthroscopically Assisted Internal Fixation of Tibial Spine Avulsion Fractures

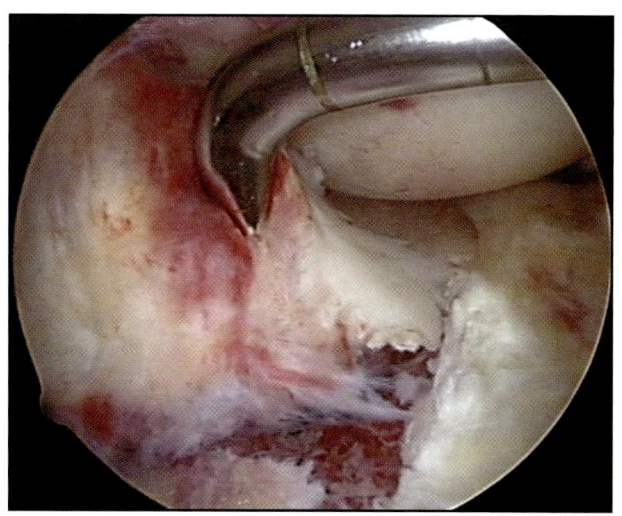

Figure 11-4. Arthroscopic view of tibial avulsion fracture reduced with microfracture pick.

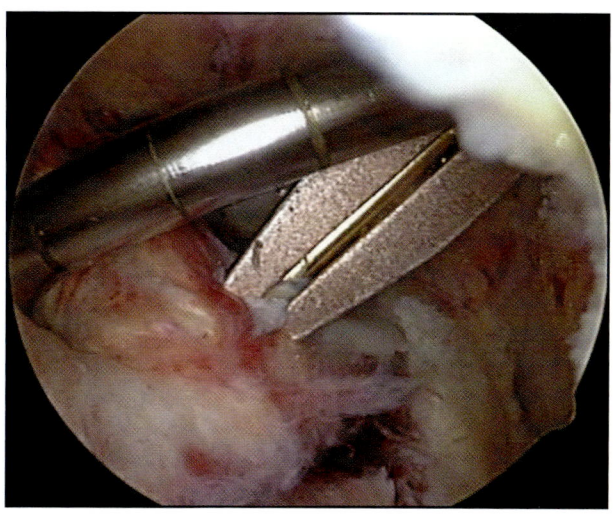

Figure 11-5. Guidepin fixation of reduced tibial spine avulsion.

* A second guidepin can then be placed if necessary.
* Fracture reduction is then confirmed by both arthroscopic visualization and fluoroscopy.
* If the guidepins are in satisfactory position, the cannulated screws can be advanced across the fracture fragment (Figures 11-6 and 11-7).
* Fluoroscopic imaging is used to confirm screw position and tibial spine reduction (Figures 11-8 and 11-9).
* We rarely employ this technique in a skeletally immature patient. A single screw is often adequate to maintain reduction and stability; however, do not hesitate to use a second screw if needed.
* In the face of a comminuted fracture, a washer is added to the construct when necessary.
* When significant damage to the ACL is present, we do not hesitate to abandon fracture fixation and directly proceed to formal ACL reconstruction. Once adequate reduction and fixation have been confirmed, the guidewires are removed, and the knee can be taken through a gentle range of motion. We visualize the knee in full extension arthroscopically to ensure there is no impingement from the screw. With this technique, we rarely see the

Figure 11-6. Cannulated screw fixation of reduced tibial spine avulsion fracture.

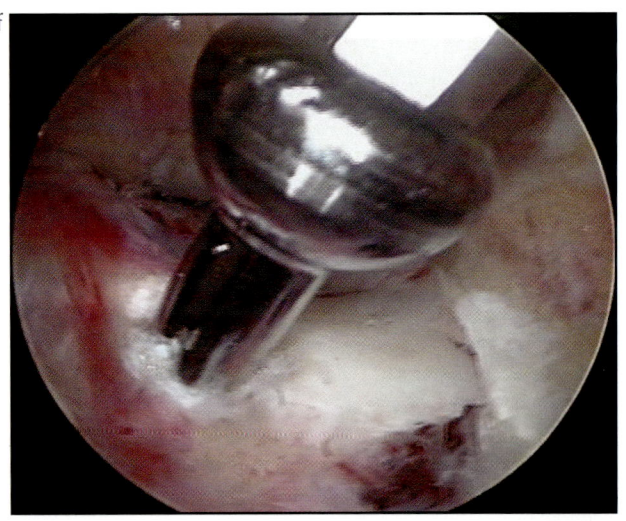

Figure 11-7. Intra-articular view of repaired tibial spine fracture with screw fixation.

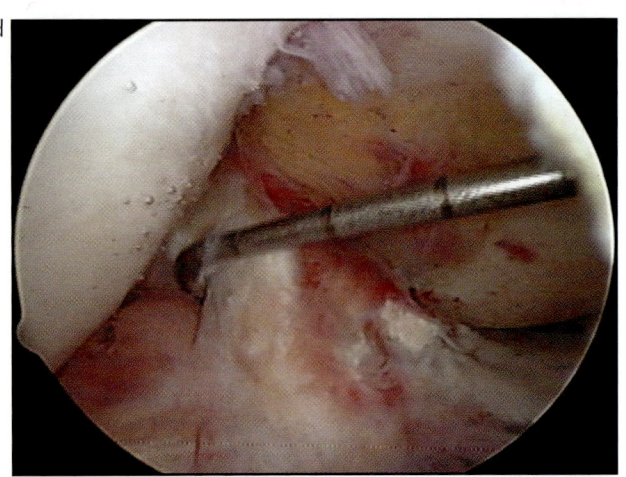

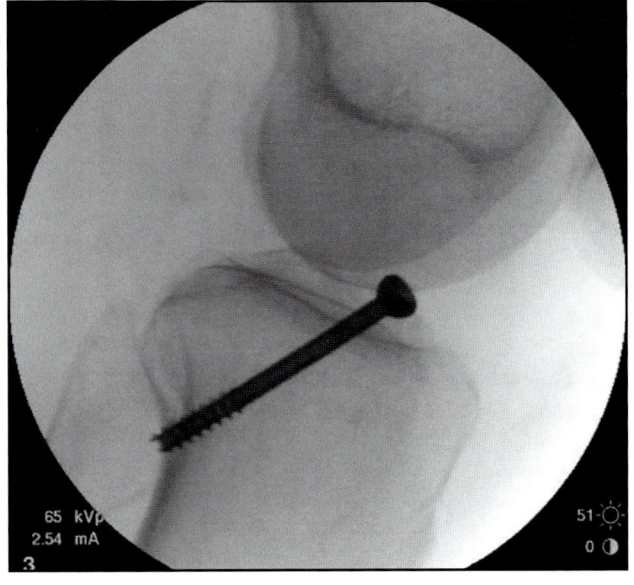

Figure 11-8. Postoperative lateral radiograph of tibial spine avulsion fracture with screw fixation.

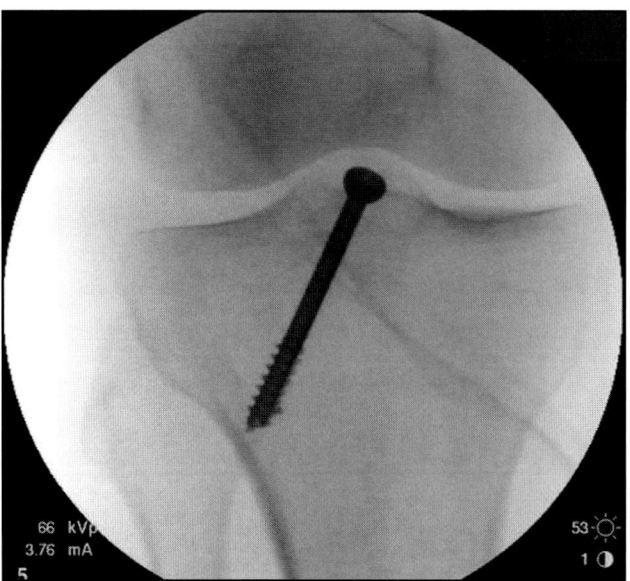

Figure 11-9. Postoperative A-P radiograph of tibial spine avulsion fracture after screw fixation.

screw creating any impingement or block to extension. The tourniquet is then deflated, and incisions are closed.

ARTHROSCOPIC REDUCTION AND FIXATION OF TIBIAL SPINE FRACTURES: SUTURE FIXATION

* Suture fixation is another treatment option for the repair of tibial spine avulsions that has been shown to be successful.[13,16,17] Ahn and colleagues showed an excellent union rate in acute and chronic cases, as well as no instability or extension limitations at minimum 2-year follow-up.[13] General or regional anesthesia is performed. A nonsterile tourniquet is applied on the upper thigh of the affected leg. The patient is placed supine with the affected leg in a leg holder. Standard arthroscopic instrumentation and set-up are used, and preoperative antibiotics are administered. The leg is exsanguinated with an Esmarch bandage. Arthroscopy is performed through the standard anterolateral viewing portal, and the anteromedial portal is used for instrumentation. The fracture hematoma is evacuated for visualization, and the fat pad is removed as necessary. A diagnostic arthroscopy is subsequently performed to evaluate any associated pathology. Any block to reduction, such as meniscal interposition or bony fragments, is removed. Often, the intermeniscal ligament prohibits reduction. We have found that, without the presence of other meniscal pathology, removal of this structure has had no adverse effects. The tibial spine avulsion fracture is then evaluated. Reduction of the fracture is performed using a 90-degree awl through the medial portal. Fluoroscopic evaluation of the reduced fragment is performed with the fluoroscopic unit positioned to view the knee in a lateral, flexed view. A 1-cm incision is made, just medial to the tibial tubercle at the level of the metaphyseal flare of the proximal tibia. In a skeletally immature patient, the incision can be made proximal to the growth plate, in a manner to allow the physis to remain undisturbed. Suture fixation should not cause growth plate disturbance, even if the sutures cross the physis.[13]

* Subsequent periosteal dissection and drilling may be performed proximal to the growth plate to minimize risk of growth disturbance, although this is technically challenging. Two medial portals are employed. With a 90-degree awl in one, the fracture is held reduced.

Figure 11-10. Postoperative suture fixation of tibial spine avulsion fracture.

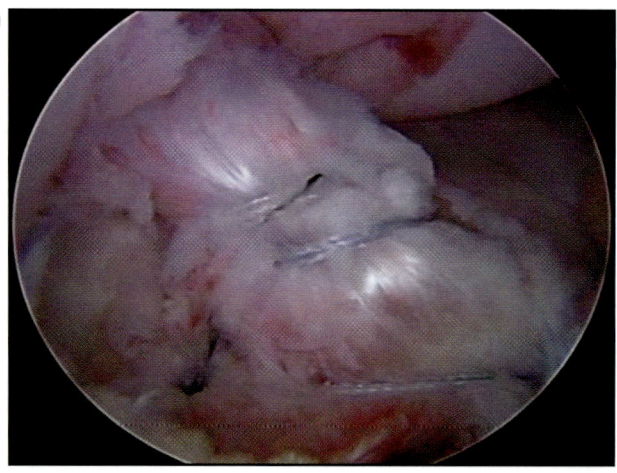

Through the second medial portal, an ACL guide set at 45 degrees (or less if avoiding the physis is being attempted) is placed into the medial half of the eminence fracture.

* A smooth 2.5-mm pin is used in this location. Using a 5- or 8-mm offset guide, a second pin is placed into the lateral half of the spine.
* A single suture end can be passed through this guide hole with a Hewson suture passer. If more than one suture is to be used, each pin can be over-drilled with a 4.5-mm cannulated drill from the EndoButton set (Smith & Nephew, London, United Kingdom).
* The Hewson suture passer is then used to pass a #1 PDS suture into the joint.
* A 90-degree Suture Lasso (Arthrex Inc, Naples, FL) is then used to capture the suture after passing through the substance of the ACL.
* In an ideal situation, 3 sutures are used. Two of these sutures will be passed through the front and back half of the ligament, respectively. A third suture is used to loop over the front of the eminence, anterior to the ligament itself. This final suture holds the front portion of the eminence into its anatomic bed (Figure 11-10).
* After pulling the 3 sutures out the anterior tibia, they can be tied over a bone bridge if appropriate.[18] Alternatively, these sutures can be tied over a screw and washer post.

POSTOPERATIVE MANAGEMENT

Following stable reduction and fixation, we aim for controlled mobility during healing. Our typical postoperative regimen allows full weightbearing in a brace locked in full extension or a knee immobilizer for the first 6 weeks. We allow the patient to remove the brace twice a day for passive range of motion, between full extension and 90 degrees of flexion, for the first 4 weeks. At the end of 4 weeks, we allow full passive and active range of motion. At the end of 6 weeks, we transition to a functional sport brace and immediately begin a more aggressive strengthening program. The first 3 weeks of strengthening are done in a closed-chain, double-leg fashion. The final 3 weeks of rehabilitation employ a more single-leg isolation program, again in a closed-chain fashion.

X-rays are taken at 2 and 6 weeks postoperatively. An x-ray is rarely taken at 12 weeks. Despite the intra-articular hardware, we rarely find the need to remove these screws, unless symptomatic.

Tips and Pearls

- ✔ Evaluate the fracture fragment, remove the hematoma, and remove some of the cancellous bone on the tibial surface to allow for countersinking of the tibial eminence without creating a step-off in the articular surface.
- ✔ Reduce the fracture under direct visualization with a 90 degrees awl.
- ✔ Feel comfortable excising the intermeniscal ligament if this is preventing reduction.
- ✔ When performing a suture technique, try to pass sutures through the ACL fibers, as well as through the anterior edge of the fracture fragment to obtain better reduction and stability.
- ✔ Always check reduction by fluoroscopy in the lateral view.
- ✔ A zone-specific meniscus suture passer can be used to pass the sutures through the ligament if desired.
- ✔ If the fracture is comminuted, use 2 screws or add a washer to the construct.
- ✔ Following fixation, evaluate the fracture dynamically with arthroscopic visualization. This will confirm a lack of impingement of the screws during extension.

Pitfalls

- ✘ Fixing the tibial spine in an excessively prominent fashion can cause extension block. Check gentle range of motion intraoperatively.
- ✘ Avoid screws crossing the physis in skeletally immature patients.
- ✘ Evaluate for concomitant ACL laxity, as there may be remaining laxity in some cases even though the tibial spine is adequately reduced.
- ✘ If significant damage to the ACL exists, proceed directly to excision of the fragment and ACL reconstruction.

References

1. Noyes FR, DeLucas JL, Torvik PJ. Biomechanics of anterior cruciate ligament failure: an analysis of strain-rate sensitivity and mechanisms of failure in primates. *J Bone Joint Surg Am.* 1974;56:236-253.
2. Meyers MH, Mckeever FM. Fracture of the intercondylar eminence of the tibia. *J Bone Joint Surg Am.* 1959;41:209-222.
3. Maffulli N. Intensive training in young athletes: the orthopaedic surgeon's viewpoint. *Sports Med.* 1990;9:229-243.
4. Kendall NS, Hsu SY, Chan KM. Fracture of the tibial spine in adults and children: a review of 31 cases. *Bone Joint Surg Br.* 1992;74:848-852.
5. Owens BD, Crane GK, Plante T, Busconi BD. Treatment of type III tibial intercondylar eminence fractures in skeletally immature athletes. *Am J Orthop.* 2003;32:103-105.
6. Prince JS, Laor T, Bean JA. MRI of anterior cruciate ligament injuries and associated findings in the pediatric knee: changes with skeletal maturation. *Am J Roentgenol.* 2005;185:756-762.
7. Kocher MS, Micheli LJ, Gerbino P, et al. Tibial eminence fractures in children: prevalence of meniscal entrapment. *Am J Sports Med.* 2003;31:404-407.
8. Monto RR, Cameron-Donaldson ML, Close MA, Ho CP, Hawkins RJ. Magnetic resonance imaging in the evaluation of tibial eminence fractures in adults. *Knee Surg.* 2006;19:187-190.
9. Zaricznyj B. Avulsion fracture of the tibial eminence: treatment by open reduction and pinning. *J Bone Joint Surg Am.* 1977;59:1111-1114.

10. McLennan JG. Lessons learned after second-look arthroscopy in type III fractures of the tibial spine. *J Pediatr Orthop.* 1995;15:59-62.
11. Lubowitz JH, Elson WS, Guttmann D. Part II: arthroscopic treatment of tibial plateau fractures: intercondylar eminence avulsion fractures. *Arthroscopy.* 2005;21:86-92.
12. Ahmad CS, Stein BE, Jeshuran W, et al. Anterior cruciate ligament function after tibial eminence fracture in skeletally mature patients. *Am J Sports Med.* 2001;29:339-345.
13. Ahn JH, Lee YS, Lee DH, Ha HC. Arthroscopic physeal sparing all inside repair of the tibial avulsion fracture in the anterior cruciate ligament: technical note. *Arch Orthop Trauma Surg.* 2008;128(11):1309-1312.
14. Hunter RE, Willis JA. Arthroscopic fixation of avulsion fractures of the tibial eminence: technique and outcome. *Arthroscopy.* 2004;20:113-121.
15. Senekovic V, Veselko M. Anterograde arthroscopic fixation of avulsion fractures of the tibial eminence with a cannulated screw: five-year results. *Arthroscopy.* 2003;19:54-61.
16. Mah JY, Otsuka NY, Mclean J. An arthroscopic technique for the reduction and fixation of tibial-eminence fractures. *J Pediatr Orthop.* 1996;16:119-121.
17. Pasa L, Visna P, Kocis J, Muzík V, Vesely R. Arthroscopic stabilization of the fractured intercondylar eminence. *Acta Chir Orthop Traumatol Cech.* 2005;72:160-163.
18. Matthews DE, Geissler WB. Arthroscopic suture fixation of displaced tibial eminence fractures. *Arthroscopy.* 1994;10:418-423.

12
Single-Bundle Posterior Cruciate Ligament Reconstruction
Arthroscopic Transtibial Technique

Luke S. Oh, MD and Thomas J. Gill, MD

OPERATIVE TECHNIQUE

EXAMINATION UNDER ANESTHESIA

* Position the patient supine on the operating room (OR) table, and perform a thorough examination under anesthesia. Note the amount of posterior drawer (Figure 12-1), anterior drawer, total anterior-posterior translation (Figure 12-2), presence or absence of an endpoint, and amount of external rotation using a dial test to assess for posterolateral corner injury (Figure 12-3).

PATIENT POSITIONING

* Adjust the patient's position to allow 360-degree circumferential access to the knee joint when the distal end of the OR table is eventually flexed to 90 degrees during the posterior cruciate ligament (PCL) reconstruction procedure. This can be accomplished by placing the patient's popliteal crease approximately 4 inches distal from the "break" in the OR table.

* In addition, we prefer to place 2 folded blankets under the thigh immediately proximal to the break in the OR table (Figure 12-4). This not only ensures circumferential access to the knee but also allows for hyperflexion of the knee required during the PCL reconstruction procedure.

* Apply a padded, nonsterile tourniquet on the thigh as proximal as possible, and place a post on the lateral side of the thigh.

PREPARATION OF THE ALLOGRAFT

* Once the decision has been made to proceed with a PCL reconstruction, then prepare the Achilles tendon allograft.

On the sterile back table, fashion the Achilles tendon allograft to fit loosely through an 11-mm spacer. First, excise a triangular portion of the Achilles tendon allograft such that a curvilinear strip of tendon remains attached to the calcaneal bone block (Figure 12-5).

Figure 12-1. Position the patient supine on the OR table, and perform a thorough examination under anesthesia of the knee. Note the amount of posterior drawer as well as the presence or absence of an end-point.

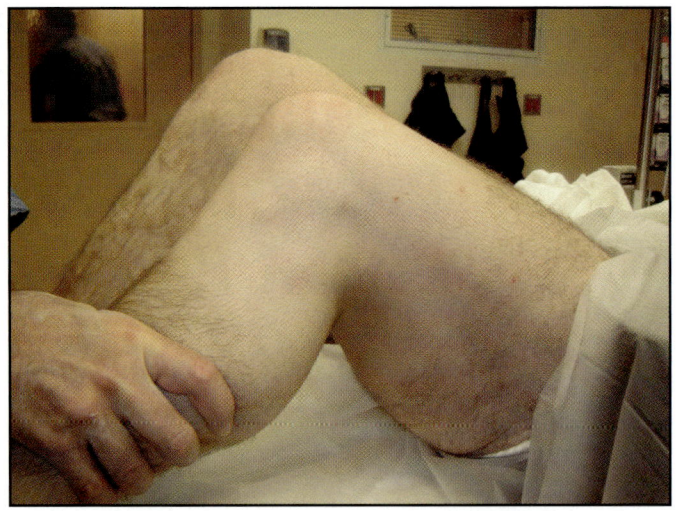

Figure 12-2. In the presence of combined ACL and PCL injury, it may be difficult to isolate and assess the degree of posterior drawer; therefore, measuring total anterior-posterior translation is useful. (A) This patient did not have an ACL tear and, therefore, a normal amount of anterior translation is noted. (B) Posterior translation consistent with PCL insufficiency.

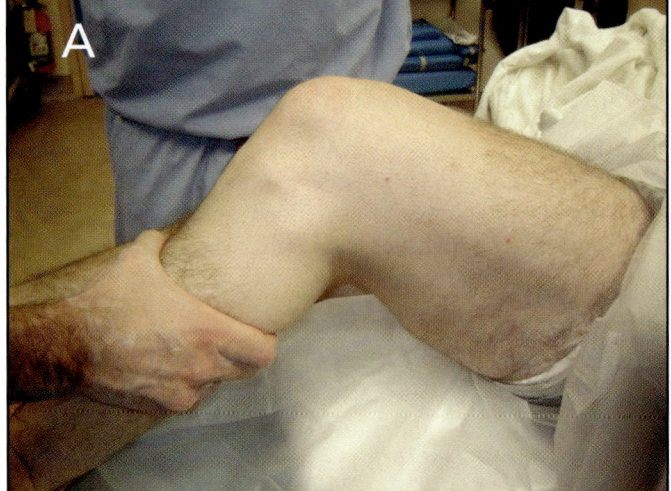

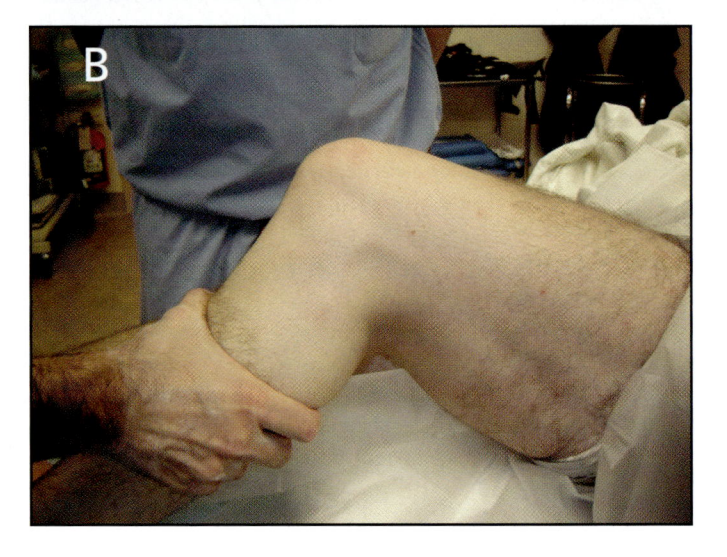

Single-Bundle Posterior Cruciate Ligament Reconstruction **149**

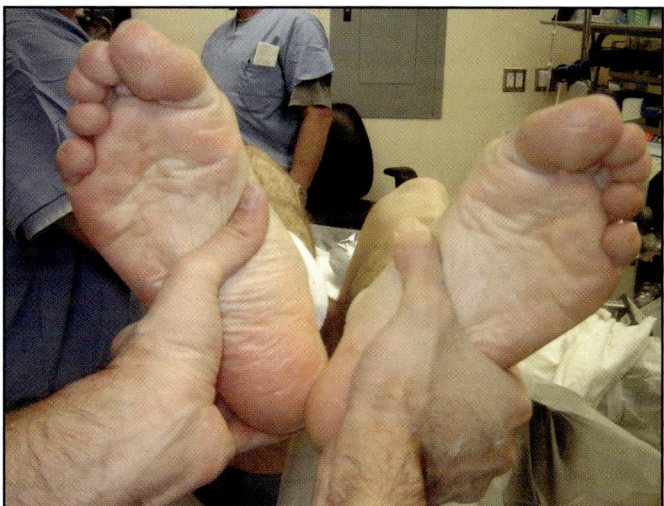

Figure 12-3. The "Dial Test" is used to assess for posterolateral corner injury. The test should be performed at both 30 and 90 degrees of knee flexion. Increased external rotation at both angles suggests injury of both the posterior cruciate ligament and the posterolateral corner. This patient had increased external rotation at 90 degrees of flexion but not at 30 degrees of flexion, which is consistent with an isolated PCL tear.

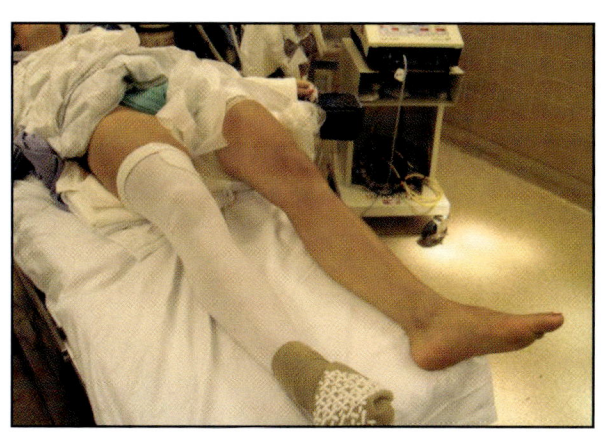

Figure 12-4. Two folded blankets are placed under the thigh immediately proximal to the "break" in the OR table. This not only ensures circumferential access to the knee but also allows for hyperflexion of the knee required during the PCL reconstruction procedure.

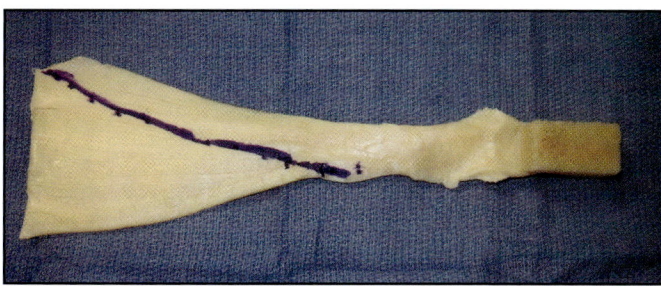

Figure 12-5. On the sterile back table, fashion the Achilles tendon allograft to fit loosely through an 11-mm spacer. First, excise a triangular portion of the Achilles tendon allograft such that a curvilinear strip of tendon remains attached to the calcaneal bone block. By leaving a strip of tendon that is curvilinear, the tendon can be rolled up into a straight tube similar to a cigar.

* By leaving a strip of tendon that is curvilinear, the tendon can be rolled up into a straight tube similar to a cigar. Whipstitches may then be placed with #2 OrthoCord (DePuy Mitek, Raynham, MA (Figure 12-6A).
* It is important to tubularize the allograft such that the tapered end of the soft-tissue tail converges to 1 to 2 mm (Figure 12-6B).
* Size the calcaneal bone block such that it fits easily through an 11-mm diameter spacer. Drill 2 holes in the calcaneal bone block, and pass a #2 OrthoCord suture through each drill hole (Figure 12-6C).

Figure 12-6. (A) Once the allograft has been tubularized, place whip-stitches using #2 OrthoCord (DePuy Mitek, Raynham, MA). (B) It is important to tubularize the allograft such that the tapered end of the soft-tissue tail converges to 1 to 2 mm. (C) Size the calcaneal bone block such that it fits easily through an 11-mm diameter spacer. Drill 2 holes in the calcaneal bone block, and pass a #2 OrthoCord suture through each drill hole

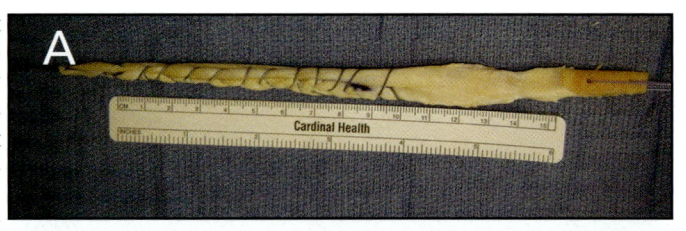

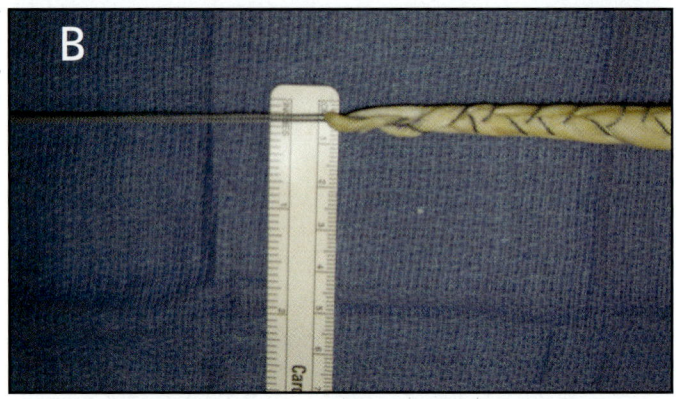

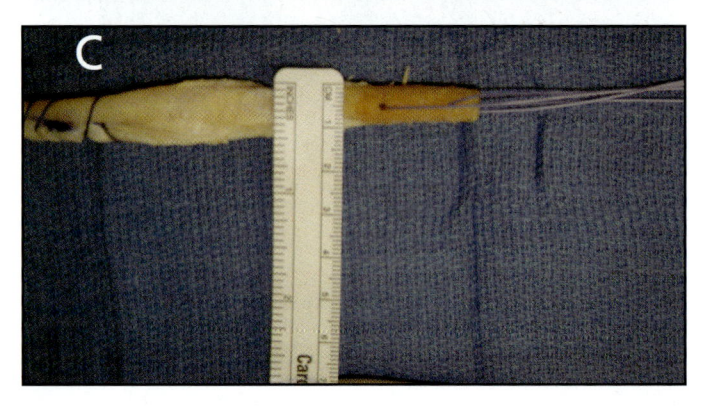

DIAGNOSTIC ARTHROSCOPY

* Prior to inflating the tourniquet, perform a diagnostic arthroscopy, and treat any meniscus tears or chondral injuries that may be present so as to limit the time under tourniquet to the critical portions of the PCL reconstruction procedure.
* Perform the diagnostic arthroscopy without flexing the foot of the OR table to 90 degrees (Figure 12-7A). If the knee needs to be flexed during the diagnostic arthroscopy or associated procedure, such as a partial meniscectomy, then drop the leg off the OR table by abducting at the hip (Figure 12-7B). Maintaining the OR table in the fully horizontal position will make it easier to maintain the leg in the figure-of-4 position while creating and working through the posteromedial portal later in the procedure.
* Inspect the PCL and tug on the PCL fibers with a probe to confirm laxity under arthroscopic visualization (Figure 12-8).

Single-Bundle Posterior Cruciate Ligament Reconstruction   151

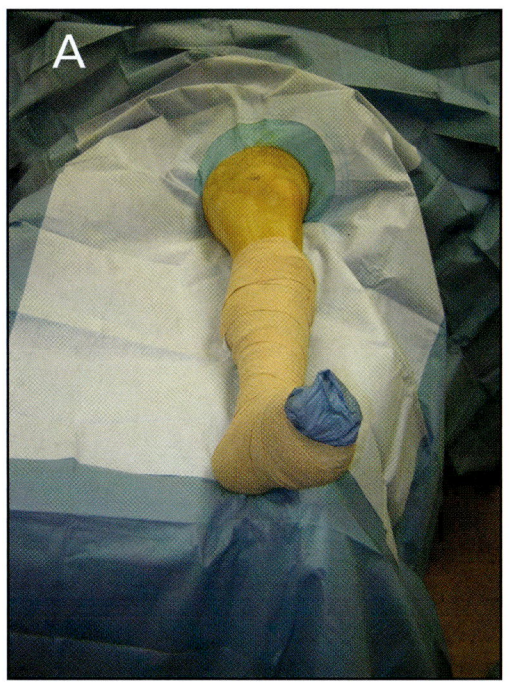

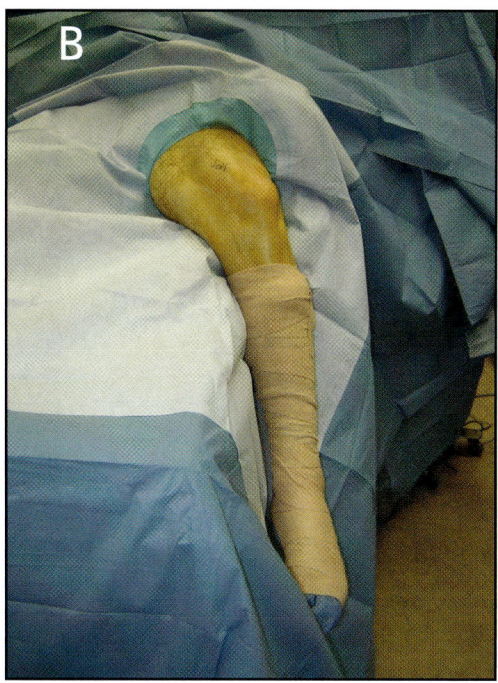

Figure 12-7. (A) Perform the diagnostic arthroscopy without flexing the foot of the OR table to 90 degrees. Maintaining the OR table in the fully horizontal position will make it easier to maintain the leg in the figure-of-4 position while creating and working through the posteromedial portal later in the procedure. (B) If the knee needs to be flexed during the diagnostic arthroscopy or associated procedure such as a partial meniscectomy, then drop the leg off the OR table by abducting at the hip.

POSTERIOR CRUCIATE LIGAMENT DÉBRIDEMENT

* When ready to work on the PCL, exsanguinate the limb with an Esmarch bandage, and inflate the tourniquet to 280 mmHg.
* Perform a thorough débridement of the PCL, starting from anterior to posterior on the lateral aspect of the medial femoral condyle (Figure 12-9). Be careful of the vascular bundle posteriorly: visualization of fat indicates the proximity of the vascular bundle.

POSTEROMEDIAL PORTAL

* While viewing through the anterolateral portal, guide the 30-degree arthroscope into the posteromedial compartment and transilluminate the joint line.
* Place the extremity in the figure-of-4 position, and palpate along the transilluminated region to determine the optimal position for the posteromedial portal (Figure 12-10).
* Place an 18-gauge spinal needle under arthroscopic visualization for localization (Figure 12-11).
* Use a #11 blade scalpel to incise the skin only. Using a hemostat clamp, gently spread and dissect bluntly down to the capsule and then puncture through under arthroscopic visualization (Figure 12-12A).
* Place a smooth cannula of choice into the posteromedial portal (Figure 12-12B). Hold the cannula in place when moving instruments in and out of this portal so as to avoid having to reinsert the cannula.

Figure 12-8. Inspect the PCL and tug on the PCL fibers with a probe to confirm laxity under arthroscopic visualization

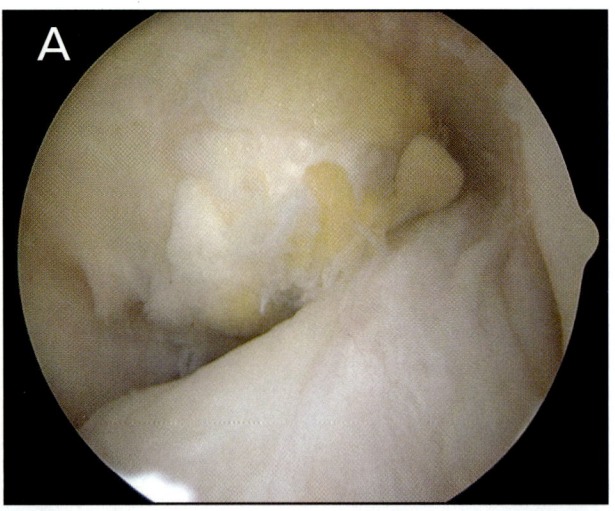

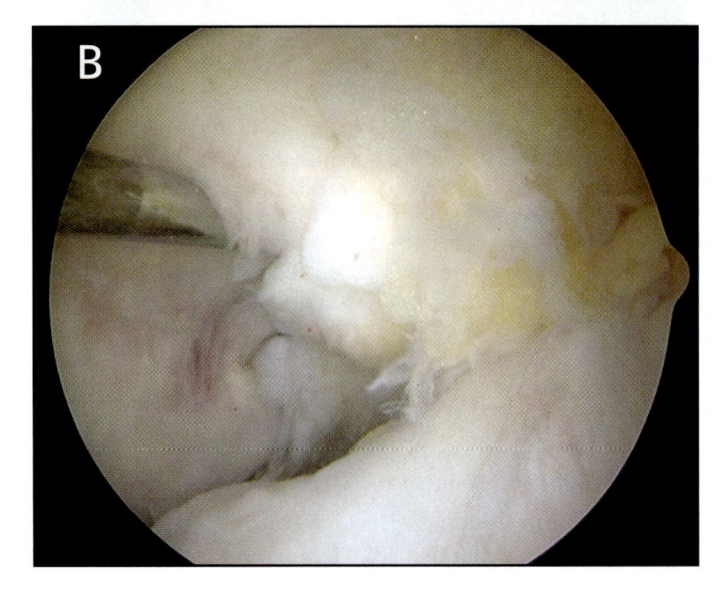

* At this time, switch the 30-degree arthroscope to a 70-degree arthroscope in the anterolateral portal.
* Place a shaver through the posteromedial portal cannula, and perform a débridement of the posterior aspect of the proximal tibia (ie, tibial insertion of PCL) until the fibers of the gastrocnemius are visible (Figure 12-13).

PREPARATION OF POSTERIOR CRUCIATE LIGAMENT TIBIAL GUIDE

* On the back table, set the PCL tibial guide to 70 degrees (Figure 12-14).
* Next, set the depth of the pin on the PCL tibial guide such that the tip of the pin passpoints 2 mm beyond the tip of the PCL guide (Figure 12-15A). While holding the pin in this position, tighten the drill over the pin flush to the PCL tibial guide such that the pin will traverse only 2 mm beyond the tip of the PCL guide before being blocked by the drill hitting the PCL guide (Figure 12-15B). This is to ensure that the pin does not inadvertently injure neurovascular structures in the popliteal fossa.

Single-Bundle Posterior Cruciate Ligament Reconstruction 153

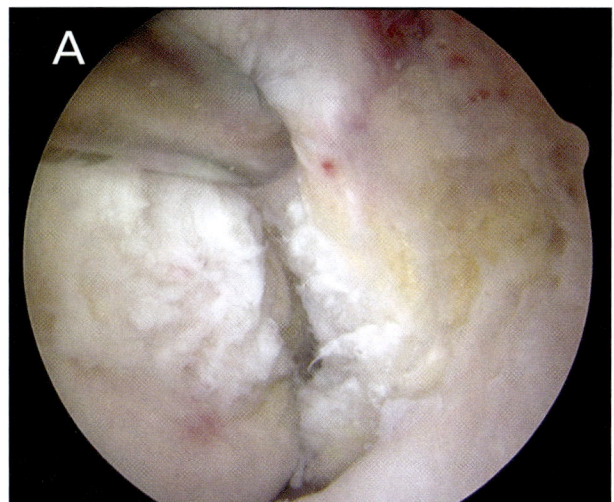

Figure 12-9. (A) Perform a thorough débridement of the PCL, starting from anterior to posterior on the lateral aspect of the medial femoral condyle. (B) Be careful of the vascular bundle posteriorly: visualization of fat indicates the proximity of the vascular bundle. (C) Arthroscopic view of the intercondylar notch after complete débridement of the PCL.

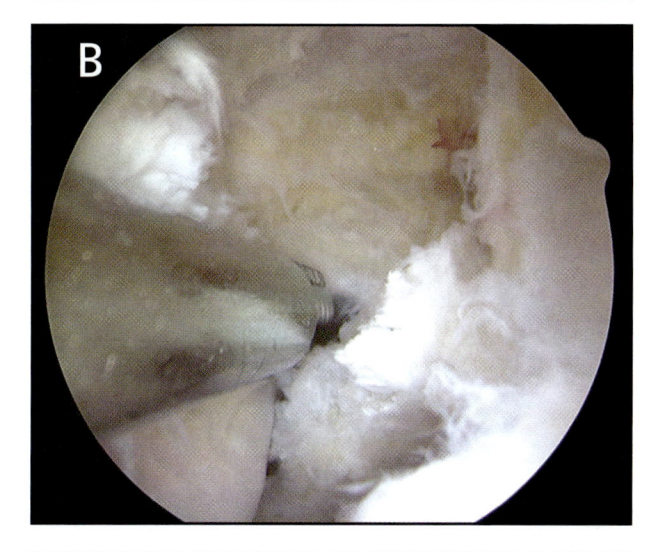

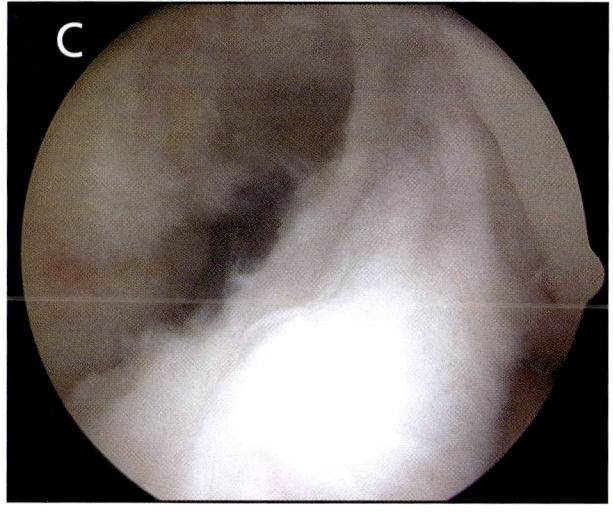

154 *Chapter 12*

Figure 12-10. While viewing through the anterolateral portal, guide the 30-degree arthroscope into the posteromedial compartment and transilluminate the joint line. Place the extremity in the figure-of-4 position and palpate along the transilluminated region to determine the optimal position for the posteromedial portal.

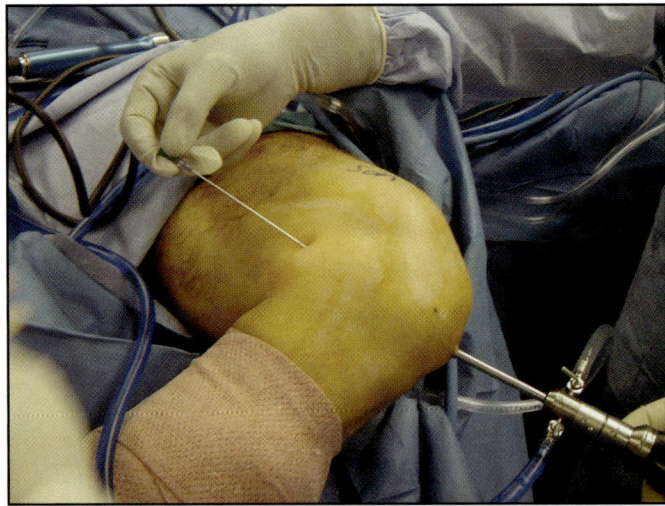

Figure 12-11. Place an 18-gauge spinal needle under arthroscopic visualization for localization.

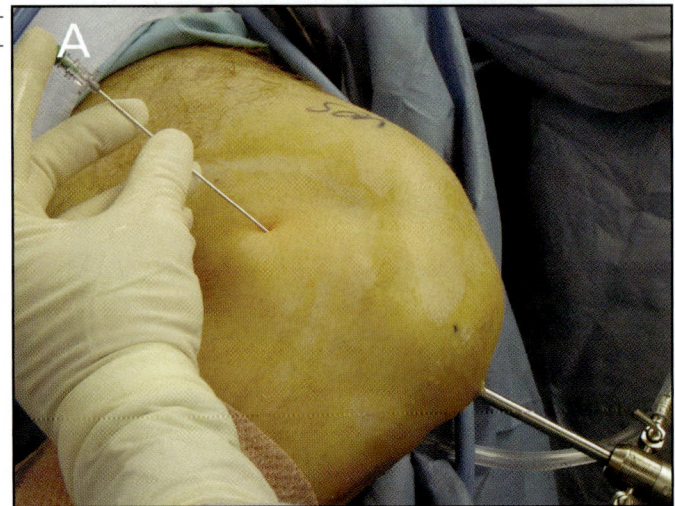

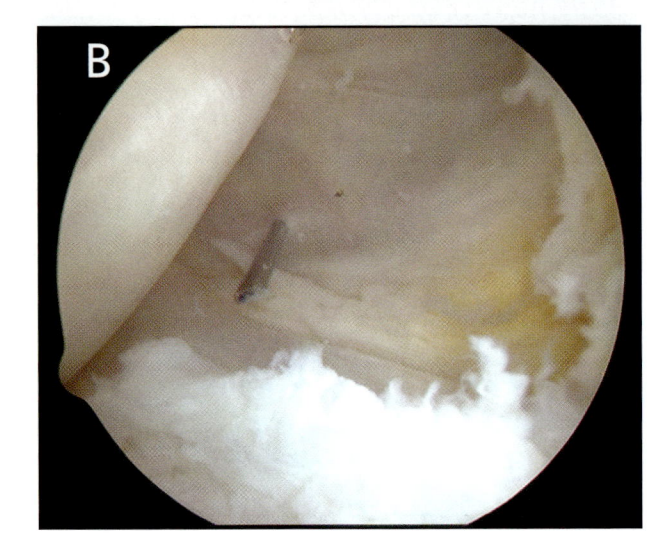

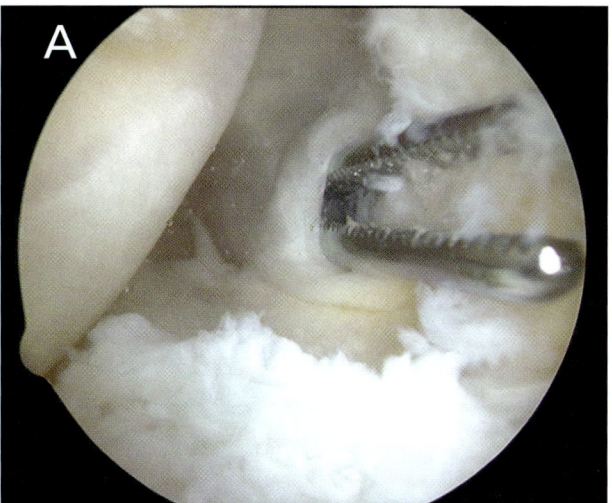

Single-Bundle Posterior Cruciate Ligament Reconstruction | **155**

Figure 12-12. Use a #11 blade scalpel to incise the skin only. (A) Using a hemostat clamp, gently spread and dissect bluntly down to the capsule and then puncture through under arthroscopic visualization. (B) Place a smooth cannula of choice into the posteromedial portal.

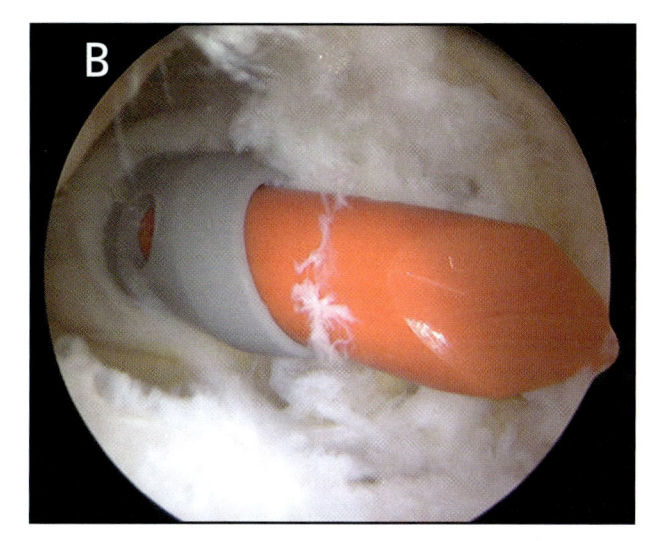

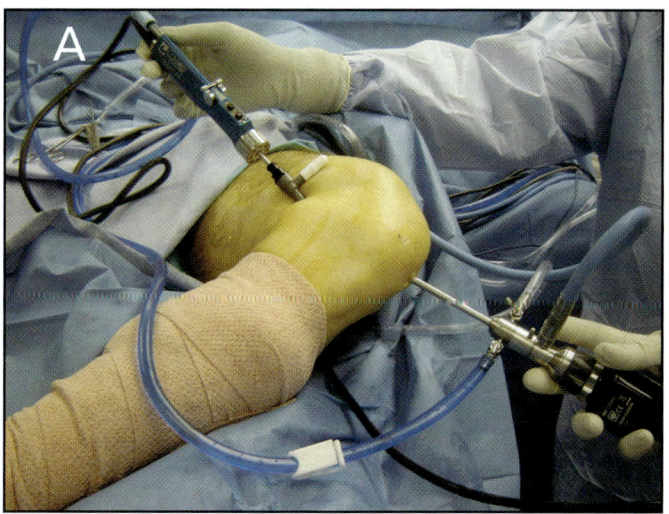

Figure 12-13. Switch the 30-degree arthroscope to a 70-degree arthroscope in the anterolateral portal. (A) Place a shaver through the posteromedial portal cannula. Hold the cannula in place when removing instruments in and out of this portal so as to avoid having to reinsert the cannula.

Figure 12-13. (B) Perform a débridement of the posterior aspect of the proximal tibia (ie, tibial insertion of PCL) (C) until the fibers of the gastrocnemius are visible.

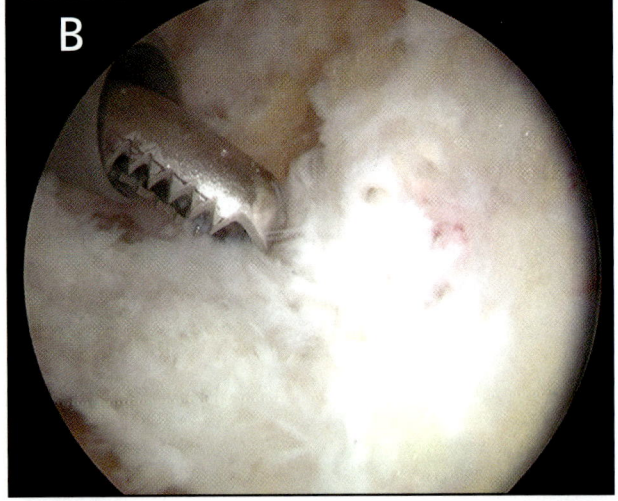

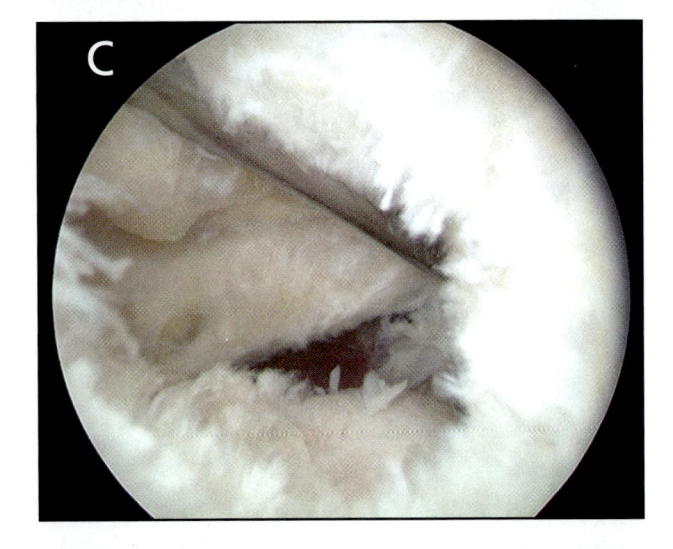

Figure 12-14. On the back table, set the PCL tibial guide to 70 degrees.

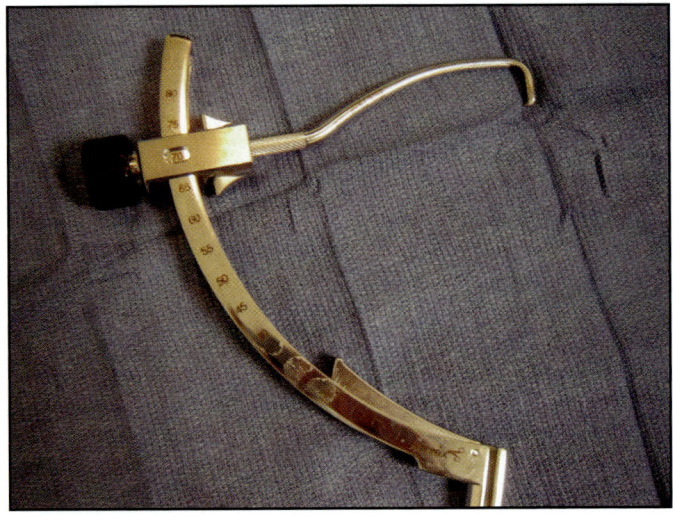

Single-Bundle Posterior Cruciate Ligament Reconstruction

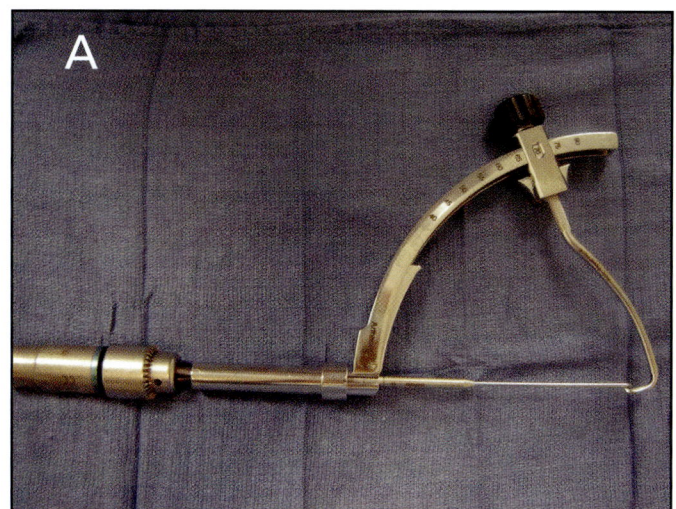

Figure 12-15. (A) Set the depth of the pin on the PCL tibial guide such that the tip of the pin pass-points 2 mm beyond the tip of the PCL guide. While holding the pin at this position, tighten the drill over the pin flush to the PCL tibial guide. (B) This ensures that the pin will traverse only 2 mm beyond the tip of the PCL guide before being blocked by the drill hitting the PCL guide. This helps to avoid injury to neurovascular structures in the popliteal fossa.

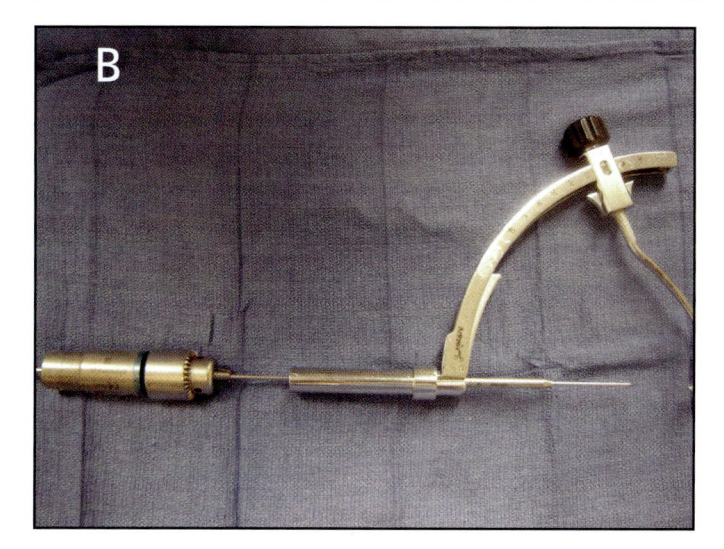

* The 2 mm of excursion of the pin beyond the tip of the PCL tibial guide allows easier visualization of the pin in those cases where the tip of the PCL tibial guide has sunk into the bone or if visualization is impaired because of inadequate débridement of soft tissues in the posterior aspect of the proximal tibia.

POSTERIOR CRUCIATE LIGAMENT TIBIAL TUNNEL

* To allow 360-degree access to the knee joint, raise the OR table, introduce Trendelenburg tilt, and then flex the distal portion of the OR table 90 degrees.
* Using the 70-degree arthroscope in the anterolateral portal for visualization, place the tip of the PCL tibial guide 1 cm distal from the proximal aspect of the posterior tibial plateau. It should be located just lateral to midline in the coronal plane, in the lateral aspect of the tibial attachment site of the PCL (Figure 12-16). This placement will help to control the increased external rotation of the tibia, seen in PCL-deficient patients.
* Position the drill sleeve for the PCL tibial guide at the estimated lateral edge of the medial collateral ligament, and make an incision for the tibial tunnel starting point.

158 Chapter 12

Figure 12-16. (A) View of the intercondylar notch as the PCL tibial guide is aimed toward the PCL tibial footprint. (B) Using a 70-degree arthroscope in the anterolateral portal for visualization, place the tip of the PCL tibial guide 1 cm distal from the proximal aspect of the posterior tibial plateau. It should be located just lateral to midline in the coronal plane, in the lateral aspect of the tibial attachment site of the PCL. This placement will help to control the increased external rotation of the tibia, seen in PCL-deficient patients.

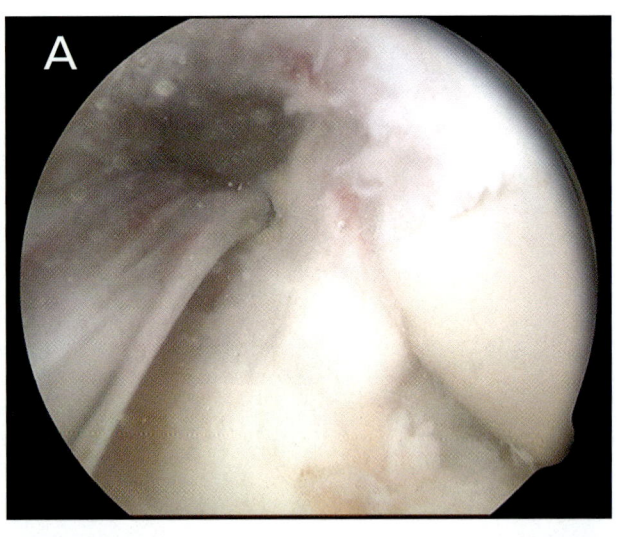

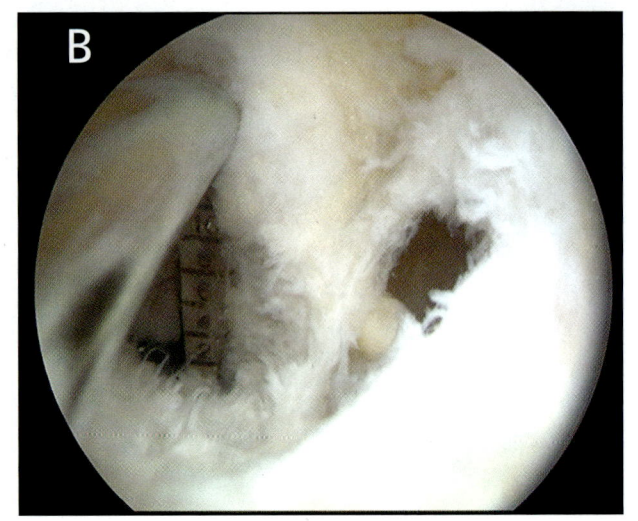

* Drill the pin to its pre-set distance by drilling until the drill itself becomes blocked by the PCL tibial guide from advancing further (Figure 12-17).
* Insert a small curette through the anteromedial portal to prevent the pin from migrating into the popliteal fossa (Figure 12-18).
* Remove the drill using a chuck key. If necessary, the pin may be tapped into the knee joint under arthroscopic visualization with protection using a curette.
* Use a 10-mm acorn reamer to drill over the pin up to but not through the posterior cortex.
* Prior to penetrating the posterior cortex, measure the tibial tunnel length using the markings on the reamer. Typically, this distance is 60 to 65 mm in length.
* Manually advance the reamer, and penetrate the posterior cortex under arthroscopic visualization (Figure 12-19).
* Use a curette to débride soft tissue in the intra-articular area surrounding the tibial tunnel.

Single-Bundle Posterior Cruciate Ligament Reconstruction 159

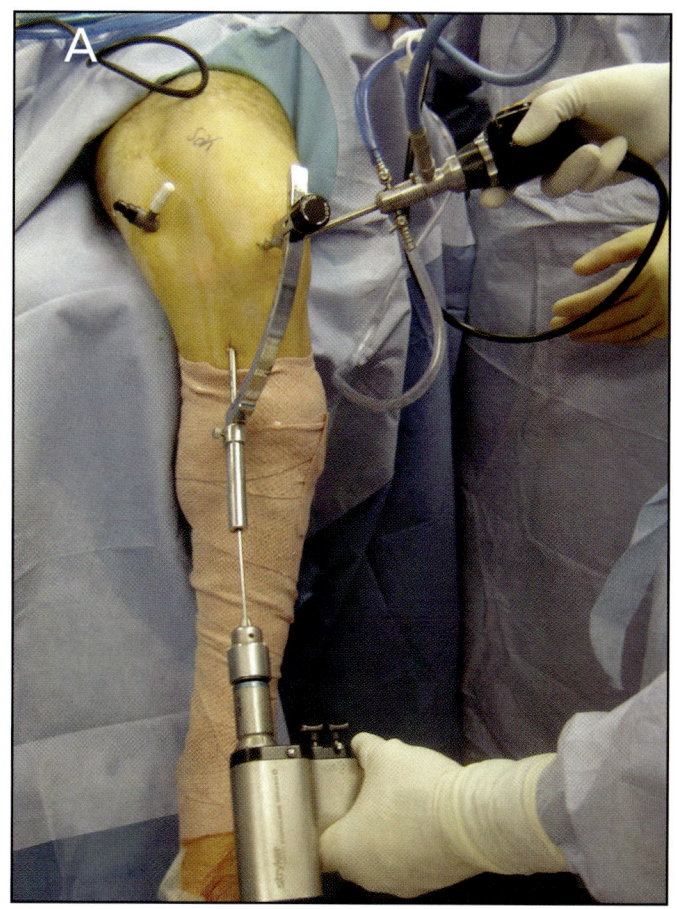

Figure 12-17. (A) Make an incision for the tibial tunnel starting point. Position the drill sleeve for the PCL tibial guide at the estimated lateral edge of the medial collateral ligament.

* Use a long depth gauge to remeasure the length of the tibial tunnel.
* Place a cannula at the entrance of the tibial tunnel to prevent loss of arthroscopy fluid and insufflation (Figure 12-20).

POSTERIOR CRUCIATE LIGAMENT FEMORAL TUNNEL

* To create a femoral tunnel, make a 3-cm longitudinal incision in line with the medial border of the patella and 2 finger-breadths superior from the superomedial corner of the patella (Figure 12-21).
* Perform blunt dissection through the vastus medialis obliquus using a snap and thyroid pole retractors down to the femur using a distal quadriceps splitting approach. Use appropriate retraction (eg, Richardson or Thyroid retractors) to aid visualization of bone. Use a Cobb elevator to ensure soft tissues have been elevated off the femur. Any remaining soft tissues at the site of the femoral tunnel will interfere with graft passage later in the procedure.
* Change from the 70-degree arthroscope to the 30-degree arthroscope.
* Set the PCL femoral guide to 70 degrees, and then insert it through the anteromedial portal.

Figure 12-17. (B) Drill the pin to its preset distance by drilling until the drill itself becomes blocked by the PCL tibial guide from advancing further.

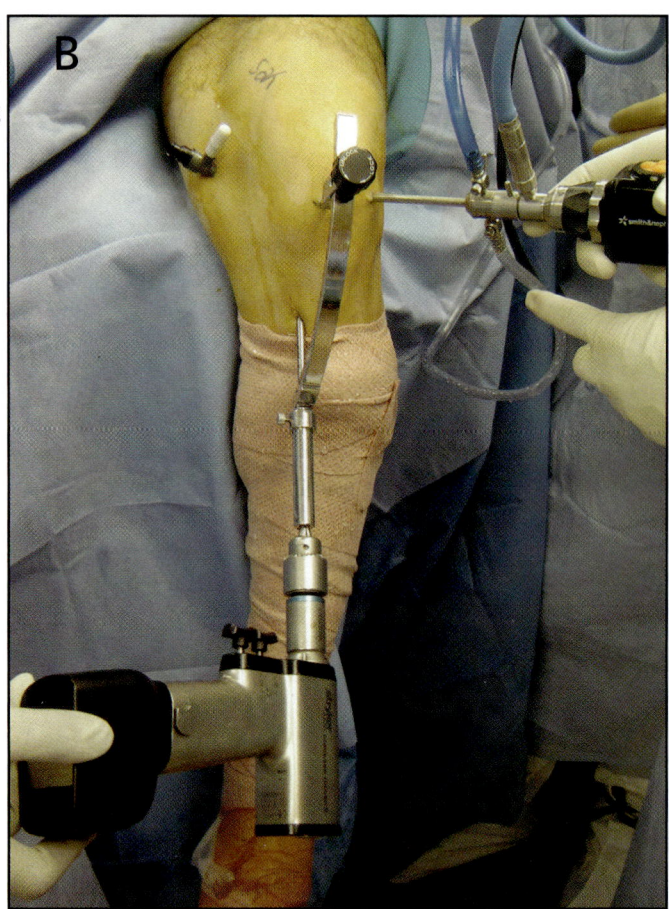

Figure 12-18. Insert a small curette through the anteromedial portal to prevent the pin from migrating into the popliteal fossa.

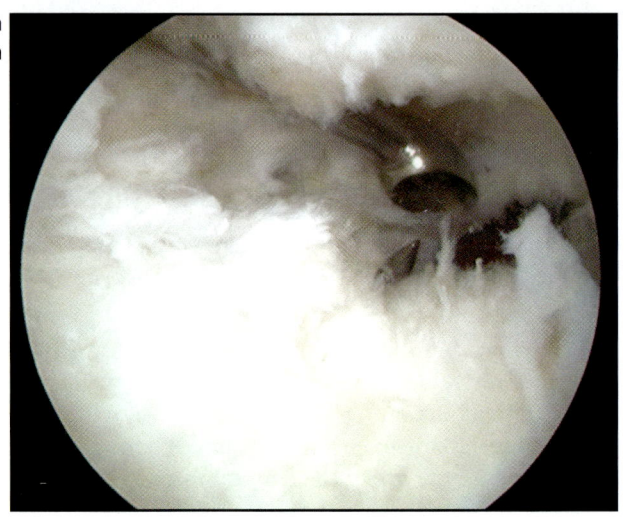

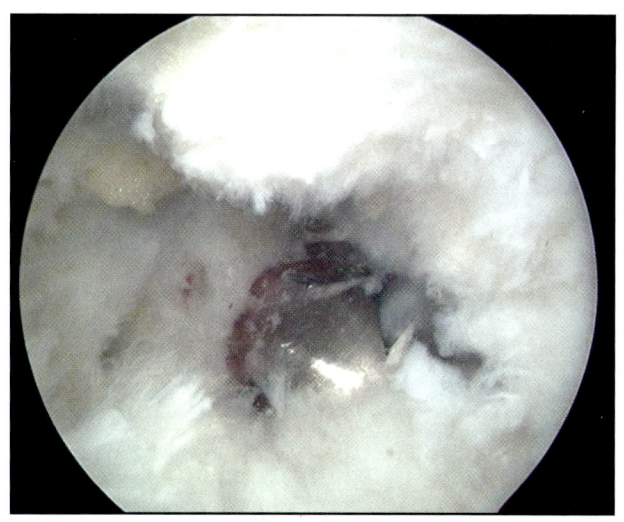

Single-Bundle Posterior Cruciate Ligament Reconstruction

Figure 12-19. Manually advance the reamer and penetrate the posterior cortex under arthroscopic visualization.

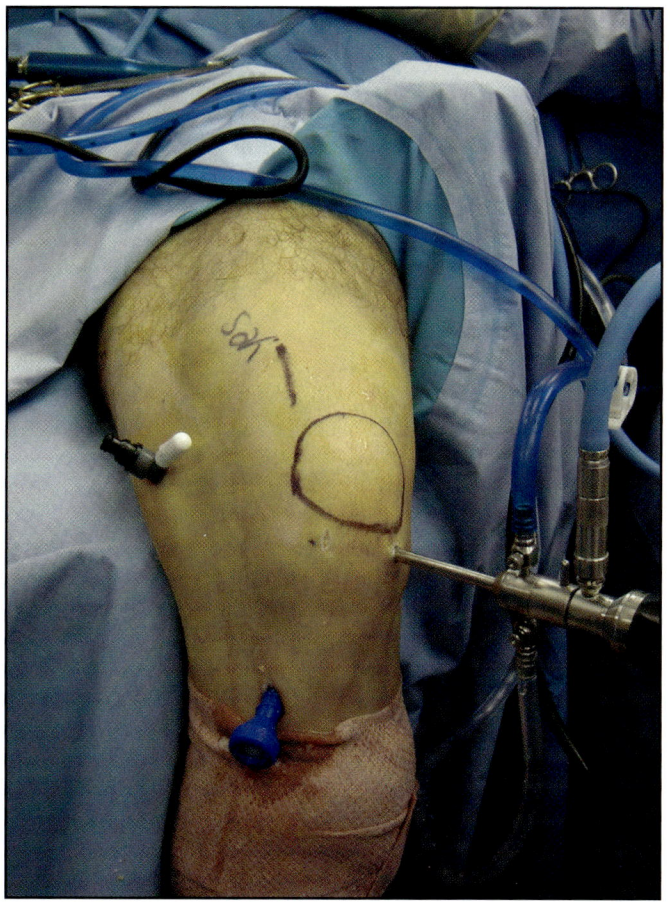

Figure 12-20. Place a cannula at the entrance of the tibial tunnel to prevent loss of arthroscopy fluid and insufflation.

Figure 12-21. To create a femoral tunnel, make a 3-cm longitudinal incision in line with the medial border of the patella and 2 finger-breadths superior from the superomedial corner of the patella. Perform blunt dissection through the vastus medialis obliquus using a snap and thyroid pole retractors down to the femur using a distal quadriceps splitting approach. Use appropriate retraction (eg, Richardson or Thyroid retractors) to aid visualization of bone. Use a Cobb elevator to ensure soft tissues have been elevated off the femur. Any remaining soft tissues at the site of the femoral tunnel will interfere with graft passage later in the procedure.

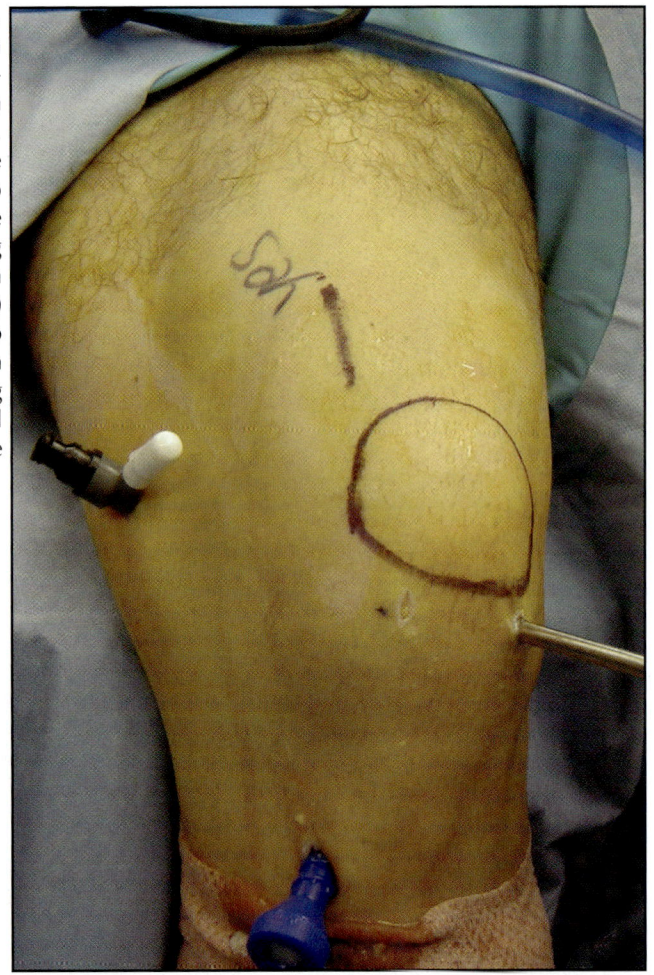

* Different from the ACL femoral tunnel, the PCL femoral tunnel should be placed quite vertical (12:30 or 1 o'clock position for right knees, 11:30 or 11 o'clock position for left knees).
* Place the tip of the PCL femoral guide at the appropriate clock position and 6 mm posterior to the articular cartilage surface (Figure 12-22).
* The extra-articular portion of the PCL femoral guide should be positioned between the medial edge of the trochlea and the medial epicondyle, and also as proximal on the femur as possible in order to decrease the risk of vascular disruption to the medial condyle and avascular necrosis (Figure 12-23).
* Place a guidepin through the PCL femoral guide and confirm location of the pin intra-articularly with the arthroscope (Figure 12-24).
* Remove the PCL femoral guide, and advance an 11-mm reamer over the guidepin up to but not through the second cortex.
* Place a shaver through the femoral tunnel to remove debris within the tunnel as well as in the joint (Figure 12-25).
* Use retractors to visualize the entrance to the femoral tunnel and ensure that there are no soft tissues that may potentially cover the tunnel or otherwise interfere with graft passage.
* Place a cannula at the entrance of the femoral tunnel to prevent loss of arthroscopy fluid and insufflation.

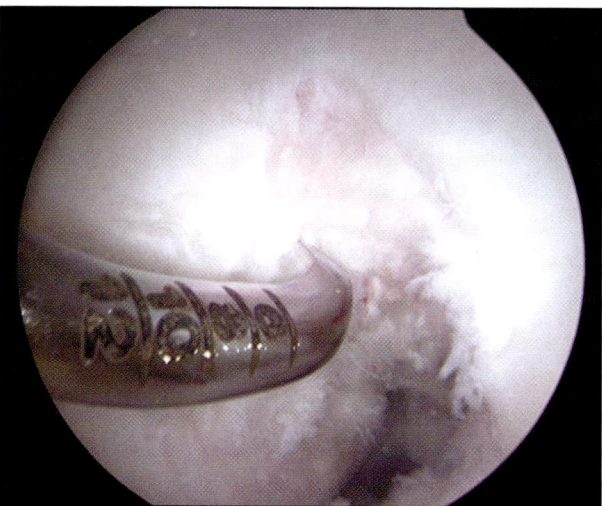

Single-Bundle Posterior Cruciate Ligament Reconstruction

Figure 12-22. Change from the 70-degree arthroscope to the 30-degree arthroscope. Set the PCL femoral guide to 70 degrees, and then insert it through the anteromedial portal. Different from the ACL femoral tunnel, the PCL femoral tunnel should be placed quite vertical (12:30 or 1 o'clock position for right knees, 11:30 or 11 o'clock position for left knees). Place the tip of the PCL femoral guide at the appropriate clock face position and located 6 mm posterior to the articular cartilage surface.

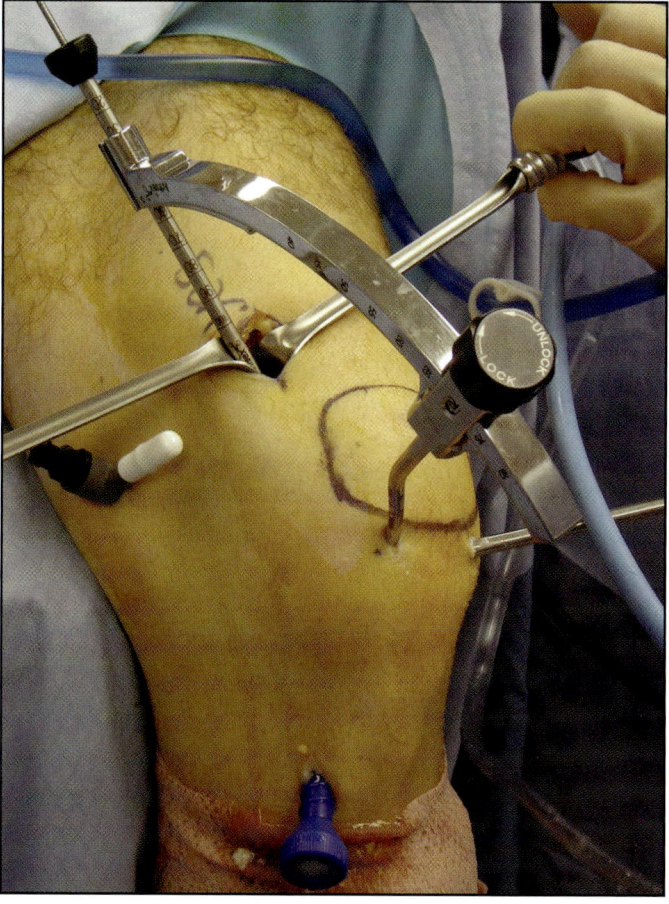

Figure 12-23. The extra-articular portion of the PCL femoral guide should be positioned between the medial edge of the trochlea and the medial epicondyle, and also as proximal on the femur as possible in order to decrease the risk of vascular disruption to the medial condyle and avascular necrosis.

Figure 12-24. Place a guidepin through the PCL femoral guide and confirm location of the pin intra-articularly with the arthroscope.

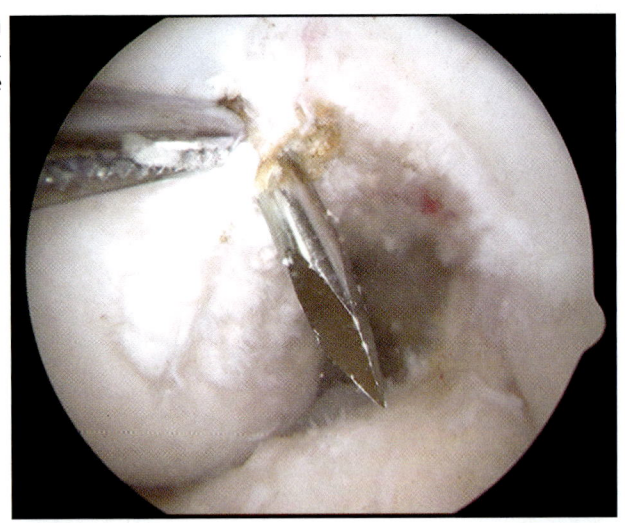

Figure 12-25. Place a shaver through the femoral tunnel to remove debris within the tunnel as well as in the joint.

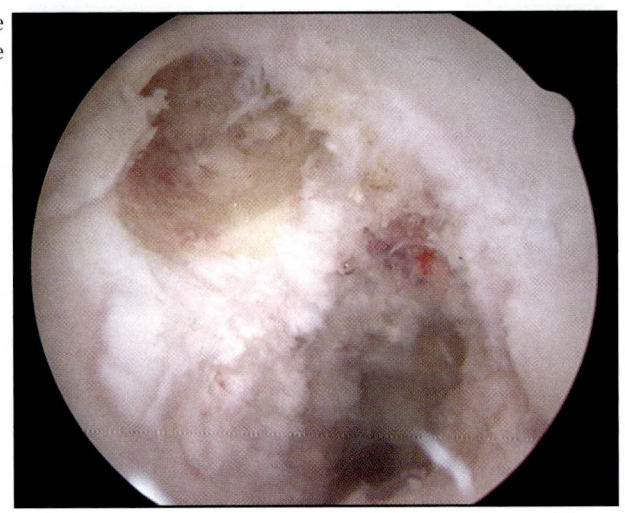

GRAFT PASSAGE

* Pass the "Worm" Curving Suture Passer (Arthrex, Naples, FL) through the tibial tunnel (Figure 12-26A). The flat edge should face anteriorly in order to ensure that the suture passer will curl toward the center of the joint (Figure 12-26B). The wire loop and passing suture will exit the tube of the suture passer and curve 180 degrees toward the intercondylar notch.
* Using a pituitary rongeur through the anteromedial portal, position the suture near the femoral tunnel. Then, insert the pituitary rongeur through the PCL femoral tunnel and grab the suture (Figure 12-27). Pull the suture out of the femoral tunnel, and tie it to the whipstitch suture on the soft-tissue end of the graft.
* Pass the graft through the knee by pulling on the passing suture (Figure 12-28).
* Palpate the bone block with a finger to keep the bone block flush with the femoral cortex.

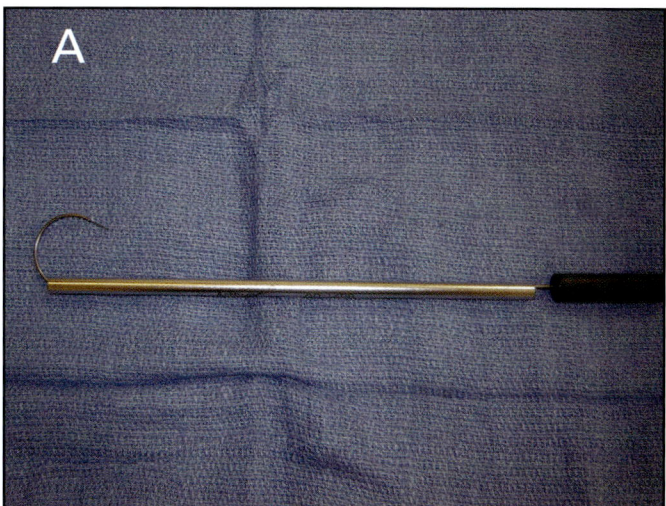

Single-Bundle Posterior Cruciate Ligament Reconstruction **165**

Figure 12-26. (A) The "Worm" Curving Suture Passer (Arthrex, Naples, FL) is a device that allows a wire loop and passing suture to exit the tube of the suture passer in the tibial tunnel and curl 180 degrees anteriorly toward the intercondylar notch. The flat edge should face anteriorly in order to ensure that the suture passer will curl toward the center of the joint. (B) Using a pituitary rongeur through the anteromedial portal, position the suture near the femoral tunnel.

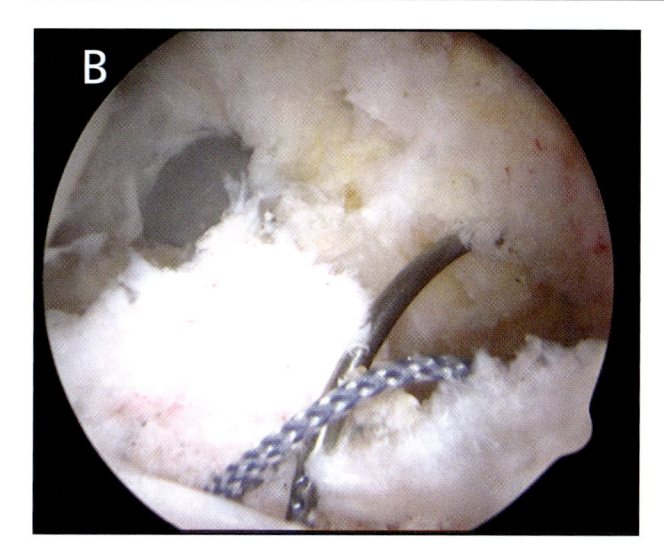

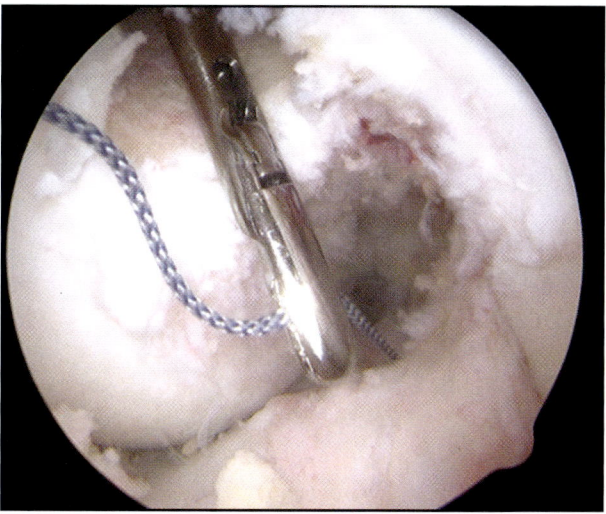

Figure 12-27. Insert a pituitary rongeur through the PCL femoral tunnel and grab the passing suture. Pull the suture out of the femoral tunnel and tie it to the whipstitch suture on the soft-tissue end of the graft.

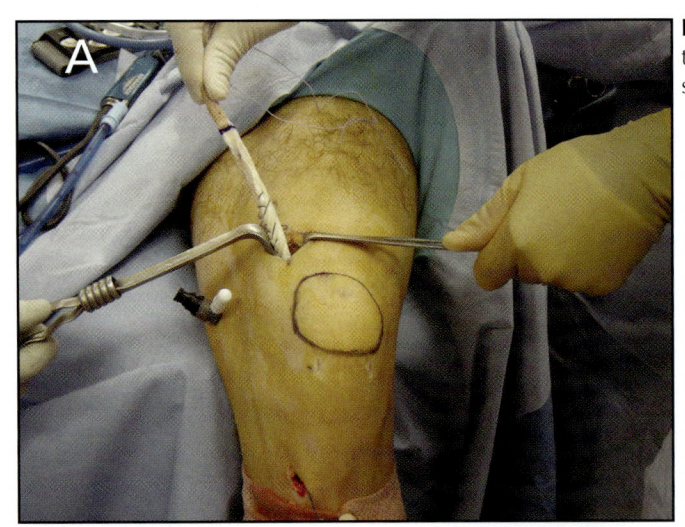

Figure 12-28. Pass the graft through the knee by pulling on the passing suture.

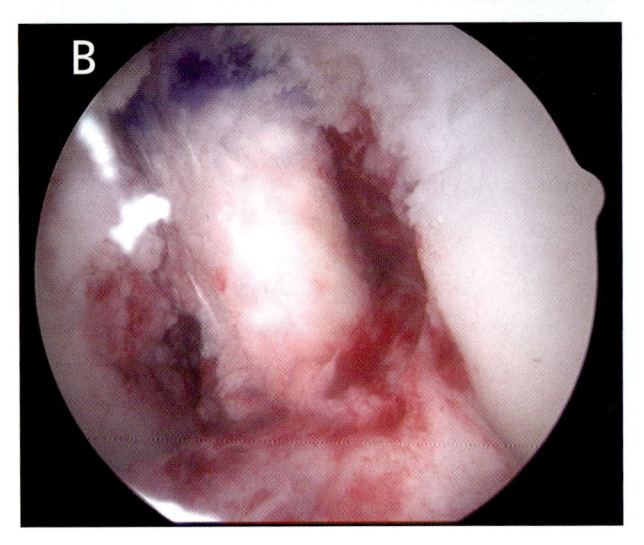

GRAFT FIXATION

* In the femoral tunnel, place a nitinol guidewire proximal to the bone block, and place an 8-mm wide bioabsorbable interference screw (eg, Milagro 8 x 30 mm) over the wire. Be careful not to sink the bone block into the femur while advancing the screw.
* Cycle the knee to assess isometry by evaluating graft motion.
* To provide aperture fixation in the tibial tunnel, place a mark on the screwdriver shaft that coincides with the measured tibial tunnel length (usually approximately 60 to 65 mm) by wrapping a Steri-Strip (3M Corp, St. Paul, MN) around the screwdriver (Figure 12-29).
* In preparation for the tibial fixation, it is important to have an assistant hold the knee at 90 degrees of flexion while performing an anterior drawer maneuver with a valgus force (Figure 12-30).
* In the tibial tunnel, place a nitinol wire inferior to the graft, and advance a 9-mm BioScrew (ConMed Linvatec, Largo, FL) (eg, Milagro 9 x 30 mm) over the wire toward the posterior and proximal aspect of the tibial tunnel, until the Steri-Strip on the screwdriver shaft

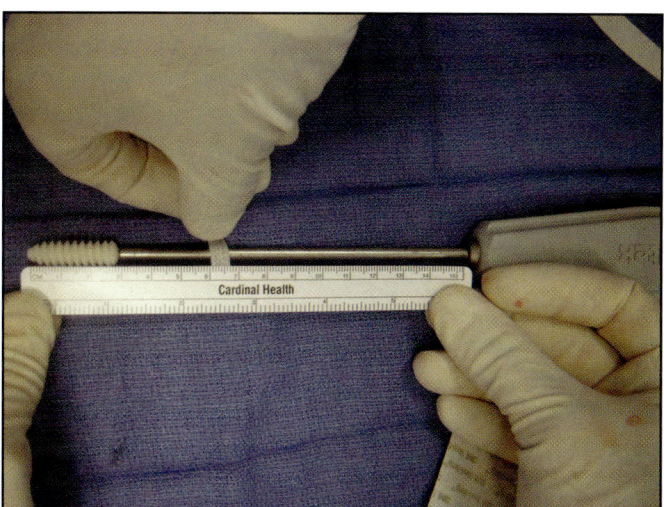

Single-Bundle Posterior Cruciate Ligament Reconstruction

Figure 12-29. To provide aperture fixation in the tibial tunnel, place a mark on the screwdriver shaft that coincides with the measured tibial tunnel length (usually approximately 60 to 65 mm) by wrapping a Steri-Strip around the screwdriver.

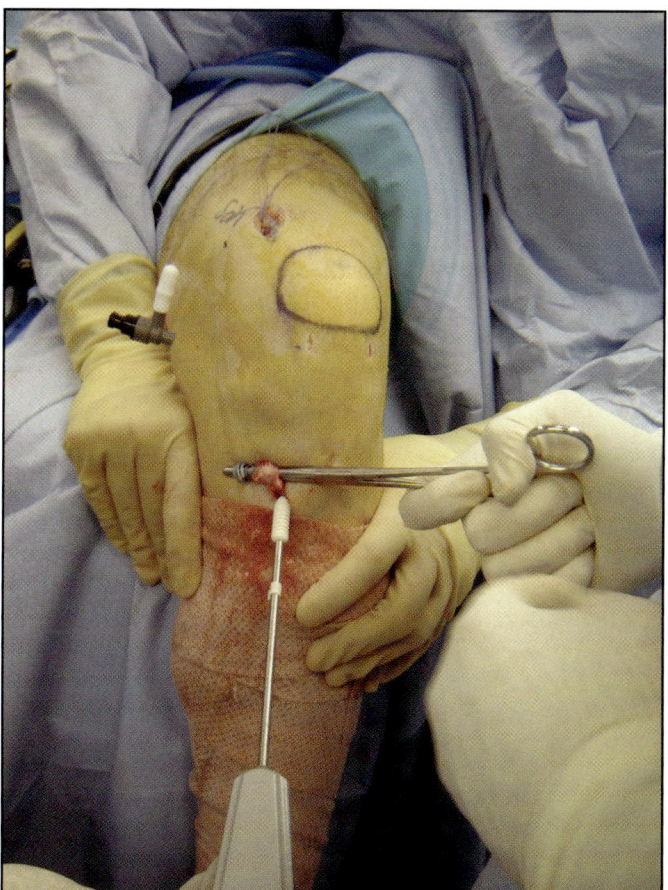

Figure 12-30. In preparation for the tibial fixation, it is important to have an assistant hold the knee at 90 degrees of flexion while performing an anterior drawer maneuver with a valgus force. Place a nitinol wire into the tibial tunnel, inferior to the graft and advance a 9-mm BioScrew (eg, Milagro screw 9 x 30 mm) over the wire toward the posterior and proximal aspect of the tibial tunnel, until the Steri-Strip on the screwdriver shaft reaches the anterior cortex of the tibia. The BioScrew is placed inferior to the graft in order to ensure that the graft does not abrade against the screw. By placing this screw at the posterior aspect of the tunnel, the effective length of the graft is shortened, producing a stiffer graft, analogous to a tibial inlay technique. It also eliminates the so-called "killer turn."

Figure 12-31. Exchange the nitinol wire with a guidewire for a 9-mm metal interference screw (eg, Guardsman 9 x 30 mm), which serves as the "back up" interference fixation of the soft-tissue portion of the graft. Be careful not to advance the metal screw too deep such that the previously placed BioScrew is not inadvertently pushed deeper. Ideally, this "back up" screw should have some purchase at the cortex by a thread or two. If there is no purchase at the cortex, the metal screw may simply sink into the softer metaphyseal bone without meaningful fixation of the soft-tissue graft.

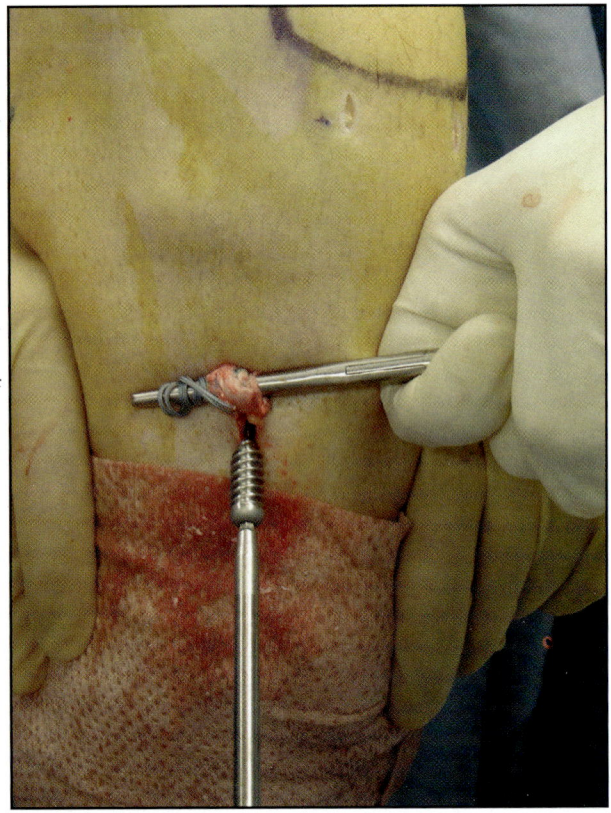

reaches the anterior cortex of the tibia. The BioScrew is placed inferior to the graft to ensure that the graft does not abrade against the screw (see Figure 12-30). By placing this screw at the posterior aspect of the tunnel, the effective length of the graft is shortened, producing a stiffer graft, analogous to a tibial inlay technique. It also eliminates the so-called "killer turn."

* Exchange the nitinol wire with a guidewire for a 9-mm metal interference screw (eg, Guardsman 9 x 30 mm), which serves as the "back up" interference fixation of the soft-tissue portion of the graft (Figure 12-31). Be careful not to advance the metal screw too deep such that the previously placed BioScrew is not inadvertently pushed deeper. Ideally, this back up screw should have some purchase at the cortex by a thread or two. If there is no purchase at the cortex, the metal screw may simply sink into the softer metaphyseal bone without meaningful fixation of the soft-tissue graft.

TIPS AND PEARLS

✔ To save time, thaw and prepare the Achilles tendon allograft prior to the patient's arrival in the OR.

✔ Make sure that the calcaneal bone block of the Achilles tendon allograft fits easily and loosely through an 11-mm spacer. If the bone block does not fit through the femoral tunnel easily and requires that the bone block be resized, then you will lose valuable

Single-Bundle Posterior Cruciate Ligament Reconstruction

operative time and tourniquet time. Moreover, allograft calcaneal bone is often quite brittle. Smaller bone blocks tend to crumble.

✔ Prior to inflating the tourniquet, perform a diagnostic arthroscopy, and treat any meniscus tears or chondral injuries that may be present so as to reserve time under tourniquet to the critical portions of the PCL reconstruction procedure.

✔ Set the depth of the pin on the PCL tibial guide such that the tip of the pin pass-points 2 mm beyond the tip of the PCL guide (see Figure 12-15A). While holding the pin at this position, tighten the drill over the pin flush to the PCL tibial guide such that the pin will traverse only 2 mm beyond the tip of the PCL guide before being blocked by the drill hitting the PCL guide (see Figure 12-17). This is to ensure that the pin does not inadvertently injure neurovascular structures in the popliteal fossa.

✔ Use retractors to visualize the entrance to the femoral tunnel, and ensure that there are no soft tissues that may potentially cover the tunnel or otherwise interfere with graft passage.

✔ To provide aperture fixation in the tibial tunnel, place a mark on the screwdriver shaft that coincides with the measured tibial tunnel length (usually approximately 60 to 65 mm) by wrapping a Steri-Strip around the screwdriver (see Figure 12-29).

PITFALLS

✘ When débriding the PCL, start from anterior to posterior on the lateral aspect of the medial femoral condyle (see Figure 12-8B). Be careful of the vascular bundle posteriorly: visualization of fat indicates the proximity of the vascular bundle (see Figure 12-9B).

✘ Immediately prior to drilling the tibial tunnel but after the pin placement through the PCL tibial guide, insert a small curette through the anteromedial portal to prevent the pin from migrating into the popliteal fossa (see Figure 12-18).

✘ To ensure safety of the posterior neurovascular structures while drilling the tibial tunnel, stop immediately prior to penetrating the cortex, and manually advance the reamer through the posterior cortex under arthroscopic visualization (see Figure 12-19).

✘ The extra-articular portion of the PCL femoral guide should be positioned between the medial edge of the trochlea and the medial epicondyle, and also as proximal on the femur as possible in order to decrease the risk of vascular disruption to the medial condyle and avascular necrosis (see Figure 12-23).

✘ In preparation for the tibial fixation, it is important to have an assistant hold the knee at 90 degrees of flexion while performing an anterior drawer maneuver with a valgus force (see Figure 12-30). Otherwise, the graft may have to be secured in a posterior drawer position, which can result in laxity of the reconstructed PCL.

✘ In the tibial tunnel, the BioScrew is placed inferior to the graft to ensure that the graft does not abrade against the screw at the site of the "killer turn" (see Figure 12-30).

✘ For back up tibial fixation, be careful not to advance the metal screw too deep such that the previously placed BioScrew is not inadvertently pushed deeper (Figure 12-31). Ideally, this back up screw should have some purchase at the cortex by a thread or two. If there is no purchase at the cortex, the metal screw may simply sink into the softer metaphyseal bone without meaningful fixation of the soft-tissue graft.

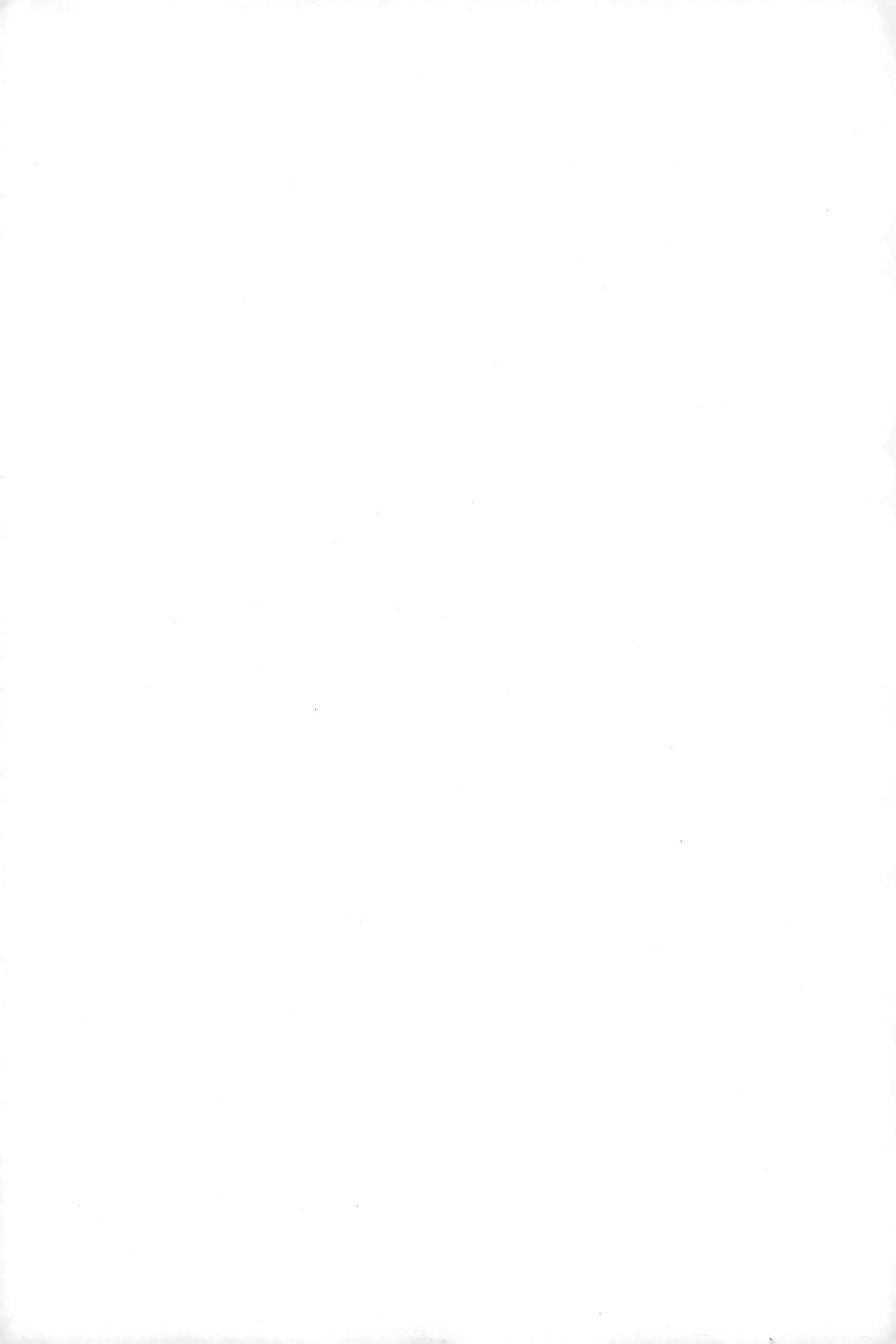

13

Posterior Cruciate Ligament Reconstruction

Single-Bundle Tibial Inlay Technique

Lutul D. Farrow, MD and John A. Bergfeld, MD

Posterior cruciate ligament (PCL) injuries occur much less frequently than anterior cruciate ligament (ACL) injuries. Likewise, the medical literature and experience with the management of PCL injuries have lagged far behind that for the ACL. Injuries to the PCL have traditionally been managed non-operatively. One of us (JAB) has previously shown that the majority of athletes with isolated tears of the PCL were able to return to athletic competition following an appropriate rehabilitation program.[1] Recent advances in our knowledge of PCL anatomy, biomechanics, and treatment have led to more aggressive surgical management of these injuries. Furthermore, our current understanding of the long-term sequelae of the PCL-deficient knee has led to a lower threshold for surgical management. In general, non-operative treatment is reserved for the asymptomatic knee with an isolated PCL tear and only mild to moderate posterior laxity (Grade I or II).[2-4]

The decision to operatively manage PCL injuries is based on several factors (Table 13-1). The primary indications for operative treatment of chronic PCL injuries are pain and symptomatic instability. The clearest indication for acute operative intervention is in the patient with a combined ligamentous injury. Injuries to the PCL in combination with injuries to the ACL, medial collateral ligament, and/or posterolateral corner complex are potentially devastating injuries that typically present with marked knee instability. These combined ligamentous injuries require surgical intervention to restore proper knee function and kinematics. However, controversy exists concerning the management of isolated tears of the PCL. Most surgeons would agree that acute bony avulsion injuries of the PCL attachment sites are best addressed with surgical fixation,[5] while Grade III injuries of the PCL involving more than 10 mm of posterior tibial displacement are typically considered for surgical management. Symptomatic, isolated Grade II tears of the PCL with less than 10 mm of posterior tibial displacement accompanied by further decrease in posterior tibial excursion after internal rotation of the tibia in the young, active patient present another treatment dilemma. Currently, most surgeons would not recommend operative management of PCL injuries in this acute subgroup of patients. Those patients with continued pain and/or instability following an adequate course of conservative management may be cautiously considered for operative intervention.

Multiple different options for PCL reconstruction have been described. The most commonly performed techniques include posterior tibial inlay and transtibial tunnel reconstruction techniques. Single-bundle and double-bundle techniques also exist. We prefer the single-bundle, posterior tibial inlay technique for reconstruction of the PCL. This technique effectively restores posterior stability of the knee by anatomically reconstructing the more substantial PCL anterolateral bundle. We do not perform double-bundle reconstruction. One of us (JAB) has previously shown no significant biomechanical differences between the two techniques.[6] The posterior tibial

> **Table 13-1**
>
> **OPERATIVE INDICATIONS**
>
> 1. Combined ligamentous injury
> 2. Grade III instability
> 3. Bony avulsion injury
> 4. Symptomatic Grade II instability in young, active patients
> 5. Failed conservative management

inlay technique also avoids the "killer curve" created at the aperture of the tibial tunnel created by the transtibial technique. One of us (JAB) previously demonstrated biomechanically that the tibial inlay technique results in less graft thinning and graft failure compared to the transtibial technique.[7] This has also been substantiated by other authors.[8] This chapter describes our technique of single-bundle, posterior tibial inlay reconstruction of the PCL.

GRAFT SELECTION

Multiple graft options exist for PCL reconstruction using the tibial inlay technique. Graft options vary with respect to anatomic donor site as well as choice of allograft versus autograft tissues. We prefer composite tendon grafts with a bony block on at least one end. The bony block is essential for rigid bone-to-bone graft fixation on the tibial side. Autograft options thus include bone-patellar tendon-bone and quadriceps tendon. Allograft options include Achilles, quadriceps, and patellar tendon grafts. Allograft tissues avoid donor site morbidity, hastening postoperative rehabilitation, and graft length mismatches. Allografts also avoid insult to the quadriceps mechanism, a dynamic inhibitor of posterior tibial translation.[9] In the knee with multiple ligamentous injury, allograft tissues theoretically avoid further insult to an already compromised knee joint. Using allograft tissue shortens total operative time. When the preoperative diagnosis is certain, the allograft tissue can even be prepared prior to patient arrival in the operative theater, further diminishing operative time in the compromised knee joint. We prefer Achilles allograft because of its versatility. It is typically longer and thicker than other allograft options, making it the ideal allograft tissue to reconstruct the robust anterolateral band of the native PCL. The benefit of bone-patellar tendon-bone allograft is the potential for bone-to-bone healing on both ends of the graft; however, there is the potential for length mismatch.

A drawback with allograft tissue is the potential for bacterial contamination and disease transmission. Although potentially devastating, both of these complications are exceedingly rare. The development of better donor screening and testing procedures have all but eliminated the risk of disease transmission. We have not experienced this complication. The risk of bacterial contamination has also been lessened by current techniques of aseptic graft harvest, antibiotic preparation, and sterilization techniques. Furthermore, the most commonly used techniques for graft sterilization do not change the biomechanical properties of the allograft tissue. The cost of allograft tissue should be considered.

Available autograft tissues include both patellar tendon and quadriceps tendon grafts. Autograft tissues are cost effective and avoid potentially devastating complications of disease transmission and bacterial contamination. There is also evidence that autograft tissues incorporate more quickly than allograft tissues. The primary downside of autograft tissue is its associated donor site morbidity. Anterior knee pain, quadriceps weakness, and patella fracture all have been documented following patellar tendon autograft. The superior pole of the patella is thicker, thus quadriceps autograft is less likely to compromise the osseous structure of the patella. Furthermore, some surgeons believe quadriceps autograft also avoids issues with anterior knee pain. Finally, with concomitant ligamentous injury, autograft harvest may further compromise an already compromised knee or require harvest from the contralateral normal knee. With respect to specific graft options, the patellar tendon autograft offers the option of bone-to-bone stabilization and healing on both ends of the graft. The downside of this graft option is its fixed length due to the attached bone blocks. Quadriceps tendon autograft offers many advantages over patellar tendon autograft. Quadriceps autograft is a much longer graft, increasing its versatility compared to patellar tendon autograft. Its increased thickness also makes quadriceps autograft favorable for reconstruction of the PCL anterolateral bundle. Quadriceps muscle function is important in the early postoperative period. Because of this, we do not use quadriceps autograft.

SURGICAL GOALS

The primary goal of PCL reconstruction is to restore normal knee kinematics and stability. With proper restoration of normal knee kinematics and stability, it is hoped that the patient will return to his or her pre-injury activity level.

OPERATIVE TECHNIQUE

* The patient is identified in the preoperative holding area, and the operative extremity is marked. The patient also receives a dose of intravenous antibiotics at this time. Once in the operating room, a time-out is taken by all personnel, and the operative extremity is once again confirmed. At this time, general anesthesia induction is begun, and an endotracheal tube is inserted and secured. We prefer formal intubation, as a laryngeal mask airway or face mask does not provide reliable control of the airway when the patient is turned to the prone position.

POSITIONING

* For the start of the case, the patient is placed in the supine position on a standard operative table. We always perform the arthroscopic portion of the procedure first. A nonsterile tourniquet is placed as proximal on the thigh as possible. The unaffected limb is then placed into a well-leg holder with the peroneal nerve free from pressure, and the operative extremity is placed into a Dyonics leg holder.
* The end of the operative table is then maximally flexed, leaving the operative limb freely suspended (Figure 13-1). The operative extremity is then prepped and draped in the usual sterile fashion (Figure 13-2).

DIAGNOSTIC ARTHROSCOPY

* A standard anterolateral arthroscopic portal is established. The anterolateral portal is made longitudinally, just lateral to the patellar tendon at the level of the inferior pole of the patella. The anterolateral portal is typically the viewing portal. The anteromedial portal is localized with a spinal needle and made in longitudinal fashion under direct arthroscopic visualization. The anteromedial portal is our working portal. A small incision is made just above the superolateral pole of the patella. A rigid outflow cannula is placed into the

Figure 13-1. Operative knee positioned in arthroscopic leg holder. The well leg is in a padded stirrup holder.

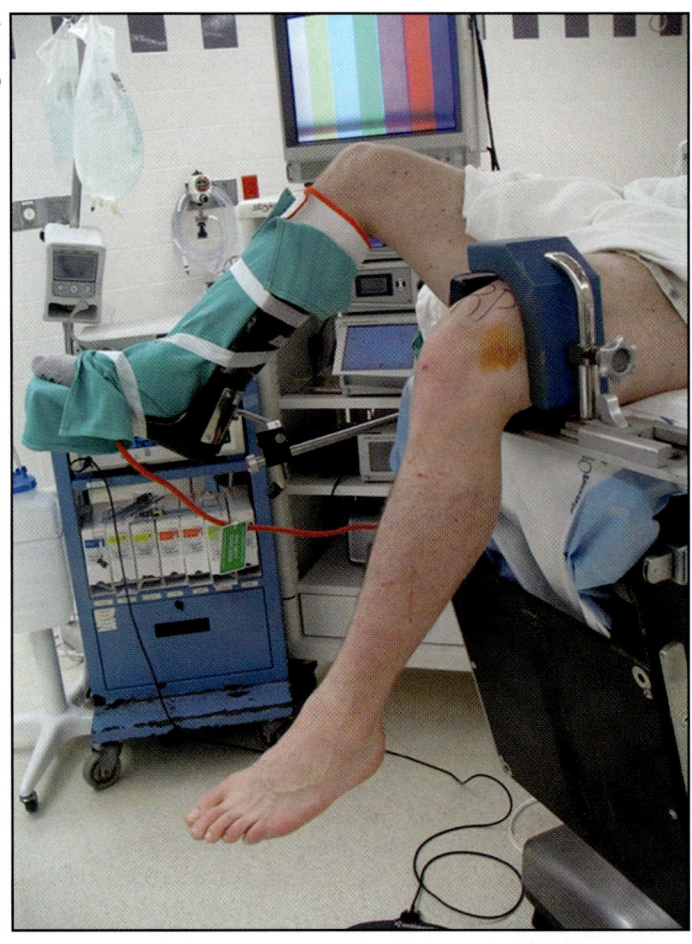

Figure 13-2. Operative extremity prepped and draped.

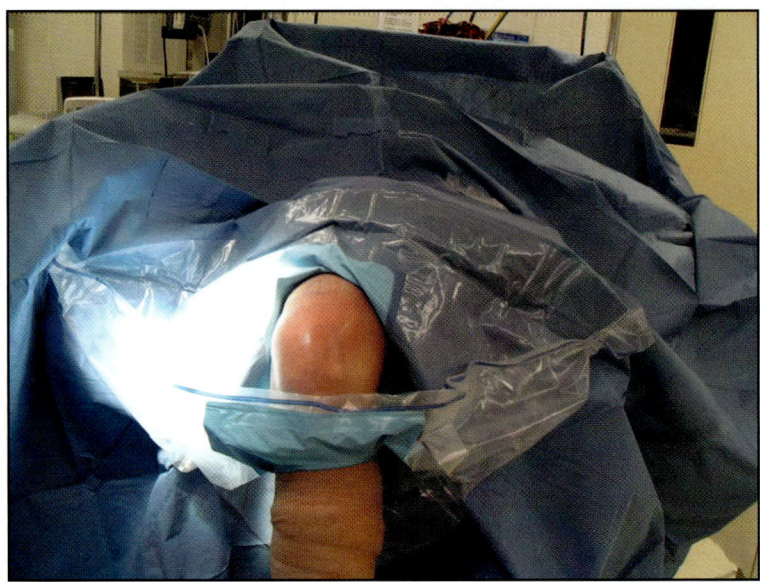

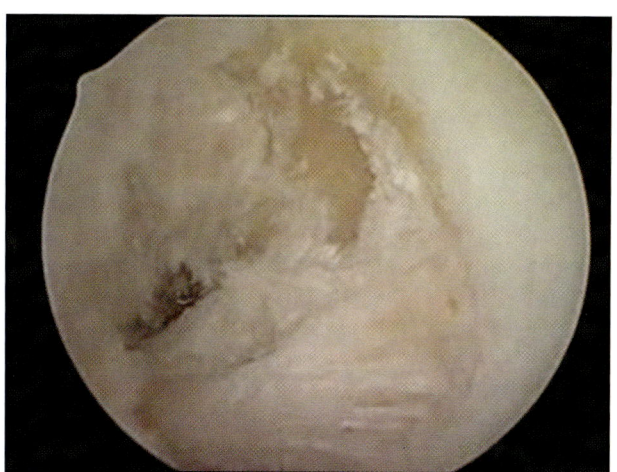

Figure 13-3. Intact anterior and posterior meniscofemoral ligaments (right knee).

suprapatellar pouch through this incision. We use an arthroscopic pump to aid with hemostasis and facilitate clear visualization.

* Diagnostic arthroscopy proceeds in a methodical, ordered fashion. Beginning in the suprapatellar pouch, we first visualize the outflow portal to ensure that it has properly entered the suprapatellar pouch. The patellofemoral articulation is examined for articular cartilage changes as this articulation may experience advanced degenerative changes with PCL deficiency. The medial gutter is then visualized. Next, the arthroscope is brought into the lateral gutter. Here, the popliteus tendon is identified, and the arthroscope is pushed gently along its course to identify any injury to this structure. At this time, the arthroscope is passed into the lateral compartment as a varus force is applied to the knee. Injury to the posterolateral ligamentous complex may manifest as excessive joint space opening when in this position. Examination of the medial compartment follows. The intercondylar notch is examined last. The ligamentum mucosa and infrapatellar fat pad are débrided as necessary to facilitate visualization of the ACL and PCL. On first viewing of the PCL, it may appear to be in continuity as many tears occur at or near the tibial attachment. An arthroscopic probe should be hooked around the deep surface of PCL, and anterior traction will typically reveal the ligamentous laxity in this situation. A large bore shaver (4.5 mm or larger) is used to débride the residual fibers of the PCL. In many cases, one of the meniscofemoral ligaments may be intact (Figure 13-3). Every effort should be made to retain this ligament as 28% of restraint to posterior tibial translation in the PCL-intact knee is accounted for by the meniscofemoral ligaments.[10]

GRAFT HARVEST

* The Achilles allograft typically comes as a long soft-tissue graft attached to an osseous block of calcaneus. We thaw the graft in its sterile packaging in warm sterile saline. Once thawed, some surgeons advocate transfer to a sterile, sealable container for serial antibiotic washes with a mixture of warm normal saline impregnated with polymyxin and bacitracin antibiotics. Gentle shaking of the container provides slight mechanical irritation for additional graft "cleansing." Eight to 10 washes are performed until 500 to 1000 cc of fluid are used.

* The Achilles bone block is prepared with an oscillating bone saw on the back table. The dimensions of the graft should be 25-mm long, 10- to 12-mm wide, and 5-mm thick. The tendinous portion of the graft should be approximately 10- to 11-mm wide and 70-mm

Figure 13-4. Achilles graft prepared with whipstitch.

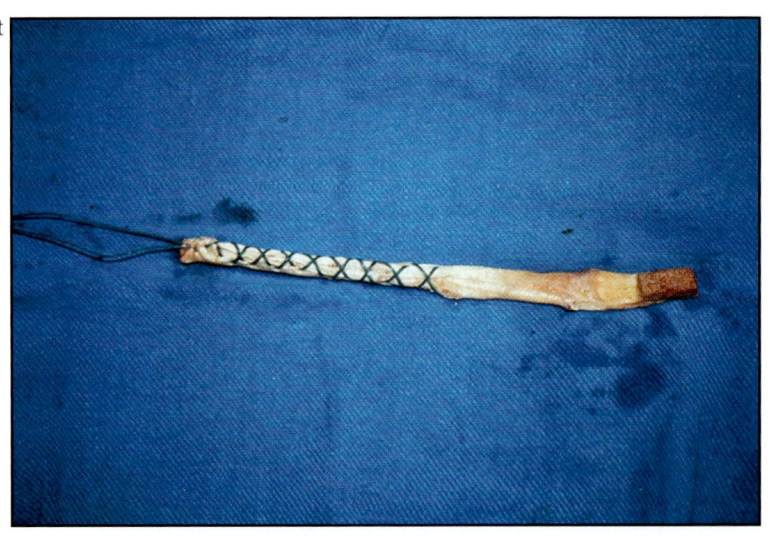

Figure 13-5. Achilles bone block with 6.5-mm cancellous screw in place.

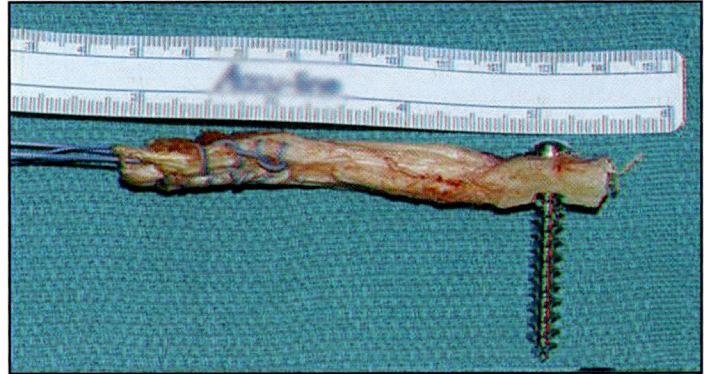

long. The distal 3 to 4 cm is then tubularized with a #5 Ethibond whipstitch (Figure 13-4). The tubularized tendon should fit snugly through a 10- to 11-mm sizing tube. The proximal Achilles tendon is fan shaped, thus some of the tendon will need to be trimmed to fit appropriately through a 10- to 11-mm sizing guide. The longer tibial bone block should then be prepared in order to accept a 6.5-mm cancellous screw with washer used for lag-type tibial fixation (Figure 13-5).

Alternative Technique—Quadriceps Autograft

* If the patient objects to allograft tissue, a quadriceps autograft may be used. A 10-mm wide bone block is taken from the central portion of the superior patella with an oscillating saw. The bone block should not be deeper than 5 to 6 mm. This bone block should measure 25 mm in length and 10 mm in width. The tendon portion of the graft should measure approximately 10 cm in length. The quadriceps tendon is 50% thicker than the patellar tendon in its anteroposterior dimension. It is composed of the superficial rectus femoris tendon and the deep vastus intermedius. The rectus femoris should be taken in its entirety. The anterior portion of the vastus intermedius should be taken, leaving only 2 mm of vastus intermedius attached to the suprapatellar pouch. The entire depth of the tendon should not be violated as the suprapatellar pouch lies just deep to it, and violation of this layer will lead to fluid extravasation, making further arthroscopy difficult. Additionally, entering the

suprapatellar pouch potentially may lead to painful scarring of the suprapatellar pouch in the postoperative period. A hemostat is now placed through the vastus intermedius at a depth of 6 mm. A narrow, curved osteotome is then used to complete the superior osteotomy at a depth of 6 mm. At this point, the bone block is prepared for later placement of the 6.5-mm cancellous bone screw with washer for tibial fixation. Seven centimeters of tendon is then harvested proximal to the bone block, taking very special care not to enter the suprapatellar pouch. The free tendon end of the graft is then whipstitched with a #5 Ethibond suture at its distal 3 to 4 cm.

* An additional graft option includes either an allograft or autograft bone-patellar tendon-bone construct.

FEMORAL TUNNEL PREPARATION

* After the tendinous portion for the Achilles graft is sized, the femoral tunnel can be prepared. Traditionally, during single-bundle PCL reconstruction, the femoral tunnel should be placed at the 11 o'clock position in the right knee (1 o'clock in the left knee), reconstructing the larger anterolateral bundle of the PCL. Various anatomic landmarks exist that assist with tunnel placement. Ideally, the guidepin should be placed in the center of the residual anterolateral bundle fibers. Alternatively, 2 osseous landmarks also exist for reference. The medial intercondylar ridge, as originally described by one of us (LDF), represents the posterior border of the native PCL.[11] As such, the femoral tunnel should lie just anterior to this landmark. The second osseous landmark, the medial bifurcate ridge, defines the junction between the PCL anterolateral and posteromedial bundles. The PCL anterolateral bundle lies superior to this landmark.[12]

* Some surgeons recommend débridement of the PCL footprint with an electrothermal device to better appreciate the osseous anatomy, as footprint débridement with an arthroscopic shaver typically obscures the osseous anatomy. We do not use cautery for this purpose.

* Once the anatomic footprint of the PCL anterolateral bundle is identified, a guidepin is placed in the center of its footprint. We prefer to use an outside-in drilling technique with a commercial PCL aiming guide (Smith & Nephew Inc, London, United Kingdom).

* Medially, the distal femoral cortex is exposed through a 3- to 5-cm longitudinal incision. The vastus medialis is identified, and its medial border is elevated to expose the distal femoral cortex (Figure 13-6).

* Once the distal femur is exposed, the tip of the targeting device is placed at the center of the PCL anterolateral bundle footprint using the medial arthroscopic portal (Figure 13-7).

* The external guidepin is advanced to the outer metaphyseal cortex. The guidepin is then advanced slightly into the joint under direct visualization to ensure that it is in the center of the anterolateral bundle footprint (Figure 13-8).

* The guide is now removed from the knee. Next, the appropriately sized reamer is used to drill the tunnel in antegrade fashion (Figure 13-9).

* The femoral drill hole will be close to the articular surface at its origin, but directed away from the articular surface as it enters the joint. We have had no problems with collapse of the articular surface. The posterior edge of the tunnel is chamfered with a bone cutting shaver or arthroscopic rasp in order to smooth the area that will contact the graft.

* After preparation of the femoral tunnel, the knee is prepared for repositioning. A DePuy graft passer (DePuy Mitek, Raynham, MA) is placed antegrade through the femoral tunnel, into the intercondylar notch, and into the posterior compartment adjacent to the medial border of the PCL tibial insertion (Figure 13-10).

Figure 13-6. Medial approach to distal femur and elevation of distal vastus medialis oblique.

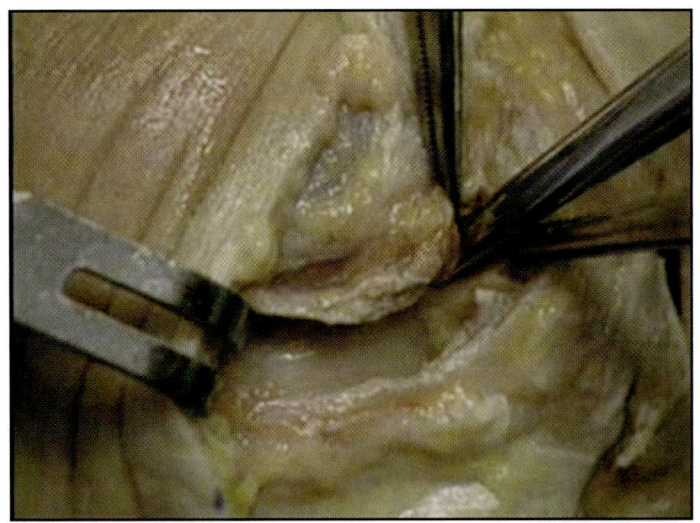

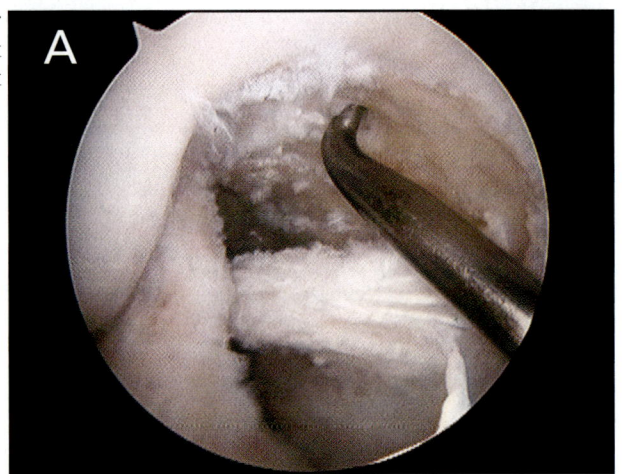

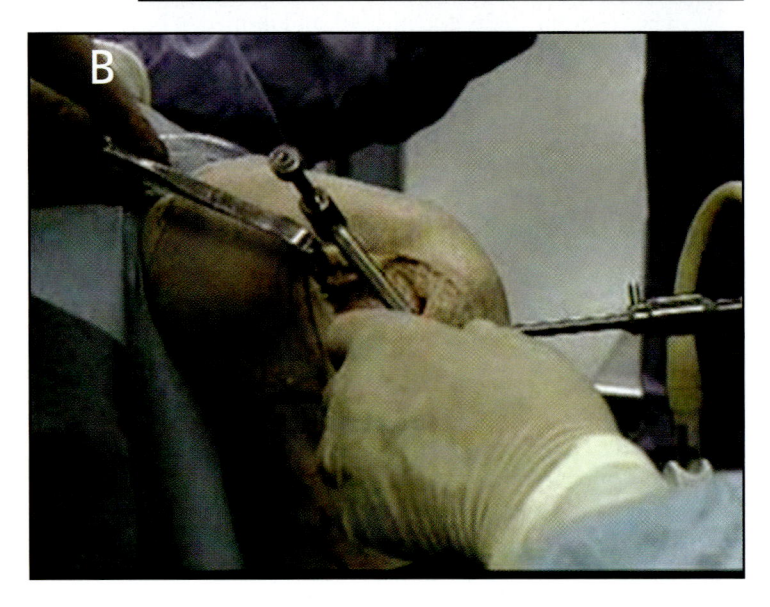

Figure 13-7. (A) PCL guide tip in center of anterolateral bundle attachment (right knee). (B) External view of PCL guide (left knee).

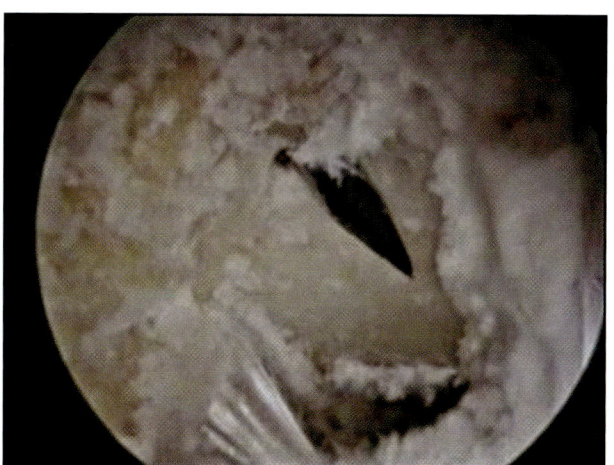

Figure 13-8. Guidepin entering joint in center of anterolateral bundle attachment (left knee).

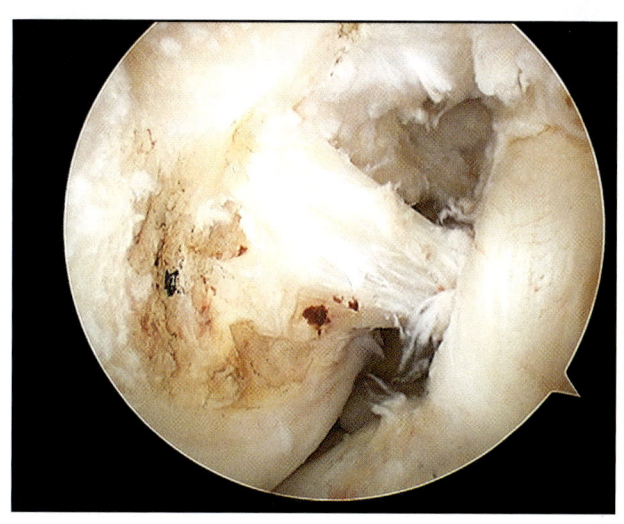

Figure 13-9. Left knee following drilling of femoral tunnel.

* Alternatively, an 18-gauge wire loop may be used for graft passage. The external portion of the graft passer is laid against the skin and secured with a sterile Coban wrap (3M Inc, St. Paul, MN). A sterile, impervious stockinette is then placed over the extremity and over-wrapped to mid thigh with another sterile Coban (Figure 13-11). This helps to ensure sterility during the turning maneuver.
* At this time, the extremity drapes are removed. Both limbs are removed from the leg holders, and the foot of the operative table is raised to its normal position.
* After clearance from the anesthesia staff, the patient is positioned in the prone position. This typically requires assistance from at least 4 people—the anesthesiologist to maintain the head and neck, 2 assistants on either side to facilitate the turn, and 1 person to manage the lower extremities. In a smaller individual, the turn can be accomplished on the same operating room table. In most individuals, it is necessary to turn the patient onto a second operative table (Figure 13-12). Turning takes approximately 8 to 10 minutes.

180 Chapter 13

Figure 13-10. (A) Graft passer being passed through the femoral tunnel. (B) Intra-articular view of the graft passer being placed next to the PCL tibial attachment.

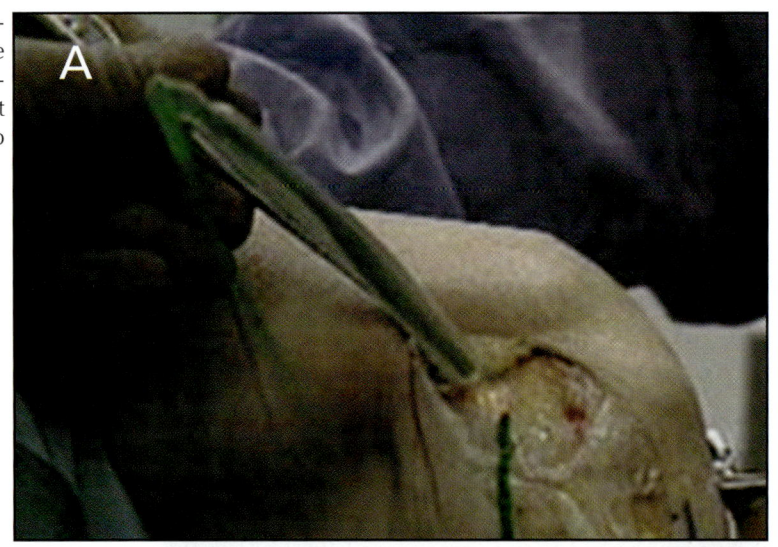

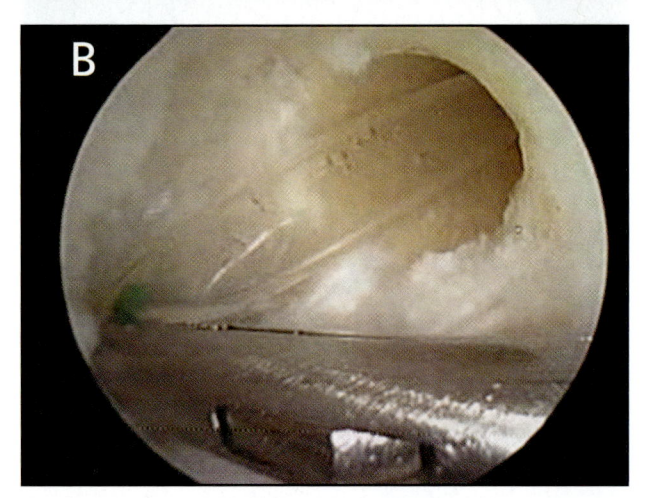

Figure 13-11. Operative extremity wrapped in sterile fashion in preparation for turn.

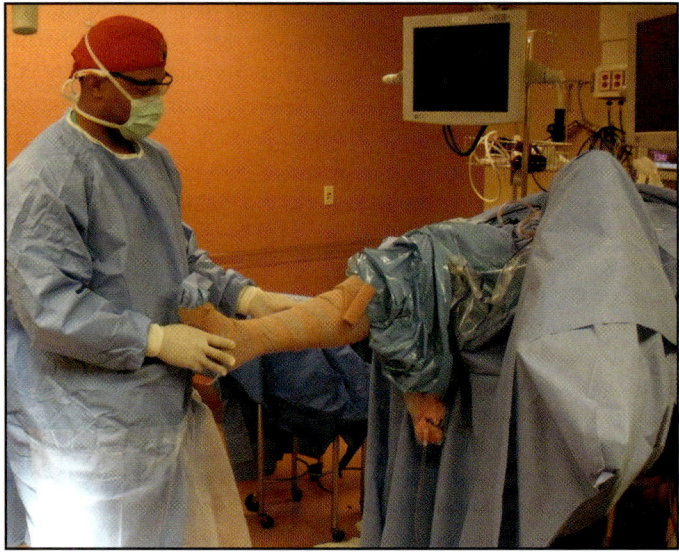

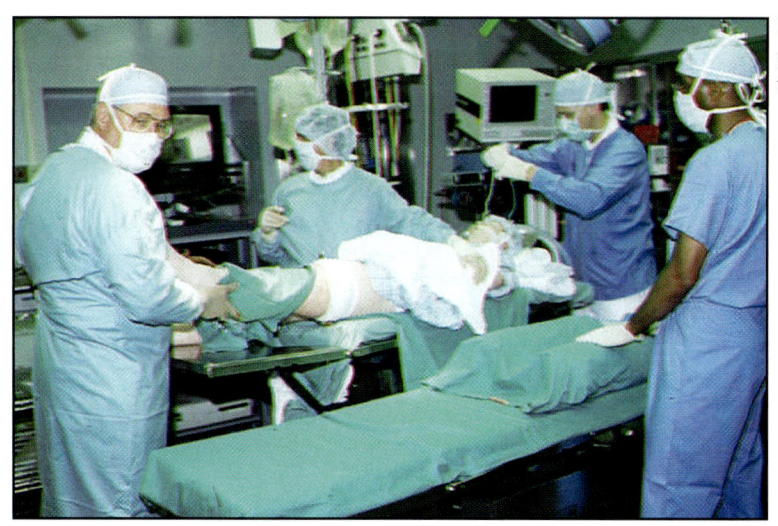

Figure 13-12. Operative personnel in place for turn to adjacent operative table.

POSTERIOR APPROACH

* The popliteal crease is identified and marked at this time. The limb is exsanguinated, and the tourniquet is inflated. We use the tourniquet here, although some surgeons may prefer not to use it.

* Starting at the popliteal crease, a 4-cm vertical incision is made distally along the medial border of the medial head of the gastrocnemius muscle (Figure 13-13).

* Once through skin and subcutaneous tissues, the fascia overlying the medial border of the gastrocnemius is incised longitudinally. Care should be taken not to injure the medial sural cutaneous nerve that perforates the popliteal fascia at this level. The interval between the gastrocnemius and semimembranosus is developed bluntly. The gastrocnemius is then retracted laterally to expose the posterior joint capsule (Figure 13-14).

* A portion of the gastrocnemius femoral insertion may be released in order to facilitate lateral retraction. A small bump may also be placed under the anterior aspect of the ankle, slightly flexing the knee, which helps to relax the gastrocnemius muscle and aid with lateral retraction. Internally rotating the tibia may also help expose the posterior tibia. Lateral retraction of the gastrocnemius muscle protects the popliteal artery, which lies lateral to it. Unicortical Steinmann pins or K-wires may be placed into the posterior tibia to function as retractors for the popliteus. We do not routinely do this.

* The PCL facet is then palpated just proximal to the superior border of the popliteus muscle belly. A window is made in the overlying posterior capsule with electrocautery (Figure 13-15).

* A curved osteotome is then used to make a 20 mm x 10 mm x 5 mm cortical window at the footprint of the PCL tibial attachment (Figure 13-16).

* The graft passer is retrieved through the posterior capsular window, and the tendinous portion of the Achilles graft is placed into the plastic sheath (Figure 13-17).

* The graft passer is then used to pull the tendinous graft through the joint and into the femoral tunnel. The Achilles bone block is now keyed into the cortical window with a 30-mm partially threaded 6.5-mm cancellous screw with a washer (Figure 13-18).

Figure 13-13. (A) Popliteal crease and skin incision drawn. (B) Posterior incision made as inverted "hockey stick" (right knee).

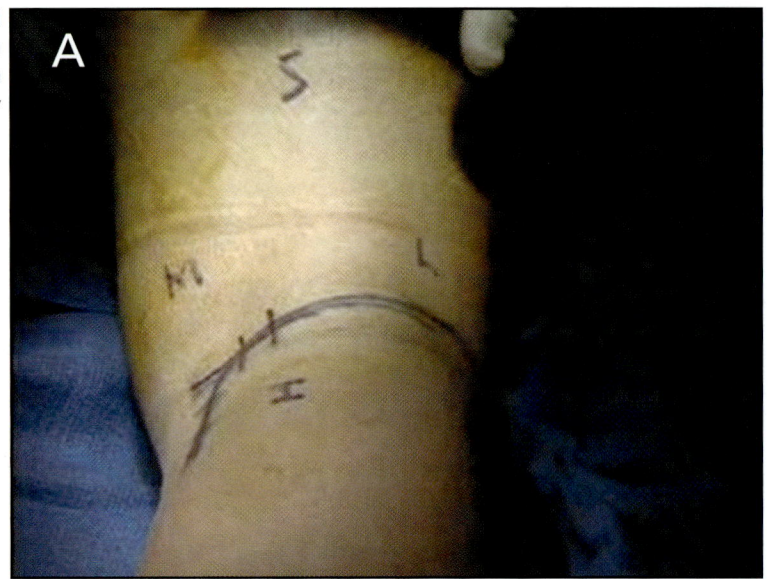

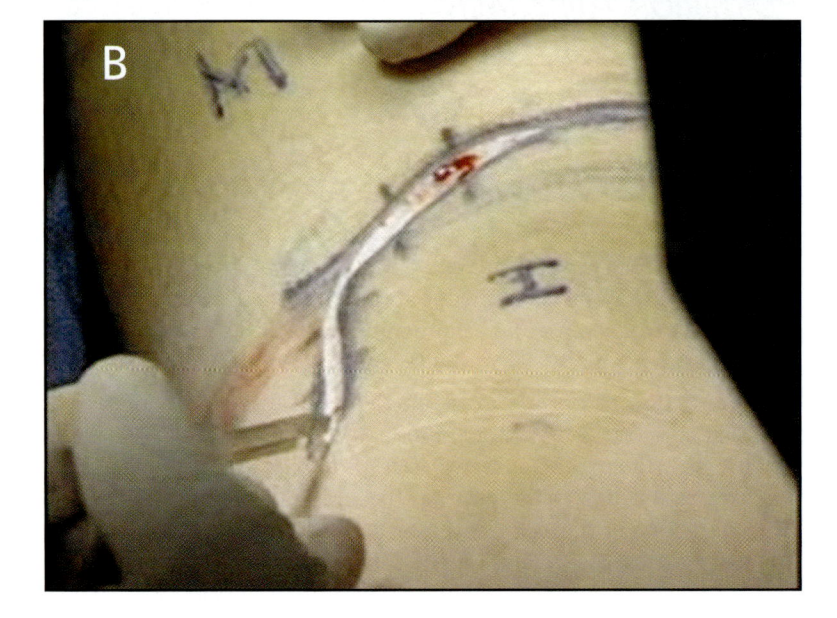

* At this time, if the tourniquet has been inflated, it is now let down, and meticulous hemostasis is obtained. The posterior wound is then closed with a 1 Vicryl suture. The investing fascia is closed, and the skin is closed with interrupted nonabsorbable sutures.
* The extremity is then prepared for the turn as described above. In this approach, one must be aware of the rare popliteal artery variants.

FEMORAL FIXATION

* Once the patient is turned to the supine position, the limb is again placed into an arthroscopic leg holder and prepped and draped.

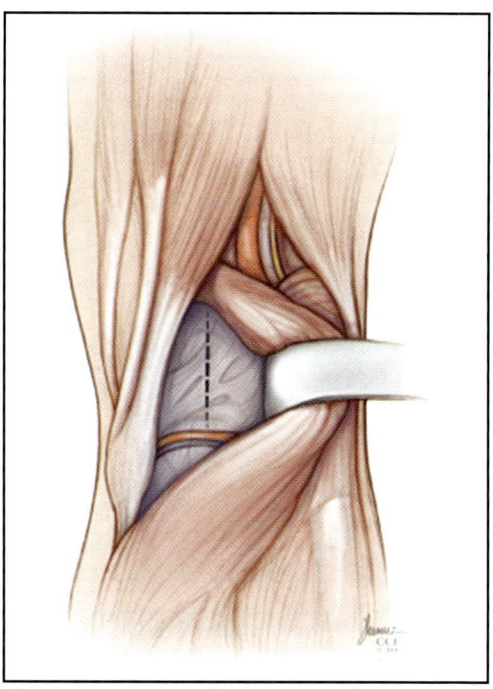

Posterior Cruciate Ligament Reconstruction 183

Figure 13-14. Lateral retraction of medial head of gastrocnemius. (Reprinted with the permission of The Cleveland Clinic Center for Medical Art & Photography © 2009. All rights reserved.)

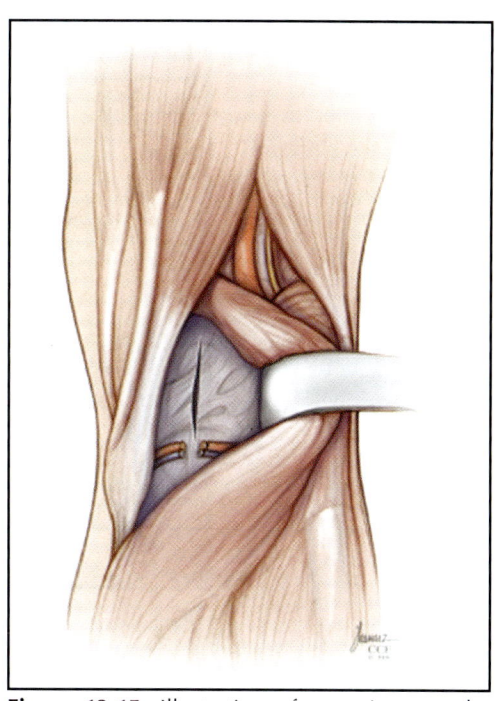

Figure 13-15. Illustration of posterior capsular incision. (Reprinted with the permission of The Cleveland Clinic Center for Medical Art & Photography © 2009. All rights reserved.)

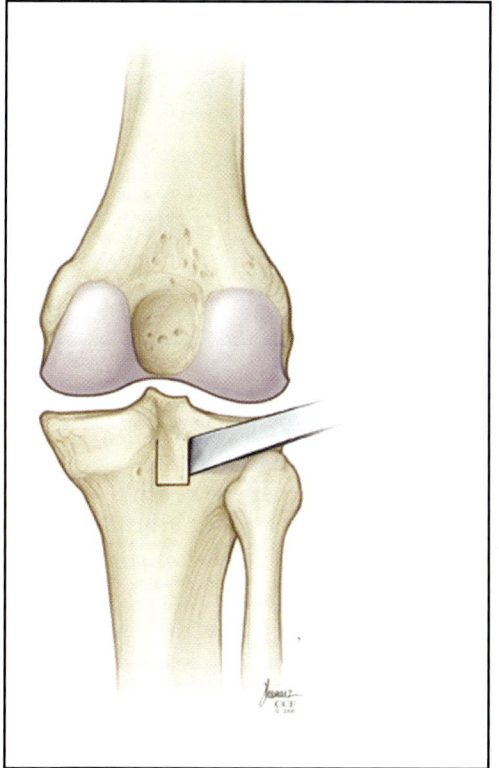

Figure 13-16. Osteotome creating posterior cortical window. (Reprinted with the permission of The Cleveland Clinic Center for Medical Art & Photography © 2009. All rights reserved.)

184 *Chapter 13*

Figure 13-17. (A) Graft passer retrieved from posterior compartment of knee through posterior capsular incision. (B) Tendinous portion of graft being passed into graft passer.

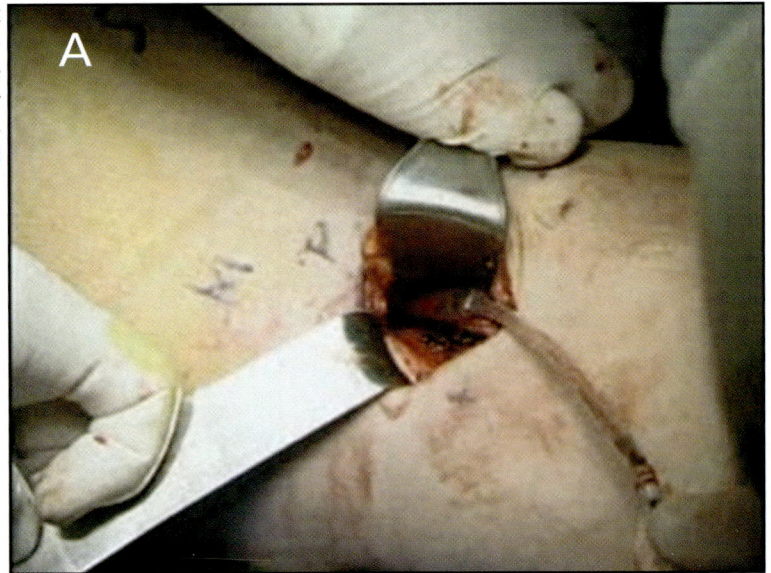

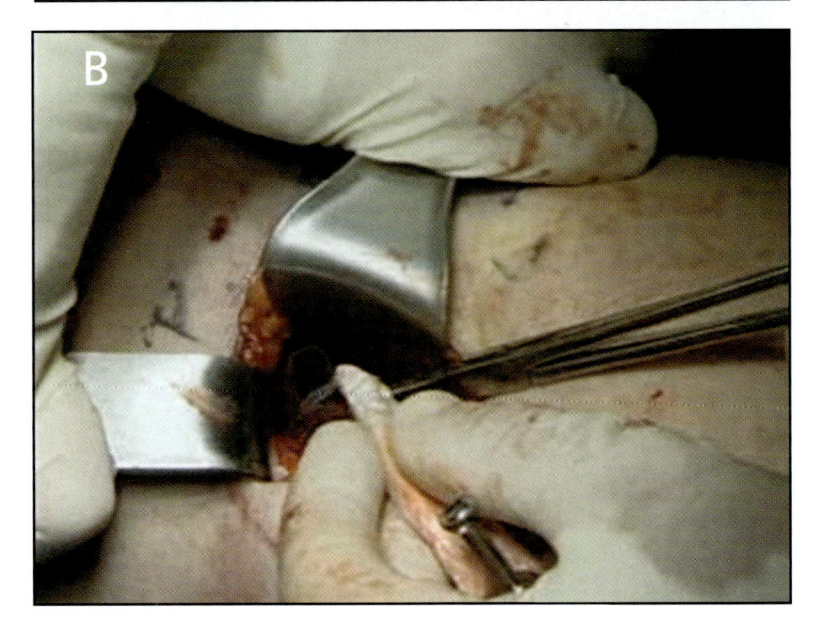

* The arthroscope is introduced through the anterolateral arthroscopic portal to confirm proper passage of the graft.
* Once proper placement of the graft is confirmed, a soft tissue interference screw is placed into the femoral tunnel from outside-in as an anterior drawer is applied to the tibia as the graft is tensioned at 70° of knee flexion (Figure 13-19).
* At this time, the knee is taken through a range of motion to ensure that full range of motion is present after graft fixation. The femoral fixation is then reinforced with a staple in the residual tendon graft. The arthroscopic portals and medial incision are closed in the usual fashion. The wounds are dressed sterilely.

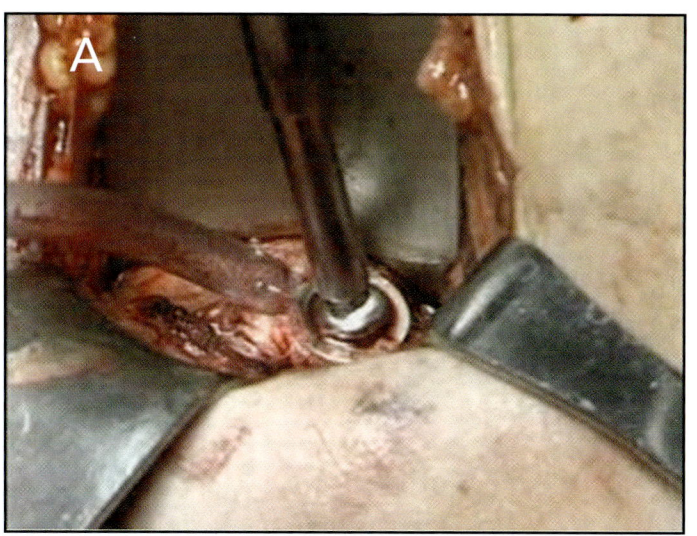

Posterior Cruciate Ligament Reconstruction | 185

Figure 13-18. Fixation of Achilles bone block into posterior cortical window. (Figure B reprinted with the permission of The Cleveland Clinic Center for Medical Art & Photography © 2009. All rights reserved.)

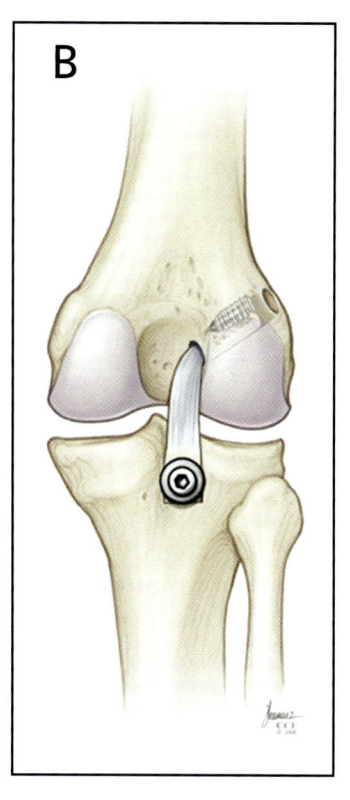

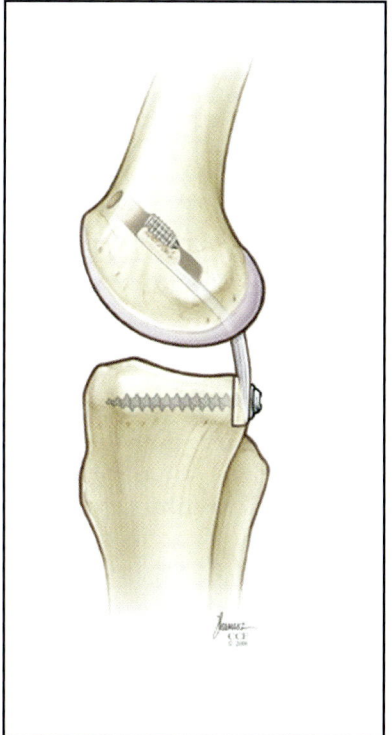

Figure 13-19. Illustration of final graft fixation. (Reprinted with the permission of The Cleveland Clinic Center for Medical Art & Photography © 2009. All rights reserved.)

Postoperative Rehabilitation

Postoperatively, the patient is placed into a full-leg, hinged knee brace locked in extension for 4 weeks. Partial weightbearing is allowed initially and advanced to full weightbearing as tolerated. Isometric quadriceps exercises are begun immediately. From 4 to 8 weeks postoperatively, the patient is advanced to active-assisted range of motion. Isotonic quadriceps exercises are added at this time. Bicycling is encouraged. Closed kinetic chain exercises are begun at 8 weeks after surgery. From week 12 through week 20, slide board exercises are progressed to agility exercises. Fast walking is progressed to jogging at 16 to 20 weeks. A knee brace with block to extension at 15° is continued for exercise. At weeks 20 to 28, running and full-speed agility exercises are instituted. The brace is discontinued for activity. At 28 weeks post surgery, the patient is allowed to return to full activity.

Tips and Pearls

- ✔ Reduction of posterior tibial sag may help with passage of the graft passer into the posterior compartment next to the remnant of the PCL tibial attachment. Avoid placement of the passer beneath the meniscus.
- ✔ Lateral retraction of the medial head of the gastrocnemius is facilitated with slight flexion of the knee and internal rotation of the tibia.
- ✔ Gynecological retractors are long and narrow and aid with deep retraction during the posterior approach.
- ✔ Once retracted, the medial head of the gastrocnemius can be temporarily held in position with a Steinmann pin placed into the lateral aspect of the proximal tibia. This provides for a wide field of view for tibial preparation and graft fixation.
- ✔ The slide board during rehabilitation is a great tool for transitioning to jogging and running.
- ✔ We find it difficult to perform the posterior tibial inlay without turning the patient. We feel that the additional 15 to 20 minutes of operative time is worth it considering the ease of posterior visualization.

Pitfalls

- ✘ Malposition of the distal femoral incision may prohibit accurate placement of the femoral guidepin. It is important to place the incision one third the distance from the medial femoral condyle to the medial border of the patella. This will allow the vastus medialis to be elevated rather than splitting the muscle fibers, which may lead to quadriceps inhibition in the early postoperative period.
- ✘ Injuries to the posterolateral ligamentous complex are commonly associated with PCL injuries. Reconstruction of the PCL could fail if the posterolateral rotatory instability is not addressed. Varus tibia osteotomy should be considered.
- ✘ Although this has not been encountered by us, osteonecrosis or subchondral collapse may occur if the femoral tunnel is placed too close to the articular surface. The distal border of the femoral tunnel should be 3 to 4 mm away from the articular cartilage border and aimed away from the joint.

- ✘ The femoral tunnel starting point at the medial aspect of the femoral metaphysis should not start too far proximal to the medial articular border. More proximal starting position will lead to a more acute angle for graft passage. We have been unable to duplicate the normal direction of the PCL tunnel by drilling from inside the femur.

- ✘ One must be aware of rare aberrant branches of the posterior tibial artery overlying the posterior tibial footprint of the PCL.

REFERENCES

1. Parolie JM, Bergfeld JA. Long-term results of nonoperative treatment of isolated posterior cruciate ligament injuries in the athlete. *Am J Sports Med.* 1986;14:35-38.
2. Fowler PJ, Messieh SS. Isolated posterior cruciate ligament injuries in athletes. *Am J Sports Med.* 1987;15:553-557.
3. Harner CD, Hoher J. Evaluation and treatment of posterior cruciate ligament injuries. *Am J Sports Med.* 1998;26:471-482.
4. Keller PM, Shelbourne KD, McCarroll JR, Rettig AC. Nonoperatively treated isolated posterior cruciate ligament injuries. *Am J Sports Med.* 1993;21:132-136.
5. Kim SJ, Shin SJ, Choi NH, Cho SK. Arthroscopically assisted treatment of avulsion fractures of the posterior cruciate ligament from the tibia. *J Bone Joint Surg Am.* 2001;83:698-708.
6. Bergfeld JA, Graham SM, Parker RD, Valdevit AD, Kambic HE. A biomechanical comparison of posterior cruciate ligament reconstructions using single- and double-bundle tibial inlay techniques. *Am J Sports Med.* 2005;33:976-981.
7. Bergfeld JA, McAllister DR, Parker RD, Valdevit AD, Kambic HE. A biomechanical comparison of posterior cruciate ligament reconstruction techniques. *Am J Sports Med.* 2001;29:129-136.
8. Markolf KL, Zemanovic JR, McAllister DR. Cyclic loading of posterior cruciate ligament replacements fixed with tibial tunnel and tibial inlay methods. *J Bone Joint Surg Am.* 2002;84:518-524.
9. Hoher J, Scheffler S, Weiler A. Graft choice and graft fixation in PCL reconstruction. *Knee Surg Sports Traumatol Arthrosc.* 2003;11:297-306.
10. Gupte CM, Bull AM, Thomas RD, Amis AA. The meniscofemoral ligaments: secondary restraints to the posterior drawer. Analysis of anteroposterior and rotatory laxity in the intact and posterior cruciate-deficient knee. *J Bone Joint Surg Br.* 2003;85:765-773.
11. Farrow LD, Chen MR, Cooperman DR, Victoroff BN, Goodfellow DB. Morphology of the femoral intercondylar notch. *J Bone Joint Surg Am.* 2007;89:2150-2155.
12. Lopes OV, Ferretti M, Shen W, Ekdahl M, Smolinski P, Fu FH. Topography of the femoral attachment of the posterior cruciate ligament. *J Bone Joint Surg Am.* 2008;90:249-255.

Transtibial Double-Bundle PCL Reconstruction

Mathew W. Pombo, MD; Brian Forsythe, MD; Randy Mascarenhas, MD; and Christopher D. Harner, MD

SURGICAL GOALS

The pathway of surgical decision making in double-bundle (DB) posterior cruciate ligament (PCL) reconstruction is complex and fraught with potential pitfalls. Not all PCL injuries are the same, and most PCL injuries do well with conservative treatment.[1,2] After deciding to pursue a surgical treatment, selecting the appropriate technique (augmentation versus single-bundle reconstruction versus DB reconstruction) can be a daunting task. DB PCL reconstructions were introduced to address the issue of residual laxity by reducing posterior tibial translation and external rotation with a more anatomic reconstruction of the PCL.[3,4] It is perhaps best indicated in surgical cases with higher grades of PCL laxity.[5,6] There are 3 keys to successfully performing a transtibial DB PCL reconstruction: 1) definition of the injury pattern based on clinical exam and imaging studies, 2) a thorough examination under anesthesia and diagnostic arthroscopy, and 3) a technically precise and anatomic DB PCL reconstruction.

The first step in management of PCL injuries lies in definition of the injury pattern. Acute, isolated Grade I or II PCL injuries usually do not require surgical intervention and are treated non-operatively with a rehabilitation program emphasizing quadriceps strengthening.[1,2] Grade II PCL injuries that fail conservative treatment can be approached with a single-bundle reconstruction or a single-bundle augmentation.[7] Careful examination of the collateral ligaments and the posterolateral corner (PLC) is essential. Acute Grade III PCL injuries in a young athlete or chronic Grade III PCL-deficient knees with associated collateral ligament or PLC injuries are good candidates for PCL reconstructions,[8-10] and we tend to recommend transtibial DB technique in these patients. The importance of defining the injury grade and pattern with respect to pursuing surgical intervention cannot be overstated.

For patients who fail conservative treatment and in whom operative intervention is pursued, the examination under anesthesia and diagnostic arthroscopy are critical factors in deciding between single-bundle PCL reconstruction, single-bundle augmentation, and DB PCL reconstruction. The examination under anesthesia is necessary to evaluate for associated injuries to the PLC, medial collateral ligament (MCL), and lateral collateral ligament (LCL). Collateral ligament injuries may heal non-operatively, depending upon their respective injury patterns. They do not need to necessarily be addressed at the time of PCL surgery. If the exam reveals a Grade II PCL injury in association with a Grade II or III PLC injury, a single-bundle augmentation or single-bundle PCL/PLC reconstruction is typically performed. If the exam reveals either an isolated Grade III PCL tear in a young patient or a chronic Grade III PCL rupture combined with a Grade II to III PLC, MCL,

Figure 14-1. Room set-up for arthroscopic DB PCL reconstruction. Notice the placement of the miniature c-arm to aid in our exam under anesthesia and several other critical steps of the procedure to be outlined later in the chapter.

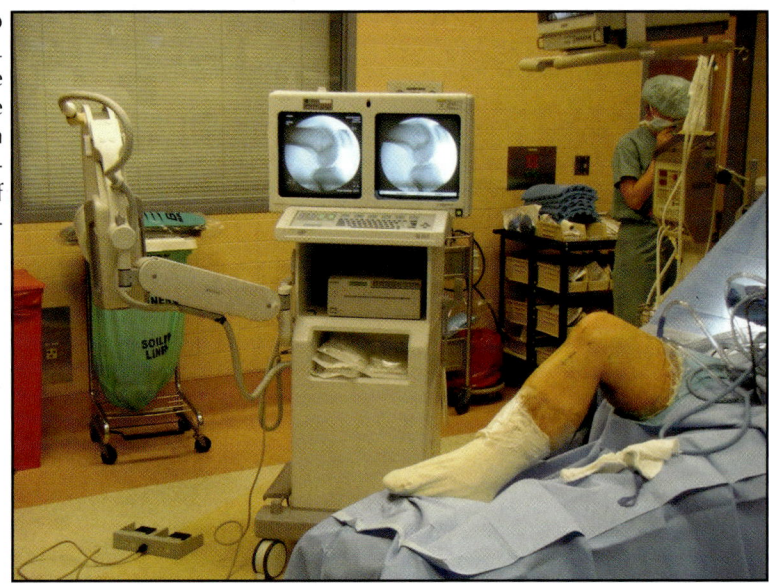

or LCL injury, a DB PCL reconstruction is performed in conjunction with appropriate surgical correction of the associated injuries. The diagnostic arthroscopy is performed in standard fashion through medial and lateral parapatellar portals. The notch is evaluated, and the anterolateral (AL) bundle, posteromedial (PM) bundle, and meniscofemoral ligaments (MFLs) are examined to note if they are intact. If fibers of any of these structures remain intact, an augmentation procedure is performed. However, if the MFLs are all that remain, a DB reconstruction is performed in the setting of increased laxity (usually Grade III PCL injuries). All efforts are made to preserve any native tissue that remains. For these reasons, the exam under anesthesia and diagnostic arthroscopy are critical steps in the surgical decision-making process when evaluating a patient for a transtibial DB PCL reconstruction.

Once the decision has been made to proceed with transtibial DB reconstruction, the procedure can be subdivided into 4 steps: 1) tibial tunnel preparation, 2) femoral tunnel preparation, 3) graft passage and tensioning, and 4) graft fixation. As mentioned previously, this procedure is usually indicated for acute Grade III PCL tears in young patients and in patients with chronic Grade III PCL ruptures with combined PLC or collateral ligament injuries who continue to be symptomatic despite conservative treatment.

Technique

* Examination under anesthesia is performed first in all circumstances for careful evaluation of associated injuries. A miniature fluoroscopy unit can be used to assist in quantifying anterior to posterior laxity. The patient is placed supine on the operating room table. No tourniquet or leg holder is used. The incisions are marked on the skin and are injected with 0.25% Marcaine with epinephrine prior to sterile prepping of the patient (Figures 14-1 and 14-2).

* Diagnostic knee arthroscopy is performed with the use of 4 portals. In addition to the 3 standard portals (medial and lateral parapatellar with a superolateral outflow), a posteromedial portal is established under arthroscopic visualization. Care must be taken to keep

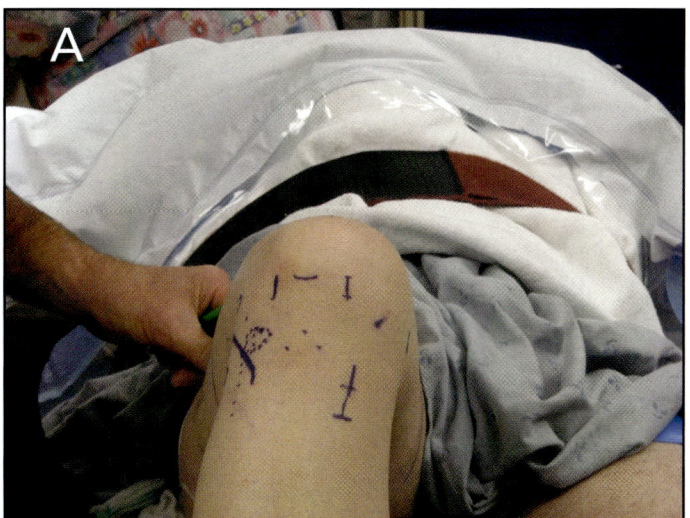

Figure 14-2. (A) Surgeon's anterior view of the knee showing the standard medial and lateral parapatellar portals. Also notice the medial and lateral tibial incisions that will be used for the preparation of the 2 tibial tunnels. (B) Medial view of the knee showing the posteromedial portal that will be used as an accessory viewing and working portal for the posterior aspect of the PCL insertion. Also, notice the incision over the vastus medialis obliquus in line with Langer's lines that will be used to fix the PCL to the femur over posts.

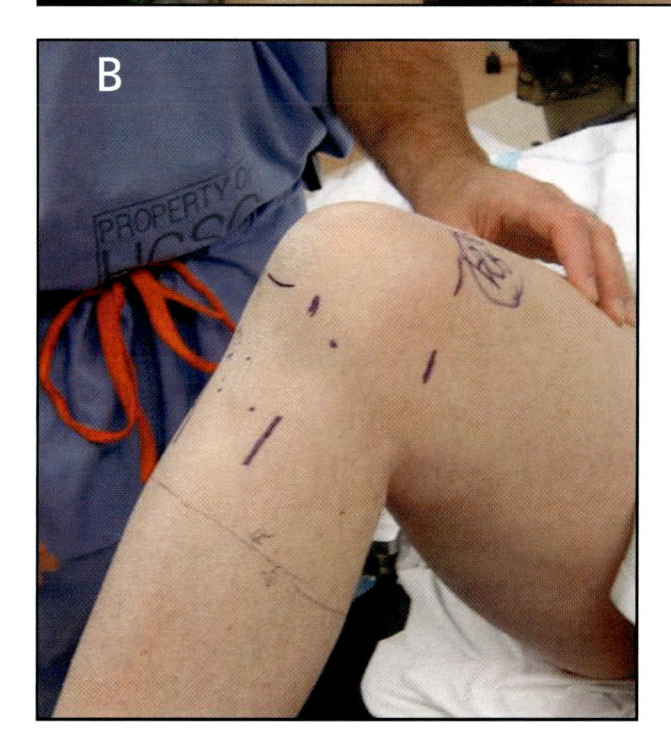

an anterior drawer force on the knee to avoid débriding the ACL secondary to diminished tension within the ligament (Figures 14-2 and 14-3).

* Next, the femoral PCL origin is visualized, and the anterolateral and posteromedial bundle origins are marked using arthroscopic cauterization. Care should be taken to preserve any native PCL tissue that remains (Figure 14-3A).

* We prefer to work on the tibial tunnels first. A PCL curette is placed in the anteromedial portal to dissect through the notch and to clear the posterior tibial insertion. After clearing anteriorly, a 70-degree scope is placed through the notch to examine the posterior aspect of the tibia as well as the posterior tibial space. The arthroscopic shaver can be placed in the

Figure 14-2. (C) This lateral view of the knee shows a case where a posterolateral corner reconstruction will be performed concomitantly. Note Gerdy's tubercle and the fibula with peroneal nerve marked preoperatively.

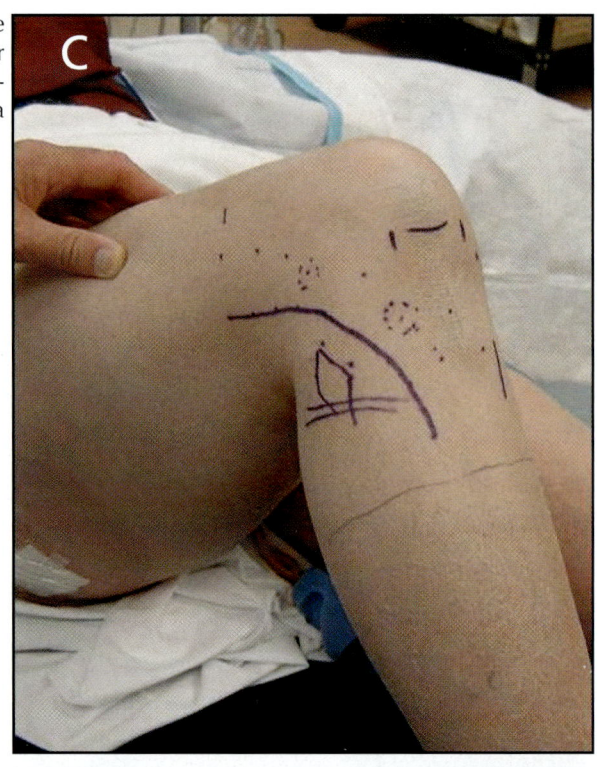

Figure 14-3. Diagnostic arthroscopy. (A) Initial arthroscopic view of the PCL insertion site on the femur as viewed from the anterolateral portal.

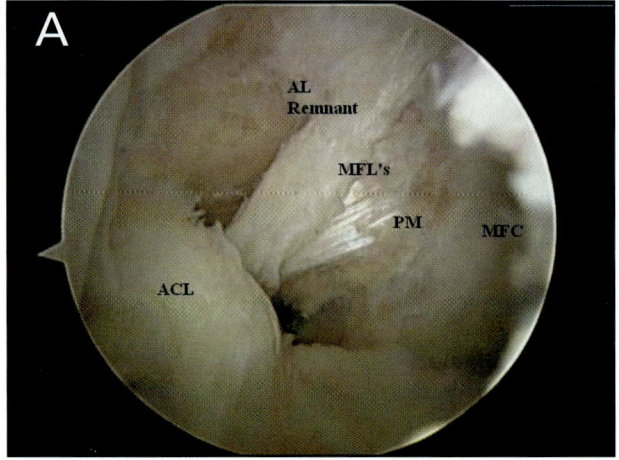

posteromedial arthroscopic portal to débride any scarred PCL remnants or debris surrounding the PCL insertion. The PCL insertion site on the tibia needs to be cleared approximately 2 to 3 cm distal to the medial joint line.

* Next, the PCL curette is re-introduced through the anteromedial portal, and the arthroscope is placed in the posteromedial portal. The PCL curette is used to clear the remainder of the tibial insertions for the 2 bundles. Adequate visualization of the anterolateral and posteromedial tibial insertions of the PCL is critical (Figure 14-3C, D).

* Place the PCL guide in the anterolateral portal while viewing with the arthroscope from the posteromedial portal. To reproduce the AL bundle insertion on the tibia, the tip of the

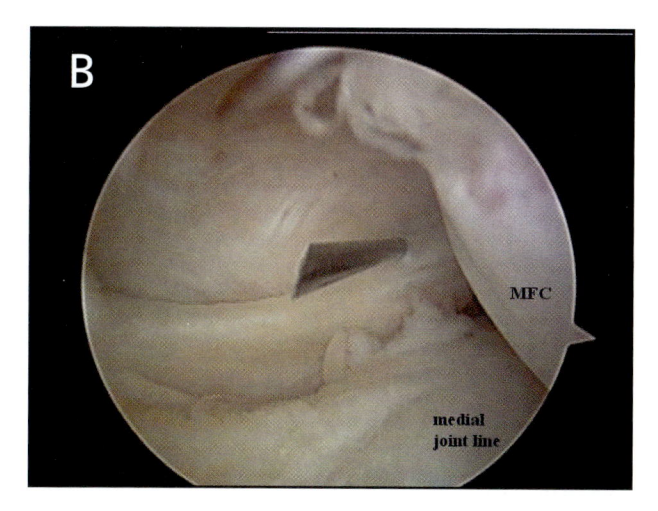

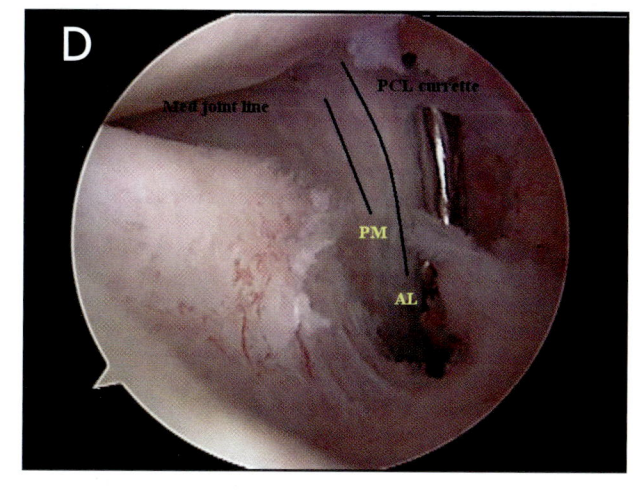

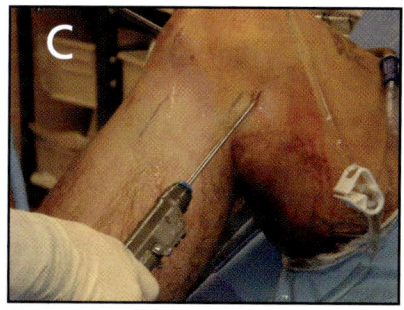

Figure 14-3. Diagnostic arthroscopy. (B) A spinal needle is used to find the location of the posteromedial portal under arthroscopic guidance. The arthroscope is looking through the notch posteromedially. (C) The arthroscopic shaver is introduced into the posteromedial portal to help débride the tibial insertion of the PCL. (D) The PCL tibial insertion is evaluated by placing the arthroscope in the posteromedial portal while the PCL curette is used to clear the insertion site.

guide is placed distal and lateral on the tibial footprint. Confirm placement with a lateral fluoroscopic view, and then place the guidepin under fluoroscopic guidance through an anterolateral incision on the tibia (use an extended approach through the same incision used to reconstruct the posterolateral corner if it is being repaired or reconstructed). The guide is set at 45 to 50 degrees for this step to avoid reaming the posterior cortex of the tibia (Figure 14-4A-C).

* For the PM bundle tibial tunnel, place the tip of the guide in the more proximal and medial anatomic location of the posteromedial bundle on the tibial footprint. Confirm placement with a lateral fluoroscopic view, and then place the guidepin under fluoroscopic guidance through an anteromedial incision on the tibia. The guide is set at 45 to 50 degrees to avoid the posterior cortex of the tibia (Figures 14-4D-I).

* Typically, the AL bundle of the PCL requires a size 8- to 9-mm graft; the PM bundle requires a size 6- to 7-mm graft. Cannulated compaction drills of appropriate size and dilators are used to drill and then manually dilate the tibial tunnels while protecting the guidepin from advancing with the PCL curette. The arthroscope is placed in the posteromedial portal while this is performed. The posterior cortex of the tibia should be drilled by hand at all times, and not by power (Figure 14-4J).

Figure 14-4. Tibial tunnel preparation. (A) The PCL drill guide is in place to guide the placement of the anterolateral PCL tunnel. Note the use of a miniature c-arm to check guidepin placement. (B) Fluoroscopic view of the anterolateral tibial guidepin in place. (C) Anterior view of AL guidepin in place.

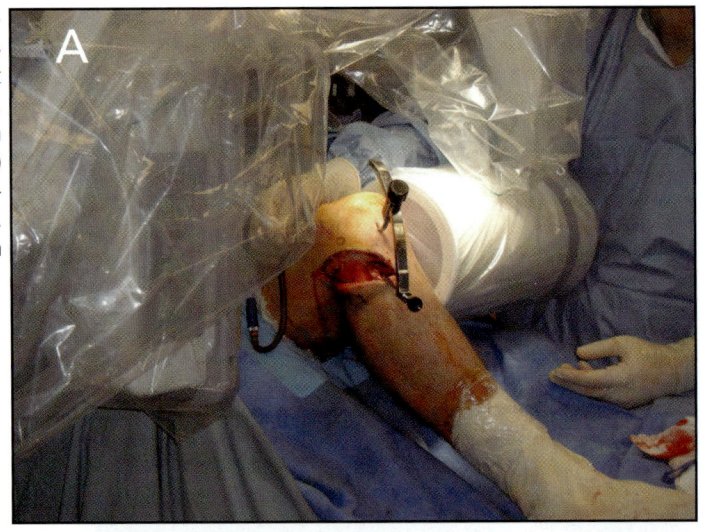

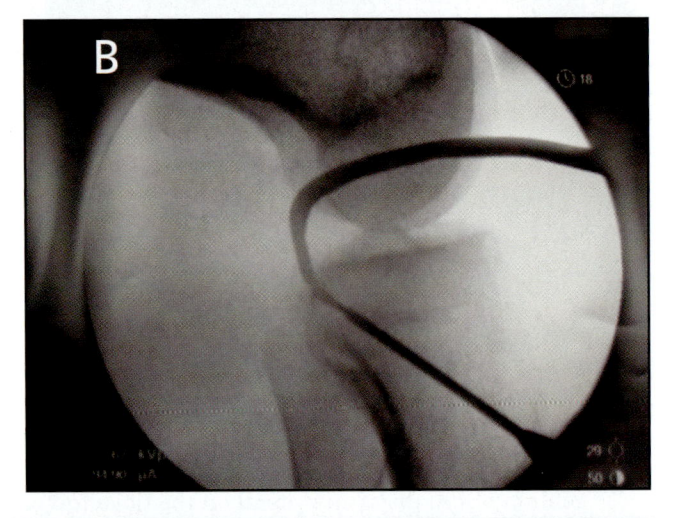

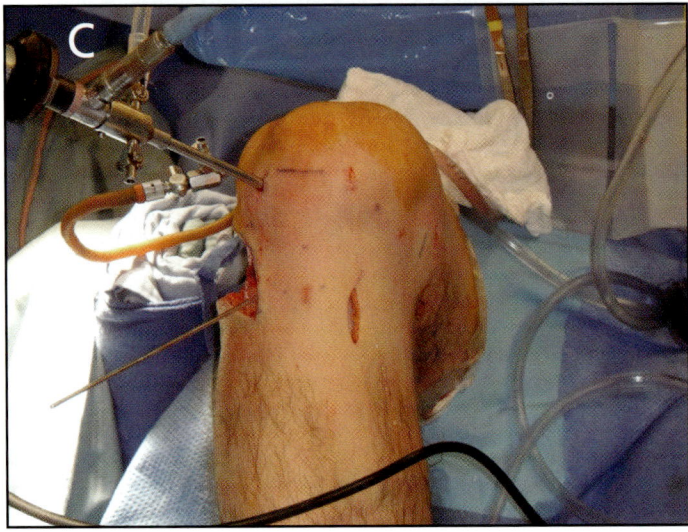

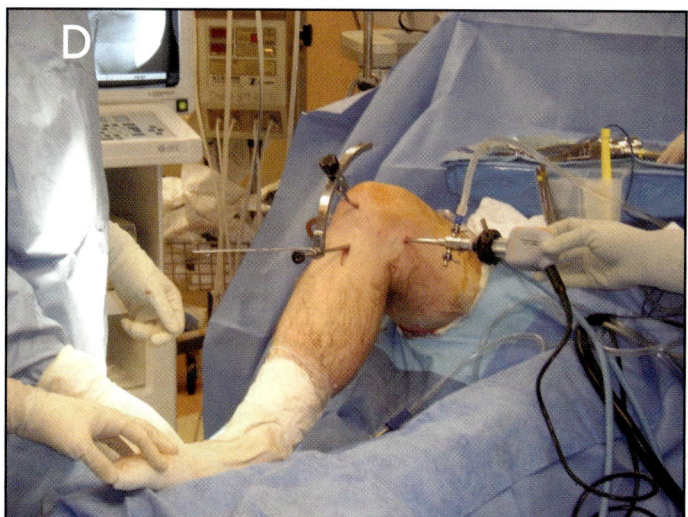

Transtibial Double-Bundle PCL Reconstruction 195

Figure 14-4. (D) The PCL guide is used to place the posteromedial tibial tunnel guidepin. Note the arthroscope in the posteromedial viewing portal to assess the pin placement in relation to the posterior tibial footprint of the PCL. (E) Drilling the guidepin under fluoroscopic guidance is an important safety step. (F) Fluoroscopic lateral knee view of the AL and PM guidepins in place.

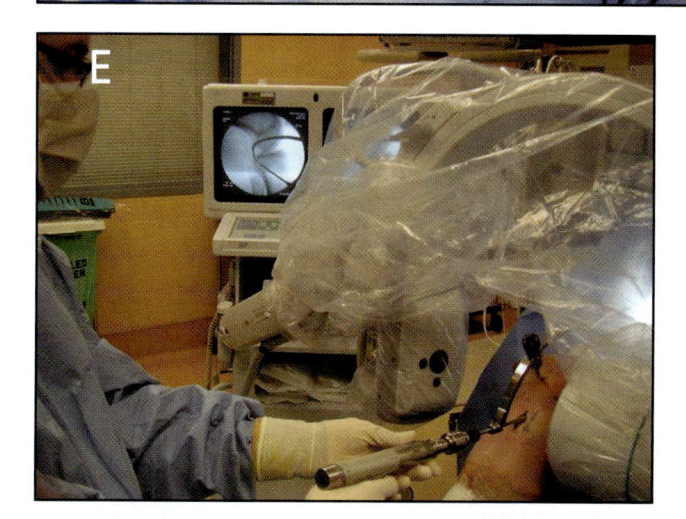

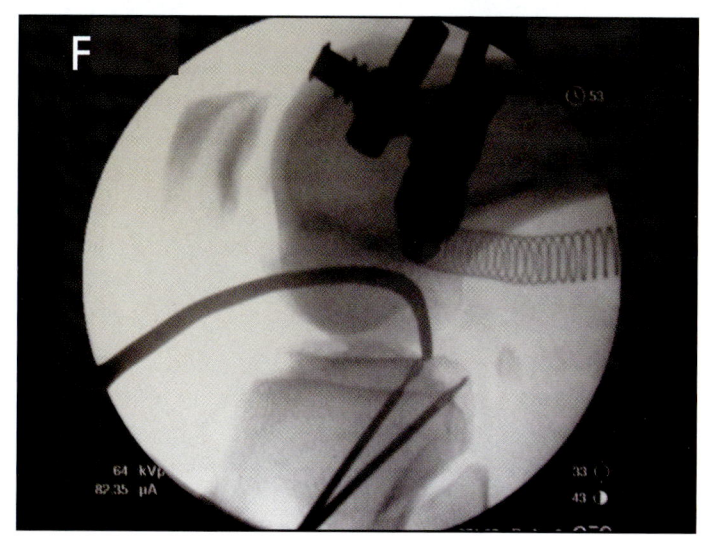

Figure 14-4. (G) Anterior view of both guidepins. (H) A view from the posteromedial viewing portal that shows the relationship of the 2 guidepins on the posterior tibial footprint of the PCL. (I) Anteroposterior fluoroscopic view of the 2 tibial guidepins.

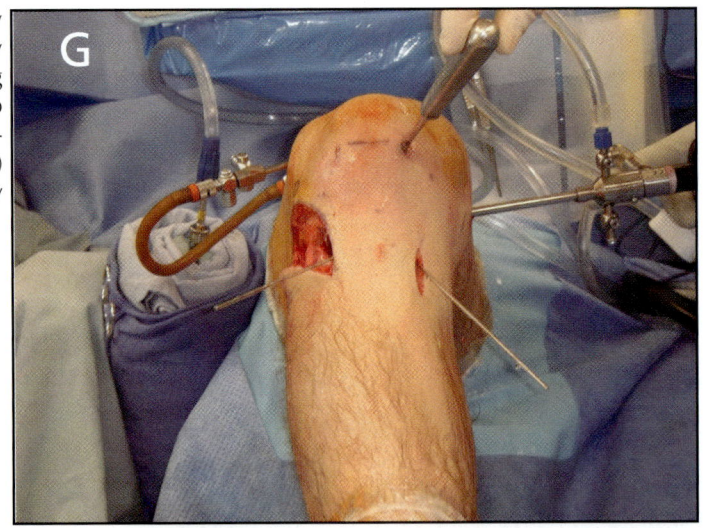

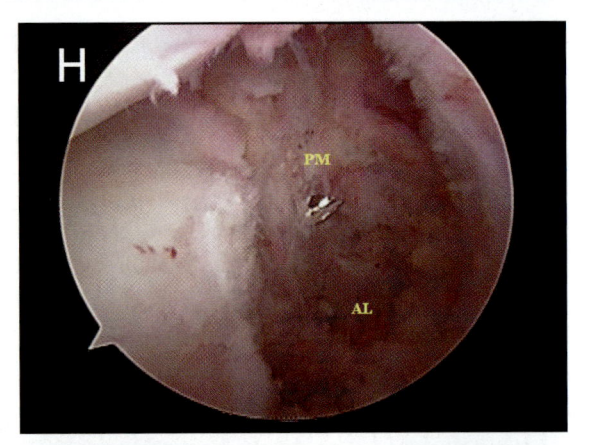

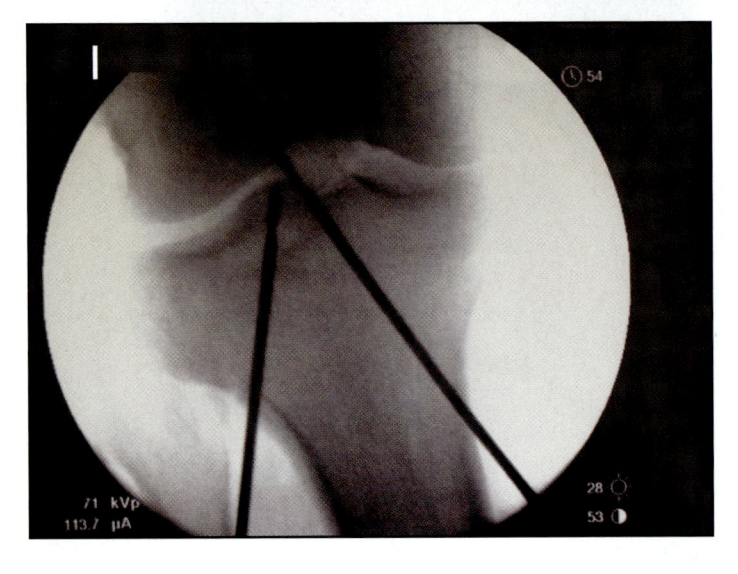

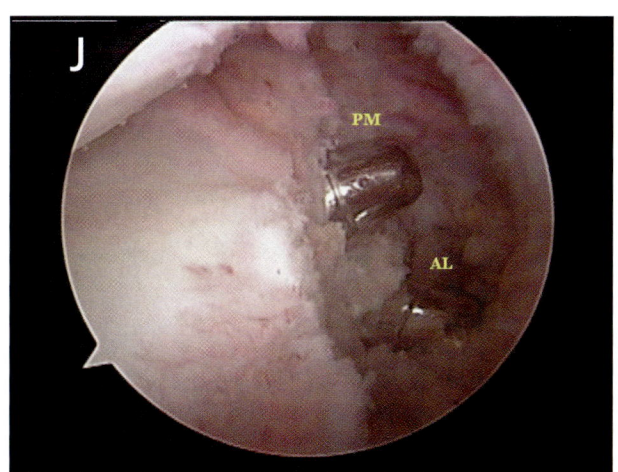

Figure 14-4. (J) A final view from the posteromedial portal showing the tibial dilators in place and the position of each bundle on the posterior tibial footprint after tunnel preparation.

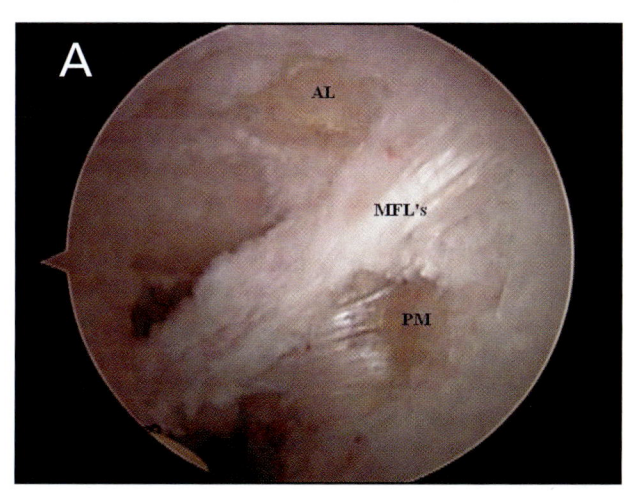

Figure 14-5. Femoral tunnel preparation. (A) The femoral insertion site of the PCL is prepared. Note the use of a bovie to mark the anterolateral and posteromedial bundle insertion sites. Also, the native AL remnant and meniscofemoral ligaments have been left intact. (B) A Steadman awl is used to mark the center of each bundle insertion site at the position on the femur where the guidepins will be placed.

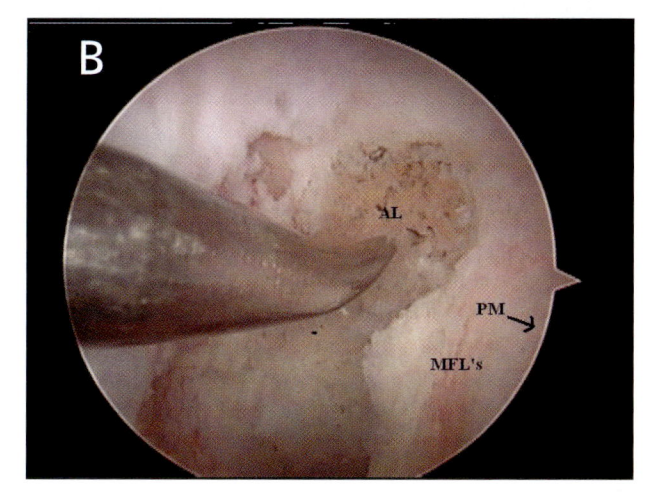

* After the tibial tunnels are prepared, the femoral tunnels are addressed. The 30-degree arthroscope is placed in the anteromedial portal, and a 30-degree Steadman awl is used to mark the femoral origins of the anterolateral and posteromedial PCL bundles for guidepin insertions (Figure 14-5A, B).

Figure 14-5. (C) A guidepin is placed at the AL insertion site with the knee flexed to 120 degrees. (D) An acorn drill is placed over the guidepin seen in C and drilled to the appropriate depth.

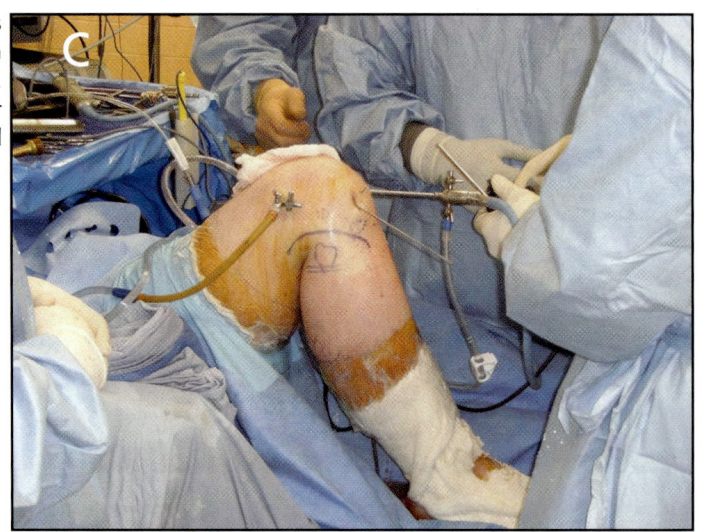

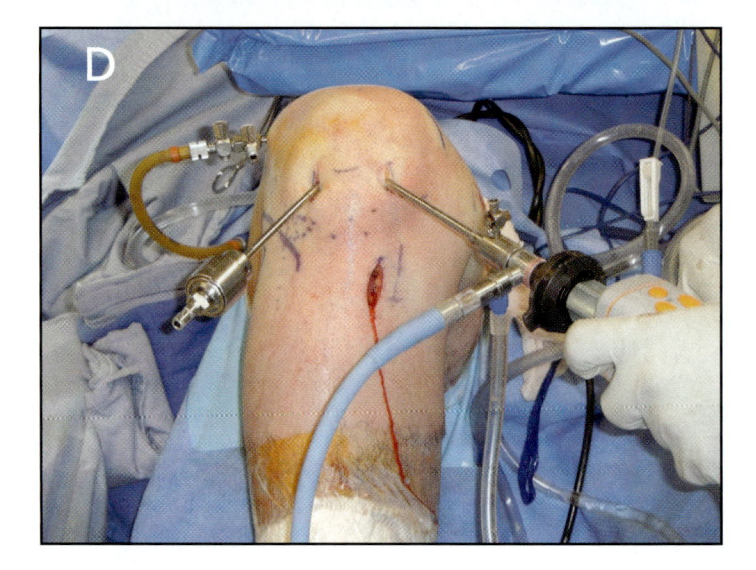

* The knee is flexed to 120 degrees, and a guidepin is placed in the femoral origin of the anterolateral PCL bundle. This is done at the same position where the awl was used to mark the tunnel site. The guidepin is tapped into place with a mallet, and the appropriate acorn reamer is used to make a tunnel approximately 30 to 40 mm deep. A dilator is used to establish the final tunnel diameter, and a 4.5-mm EndoButton drill bit is then used to drill the remainder of the tunnel and medial femoral cortex (Figure 14-5C, D).
* The knee is flexed to 110 degrees, and the posteromedial bundle femoral tunnel is drilled in a manner similar to that described in step 10. The only difference is that the tunnel depth in this case should be roughly 25 mm (Figure 14-5E).
* The tibial and femoral tunnels are now prepared, and the grafts are ready to be passed. We prefer tibialis anterior allograft tissue as it matches the demands required of a successful PCL substitute with its high tensile strength. The timing and extent of injury, availability of allograft, prior history of surgery, and surgeon/patient preference all contribute to graft selection. Autograft choices include patellar tendon, quadriceps tendon, and hamstring tendons (Figure 14-6A).

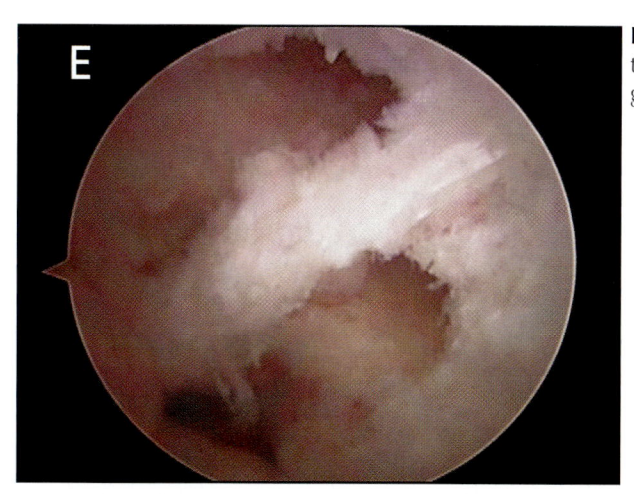

Figure 14-5. (E) Both femoral tunnels after they have been drilled and prepared for graft passage.

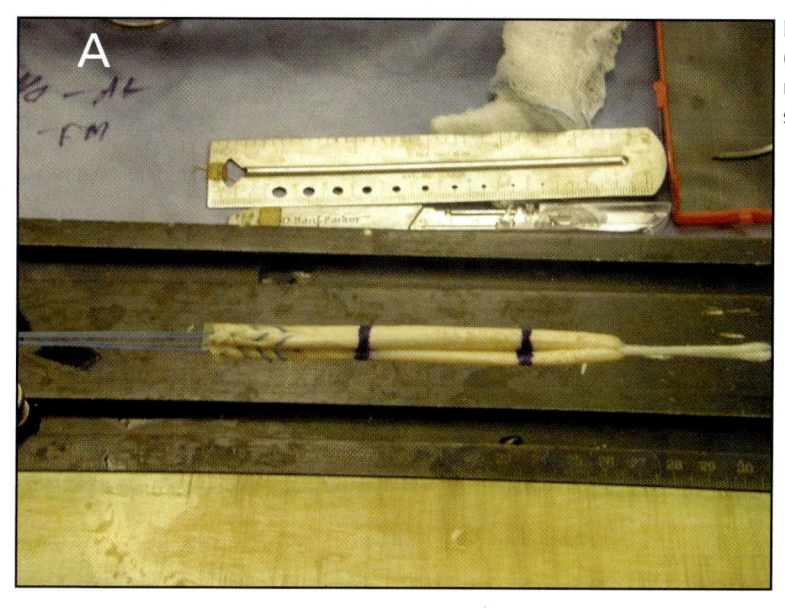

Figure 14-6. Graft passage. (A) We prefer tibialis anterior allograft for our reconstructions.

* To prepare our tunnels for graft passage, we place two 8 French pediatric feeding tubes in a retrograde fashion through each tibial tunnel, exiting the anterolateral portal to assist with graft passage. If the meniscofemoral ligaments remain, the anterolateral bundle will pass over the ligaments, and the posteromedial bundle will pass below the ligaments (Figure 14-6B).

* The anterolateral graft is passed first by tying the free ends of the whipstitched graft tails to the shuttle suture exiting the anterolateral parapatellar portal. This allows the tibial side of the graft to pass anterograde through the anterolateral parapatellar portal and retrograde into the tibial tunnel. Next, the femoral side of the graft is passed anterograde into the femoral tunnel. We prefer to use a 40-mm EndoLoop (Smith & Nephew, Inc, London, United Kingdom) (with the EndoButton removed) to secure the graft over a post to provide femoral fixation. A beath pin is thus placed in the corresponding anterolateral femoral tunnel to facilitate passage of the femoral EndoLoop and suture through the anteromedial aspect of the knee (Figures 14-6C-F).

Figure 14-6. (B) An 8 French pediatric feeding tube is used to facilitate graft passage. (C) The tails of the AL graft are passed retrograde through the anterolateral portal and out of the anterolateral tibial tunnel. (D) A beath needle is passed up the anterolateral bundle femoral tunnel, and the graft is passed anterograde into the femoral tunnel.

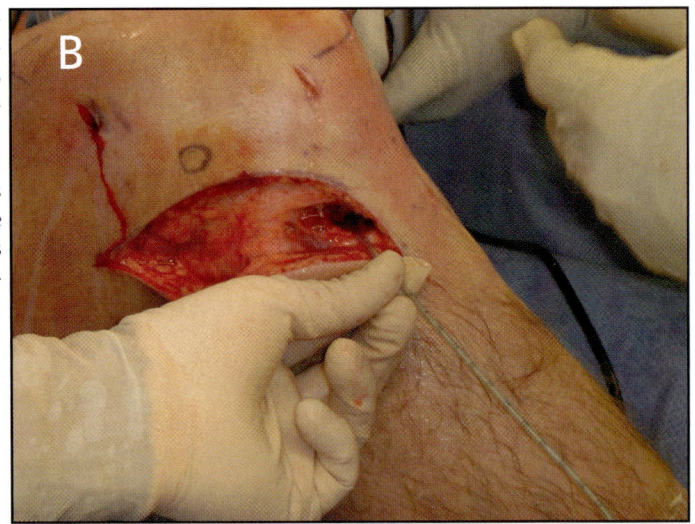

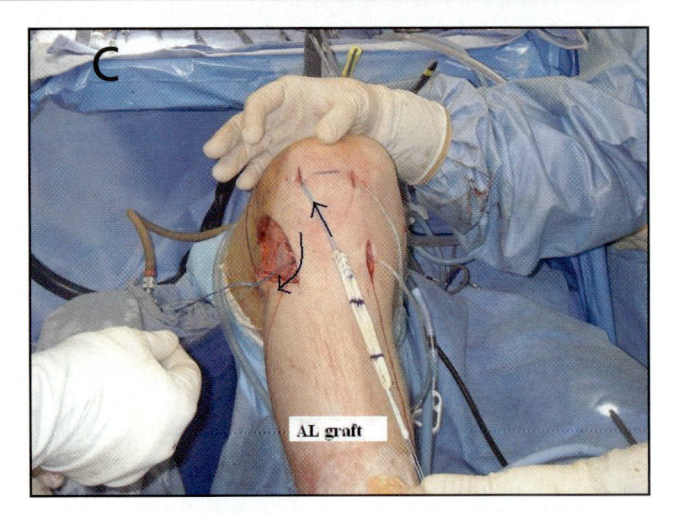

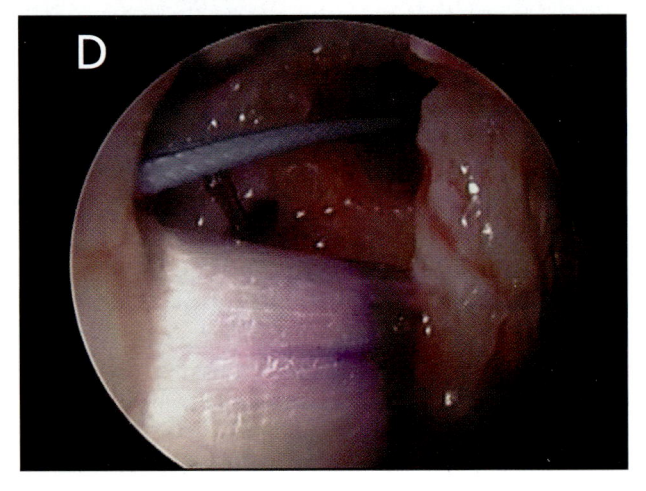

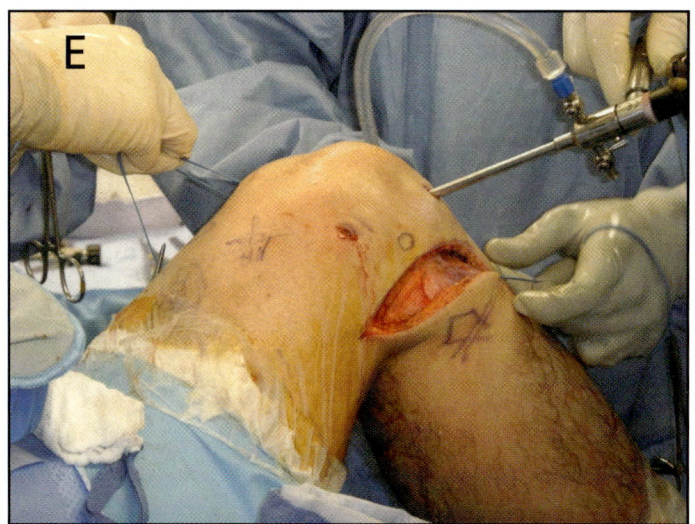

Figure 14-6. (E) The suture is pulled to pass the graft into the femoral tunnel. (F) Arthroscopic view of the AL graft after passage. Note the other 8 French pediatric feeding tube under the meniscofemoral ligaments that will be used to facilitate passage of the PM graft.

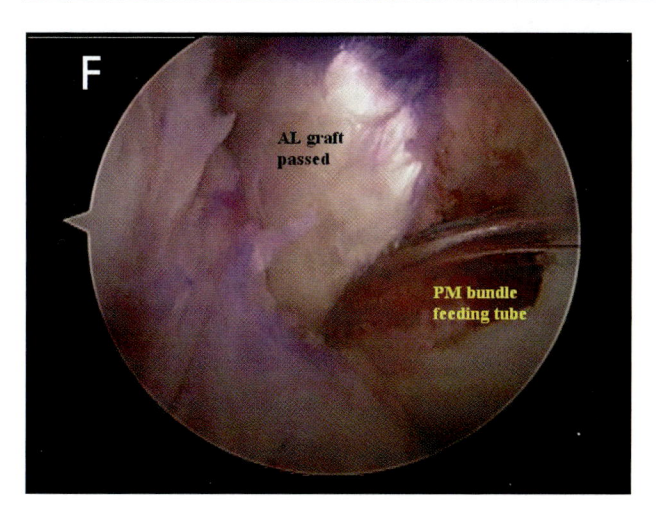

* The posteromedial bundle graft is passed in the same fashion as the anterolateral graft, as described in step 14. We use a 50-mm EndoLoop for the posteromedial bundle (Figures 14-6G-I).
* The grafts are then fixed on the femoral side with 2 AO 6.5-mm cancellous screws and washers that function as posts for the EndoLoops. There are a wide range of options for femoral graft fixation that include interference screw fixation as well as EndoButton fixation.
* If a posterolateral reconstruction or collateral ligament repair is required, it is performed and tensioned at this time.
* The knee is then cycled, and the 2 PCL bundles are tensioned and secured on the tibial side. The anterolateral PCL bundle is tensioned first with the knee at 90 degrees of flexion and an anterior drawer force placed on the knee. We prefer to tie grafts over posts (AO 4.5-mm bicortical screws with washers), although other fixation choices are available.
* Next, the PM component is tensioned and fixed with the knee at 30 degrees of flexion while an anterior drawer is being placed on the knee (Figure 14-7).

Figure 14-6. (G) The PM bundle graft is passed retrograde into the posteromedial tibial tunnel. (H) Arthroscopic view showing the PM graft after it has been passed retrograde into the tibial tunnel. Notice the femoral side of the PM graft coming out of the anteromedial portal. A beath needle will be passed to pull the femoral side into the femoral tunnel of the PM bundle. (I) Arthroscopic view of both bundles passed into their respective femoral tunnels.

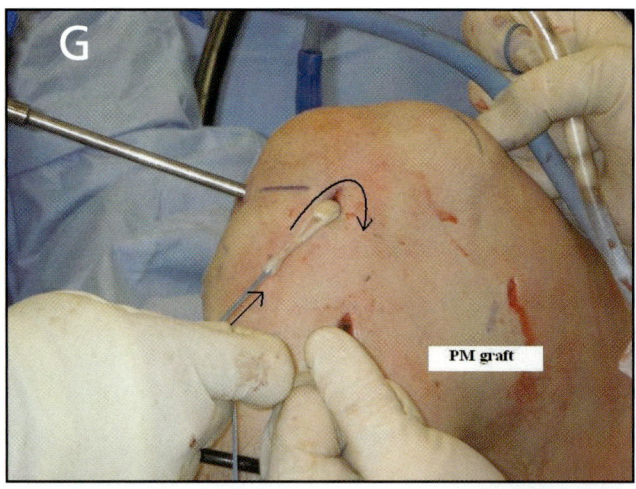

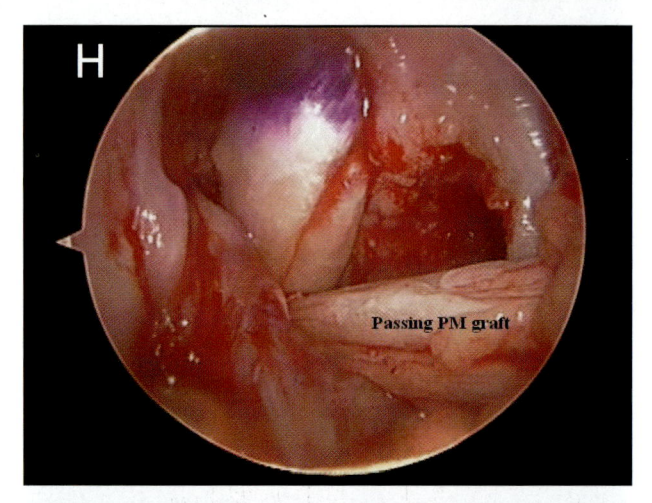

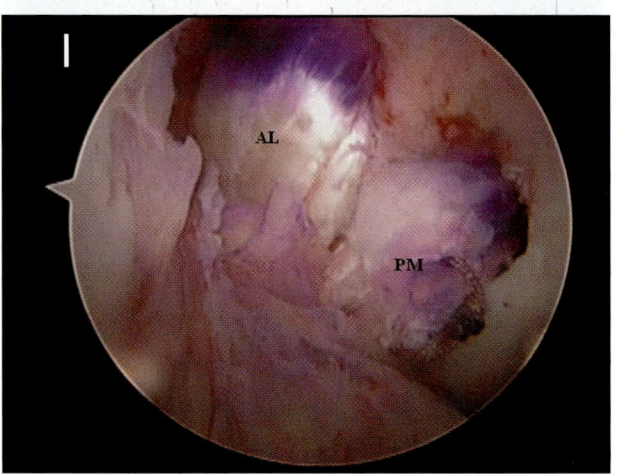

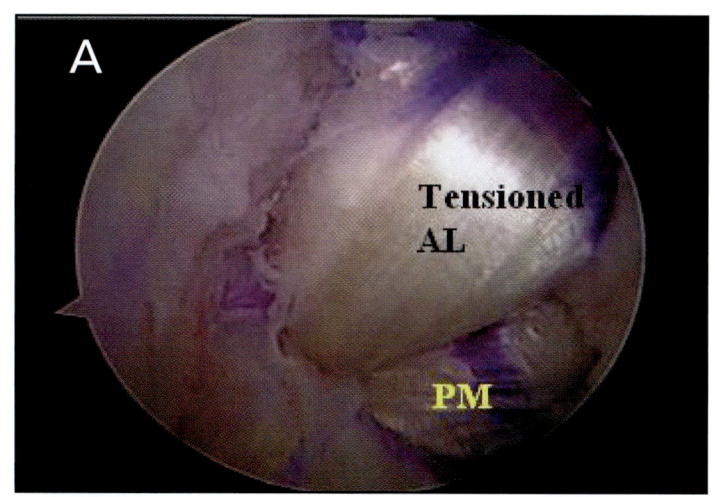

Figure 14-7. (A) Final arthroscopic view from the anterior lateral parapatellar portal showing the tensioned DB reconstruction at the femoral origin. (B) Final arthroscopic view from the posteromedial portal showing the tensioned DB reconstruction as it passes posteriorly to the tibia.

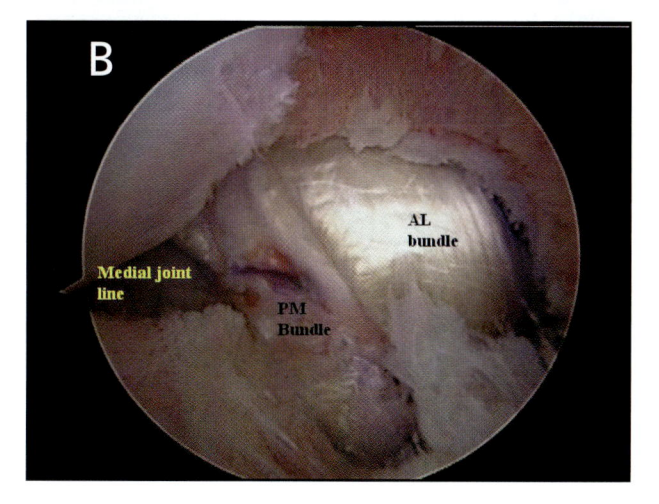

PORTALS AND INCISIONS (SEE FIGURE 14-2)

* Standard medial and lateral parapatellar portals are used. An additional posteromedial portal is made under arthroscopic guidance to better visualize and identify the PCL insertion site anatomy on the posterior aspect of the tibia. This portal also aids in the débridement of the insertion site and functions as a working and viewing portal.

* The incisions include an anterolateral incision and an anteromedial incision on the proximal tibia for tibial tunnel placement. The anteromedial incision is marked with the PCL guide on the skin to dictate the placement of the 3-cm incision. The anterolateral incision is marked in a similar fashion, and a 3-cm incision is made with dissection through the anterior compartment fascia to the anterolateral aspect of the tibia. Alternatively, if a posterolateral corner reconstruction is being performed in addition to the PCL reconstruction, the anterolateral incision for the tibial tunnel can be incorporated into the posterolateral corner incision by extending the PLC exposure distally.

* For femoral graft fixation, our preferred technique is to tie our femoral EndoLoops over a post. To accomplish this, we make an incision on the proximal medial aspect of the knee along Langer's lines. We dissect through the fascia over vastus medialis obliquus and bluntly

204 Chapter 14

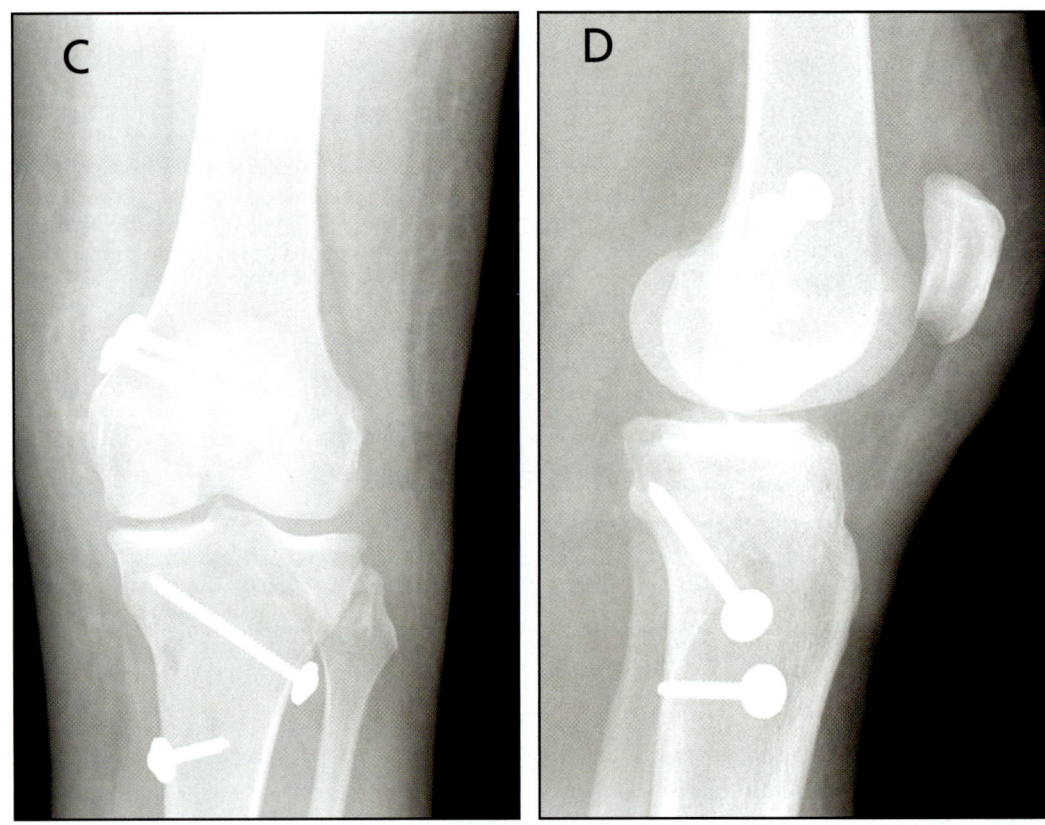

Figure 14-7. (C) AP and (D) lateral radiographs showing the fixation and tunnel positions postoperatively.

dissect in line with its fibers until the femur is encountered. This allows us to locate our EndoLoops and secure them over posts.

TIPS AND PEARLS

✔ During initial arthroscopy of the knee, have an assistant provide an anterior drawer to the knee to establish ACL tension. This will ensure that it is not suctioned into the shaver and inadvertently débrided.

✔ Take the time to curettage and débride the posterior tibial PCL insertion to gain adequate visualization of the bundle insertions.

✔ During our 10-year experience with DB PCL reconstructions, we have moved away from stacking our tibial tunnels on the medial side of the tibia. Currently, we converge the guidepins by using an anteromedial incision for the PM bundle and an anterolateral incision for the AL bundle. This has significantly simplified preparation of the tibial tunnel and prevented tunnel coalescence. As a result, graft passage and fixation are much easier.

✔ Use fluoroscopic imaging to verify and monitor guidepin placement. It will confirm anatomic bundle reconstruction and will provide additional safety for the patient.

✓ Graft passage and the "killer turn" have always posed a challenge for surgeons performing PCL reconstructions.[11-13] Of late, we have incorporated the use of 8 French pediatric feeding tubes to navigate the posterior aspect of the tibia. We have found this aforementioned technique to have significantly simplified graft passage.

PITFALLS

✗ A DB PCL reconstruction is not a simple procedure and should not be performed in an ambulatory surgery center, where vascular surgery back-up is not present. A vascular surgeon should be on call at all times during this procedure. Several technical tips are important to prevent neurovascular injury. These include the following:
  - The avoidance of a tourniquet to allow immediate identification of vascular injury
  - The use of a PCL curette to protect the guidepin tip from advancing into the popliteal fossa
  - The use of fluoroscopy throughout the case
  - Always drilling the posterior cortex of the tibia by hand.

✗ When débriding the posterior tibial insertion of the PCL, keep the shaver blade pointed anteriorly, and take care that suction does not pull the popliteal fat and neurovascular structures into the shaver.

✗ Careful lateral fluoroscopic evaluation of guidepin placement for the 2 tibial tunnels is critical to ensure anatomic placement of the bundles and to verify that there will be a bony bridge between the 2 tunnels, preventing them from coalescing.

REFERENCES

1. Harner CD, Hoher J. Evaluation and treatment of posterior cruciate ligament injuries. *Am J Sports Med.* 1998;26(3):471-482.
2. Shelbourne K, Davis T, Patel D. The natural history of acute, isolated nonoperatively treated posterior cruciate ligament injuries. *Am J Sports Med.* 1999;27:276-283.
3. Race A, Amis AA. PCL reconstruction: in vitro biomechanical comparison of "isometric" versus single and double-bundled "anatomic" grafts. *J Bone Joint Surg Br.* 1998;80:173-179.
4. Valdevit A, Kambic H, Lilly D, Graham S, Parker B, Bergfeld J. Non-linear fitting of mechanical data for efficacy determination of single versus double bundle Achilles tendon grafts for PCL reconstructions. *Biomed Mater Eng.* 2002;12(3):309-317.
5. Petrie RS, Harner C. Double bundle posterior cruciate ligament reconstruction technique: University of Pittsburgh approach. *Oper Tech Sports Med.* 1999;7:118-126.
6. Chhabra A, Kline AJ, Harner CD. Single-bundle versus double-bundle posterior cruciate ligament reconstruction: scientific rationale and surgical technique. *Instr Course Lect.* 2006;55:497-507.
7. Klimkiewicz JJ, Harner CD, Fu FH. Single bundle posterior cruciate ligament reconstruction: University of Pittsburgh approach. *Oper Tech Sports Med.* 1999;7:105-109.
8. Boynton M, Tietjens B. Long-term followup of the untreated isolated posterior cruciate ligament deficient knee. *Am J Sports Med.* 1996;24:306-310.
9. Cross MJ, Powell JF. Long-term followup of posterior cruciate ligament rupture: a study of 116 cases. *Am J Sports Med.* 1984;12(4):292-297.
10. Keller PM, Shelbourne KD, McCarroll JR, Rettig AC. Nonoperatively treated isolated posterior cruciate ligament injuries. *Am J Sports Med.* 1993;21(1):132-136.
11. Cooper D. Treatment of combined posterior cruciate ligament and posterolateral injuries of the knee. *Oper Tech Sports Med.* 1999;7:135-142.

12. Fanelli GC, Giannotti BF, Edson CJ. The posterior cruciate ligament arthroscopic evaluation and treatment. *Arthroscopy.* 1994;10(6):673-688.
13. Miller M, Gordon W. Posterior cruciate ligament reconstruction: tibial inlay technique—principles and procedure. *Oper Tech Sports Med.* 1999:127-133.

Arthroscopic Treatment of Arthrofibrosis of the Knee

J. Richard Steadman, MD

Arthrofibrosis is a term used to describe a wide variety of disorders.[1-7] Its symptoms include joint tightness, loss of mobility, and pain, and these symptoms can range from mild to severe in intensity. The treatment depends on the extent of the problem. A relatively new concept is that motion loss associated with degenerative arthritis is a type of arthrofibrosis, and we have found that this motion loss in the affected joint can be corrected or improved with the use of certain treatments.

Another type of arthrofibrosis is the loss of patellar mobility after arthroscopic surgery. Even minor procedures can produce scarring in the infrapatellar or suprapatellar area, resulting in loss of patellar mobility. Restricted patellar mobility can produce pain and joint compression, which leads to articular cartilage compression,[8] loss of function, and eventually to articular cartilage injury. The physical examination finding of decreased patellar or patellar tendon mobility should alert the physician to the likelihood of arthrofibrosis.

More severe contractures usually result from surgery. These contractures are seen rarely and are much more severe than normal postoperative stiffness associated with surgery. Arthroscopic surgery with soft-tissue releases can usually correct these contractures.

Understanding the role of the normal infrapatellar and suprapatellar anatomy is important in correcting arthrofibrosis. The infrapatellar area has a normal opening between the patellar tendon and the tibia that we call the "anterior interval."[9] This space closes with flexion and opens with extension. The patellar tendon sits on the tibia in flexion and separates approximately 1.5 cm in extension. Loss of this "slack" in the system creates cartilage compression. Closure of the interval also results in a subtle deficiency in terminal extension. The normal suprapatellar pouch is an open area that allows for flexion and extension. Loss of this space from scarring or suprapatellar compartmentalization results in increased compression forces on the patellofemoral joint and femorotibial joint.[8] Stiff infrapatellar plica causing compartmentalization can lead to this type of arthrofibrosis.

In summary, arthrofibrosis of the knee can have multiple etiologies and is a complex and difficult clinical problem to treat. It is usually manifested by loss of motion accompanied by knee pain. Contractures that close spaces due to compartmentalization or adhesions in the joint can be a significant contributor to knee pain. There are a variety of definitions and causes of arthrofibrosis that have been reported in the literature.[1-7,10-14] In most patients, early recognition and successful treatment of the problem can effectively restore motion and alleviate pain, thus allowing patients to regain function and improve their activity levels.

Nonoperative Treatment

Nonoperative treatment includes nonsteroidal anti-inflammatory drugs (NSAIDs), physical therapy, corticosteroid injections, and cryotherapy. Deep tissue massage can be helpful, as is the use of devices to improve motion during physical therapy.

An extensive course of modalities to include muscle stimulation, iontophoresis, ultrasound, and a combination of heat and cold should be carried out initially. If symptoms persist even after these measures have been fully tried, surgery becomes the next treatment option. It must be emphasized that any gain from Nonoperative therapy can make surgical treatment easier, less invasive, and more effective. Preoperatively, an attempt should be made to decrease inflammation, if present. Inflammation creates heat within the joint, and the excessive warmth can be felt on the skin. Treatment measures include NSAIDs, corticosteroid injections, and cold or heat applications, whichever is more effective.

Surgical Treatment

Most knee arthrofibrosis can be treated arthroscopically. Surgical treatment depends on the severity of the contractures and the state of the tissues involved in the problem. A tourniquet is rarely used, so hemostasis should be maintained with the use of an arthroscopic pump or gravity flow device. Portal placements are important in visualizing the suprapatellar and infrapatellar area. A superomedial inflow portal is first established, followed by an anterolateral viewing portal and anteromedial working portal. If the severity of the arthrofibrosis is so great that it decreases inflow from the separate inflow cannula, then fluid flow should be routed through the arthroscope with a separate outflow portal established. The position of the viewing portal is more proximal than a standard lateral portal, thus permitting better visualization of the suprapatellar and infrapatellar areas.

Surgery for Mild to Moderate Arthrofibrosis

Capsular Distention

The first step in treating arthrofibrosis with arthroscopy is to re-establish joint volume using insufflation.[15] In the severely arthrofibrotic knee, the joint volume is contracted, with a volume of only 60 to 90 mL, whereas a normal knee has about 180 mL of volume. An 18-gauge needle and a 60-mL syringe are used to insufflate and expand the joint with a saline solution (Figures 15-1 and 15-2). The goal is to insufflate with as much fluid as possible, releasing adhesions and stretching the capsule. It is preferable not to rupture the capsule during insufflation, but if the capsule does rupture, it is possible to proceed with the arthroscopy. In the event of rupture, the thigh should be monitored for distension secondary to capsular leakage.

Anterior Interval

The anterior interval is the space between the infrapatellar fat pad and patellar tendon anteriorly, and the anterior border of the tibia and the transverse meniscal ligament (anterior intermeniscal ligament) posteriorly.[9] No bridging scar tissue is normally present in this region. To have proper kinematics in the joint, the anterior interval must be open. The infrapatellar fat pad is often scarred or hypertrophied. If there is scarring in this interval between the patellar tendon and the tibia, the normal separation of tissues (described previously) cannot occur, and painful joint compression results. The anterior interval is opened by releasing the area just anterior to the

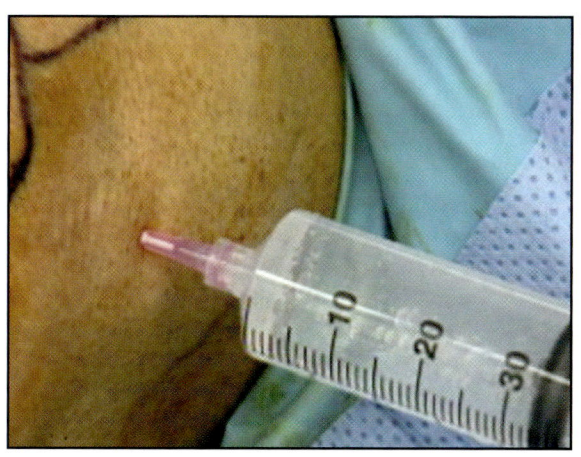

Figure 15-1. A large-gauge needle is placed in the suprapatellar pouch to allow for tactile feedback to ensure that fluid is flowing freely into the true joint space.

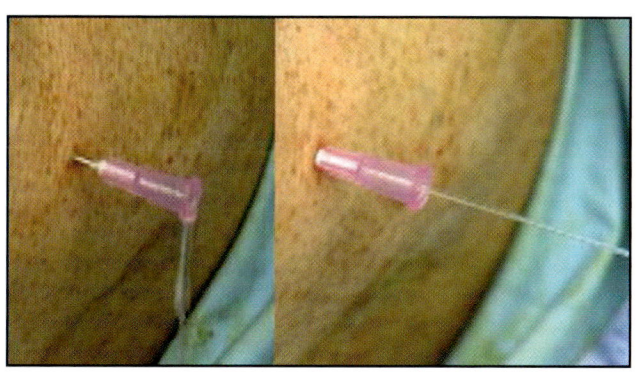

Figure 15-2. As the joint is expanded with fluid, back flow from the needle indicates a full capsule.

intermeniscal ligament (Figures 15-3 through 15-6). This release is done from medial to lateral, just anterior to the peripheral rim of the anterior horn of each meniscus. It is of critical importance that care is taken to avoid destabilizing the menisci. The release can be performed with a 70-degree thermal ablation device (Arthrocare, Arthrocare Corp, Sunnyvale, CA). It is important to have a fluid outflow on this device. The release should also proceed distally from proximal (at the level of the meniscus) to approximately 1 to 1.5 cm distal along the anterior tibial cortex or until normal fat is visualized. Meticulous hemostasis must be obtained after the release using the thermal ablation device or an arthroscopic electrocautery device.

Suprapatellar Pouch

Adhesions in the suprapatellar pouch can restrict knee mobility, and a shortened pouch can limit normal knee flexion. We use the thermal ablation device described previously to lyse adhesions and release scarring to re-establish the pouch. It is important to realize that the pouch is quite large, and ideally it should extend 3 to 4 cm proximal to the patella. Releases should continue until this measurement is achieved (Figures 15-7 and 15-8). Compartmentalization with increased stiffness may be caused by suprapatellar scarring or plica. This condition can be identified by observing the quadriceps tendon arthroscopically when finger pressure is placed onto the quadriceps tendon through the skin. The arthroscopic view of the pouch at this point should show it extending approximately 4 finger-breadths above the patella. If this volume is not present, the abnormal tissue is removed. It is difficult to recognize the loss of volume in the pouch due to compartmentalization from a thickened plica. The tissue appears similar to the normal pouch. The identifying factor that helps one appreciate this process is that as the suprapatellar

Figure 15-3. Scarring in the interval between the patellar tendon and the tibia.

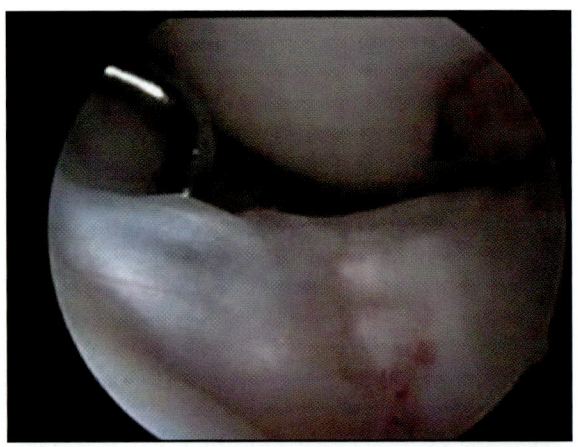

Figure 15-4. A thermal ablation device starts the release of the scarring from medial to lateral, just anterior to the peripheral rim of the anterior horn of each meniscus.

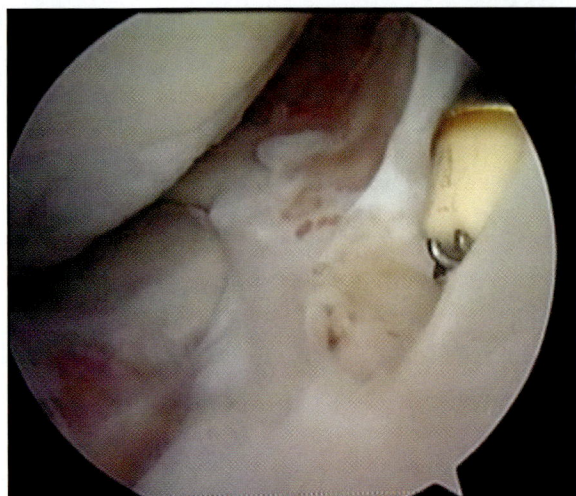

Figure 15-5. The release should also proceed distally from proximal (at the level of the meniscus) to approximately 1 to 1.5 cm distal along the anterior tibial cortex, or until normal fat is visualized.

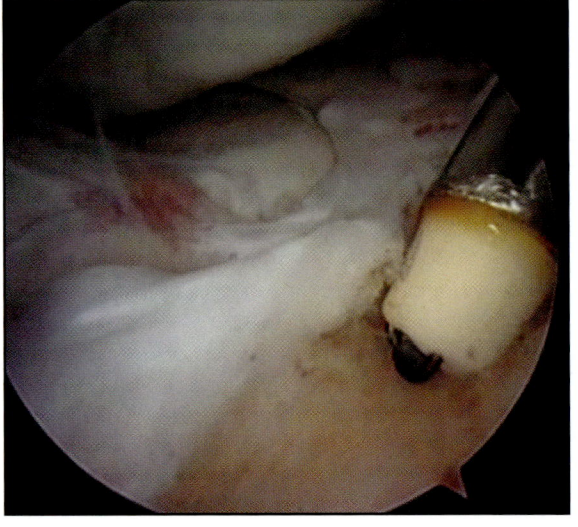

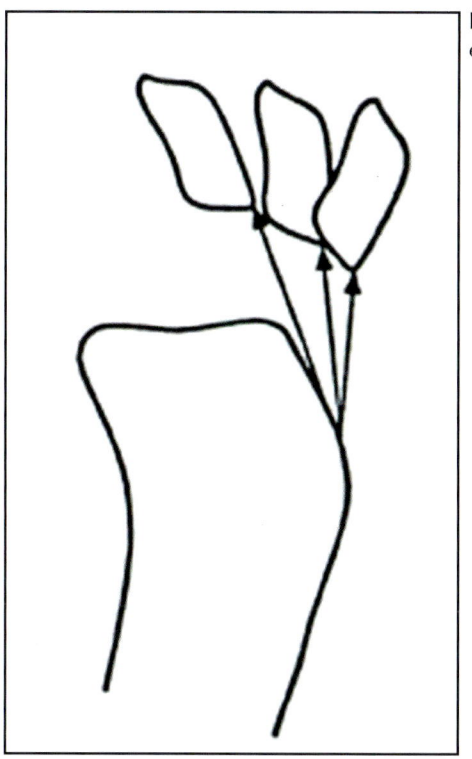

Figure 15-6. Anterior interval should widen with full extension and close with flexion after successful release.

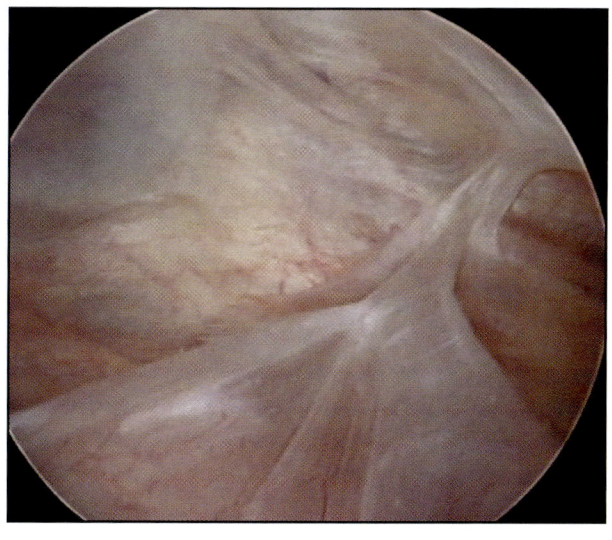

Figure 15-7. Scarred suprapatellar pouch.

area is visualized, the patellar tendon cannot be seen directly because the view is obstructed by the compartmentalization. Once the compartmentalization is released, a normal-sized pouch is restored, and the patella tendon can be visualized.

Medial and Lateral Gutters

Adhesions are frequently found in the medial and lateral gutters. An important aspect of surgical treatment is to remove these adhesions so they will not cause stiffness, motion loss, or restricted volume.

Figure 15-8. (A) Suprapatellar pouch is released using a thermal device. (B) Following release of scar tissue, additional knee volume can be visualized.

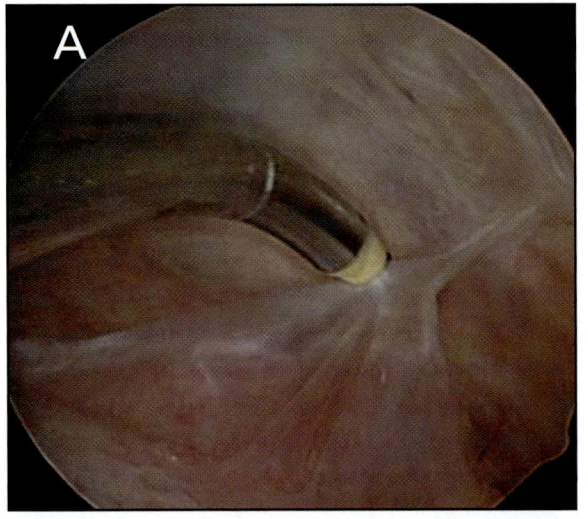

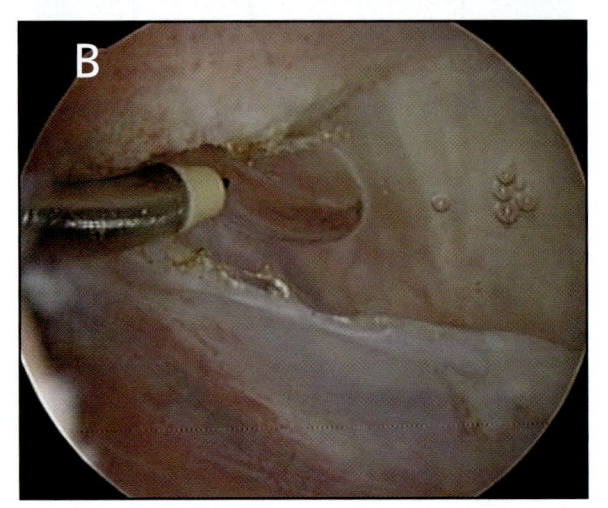

Combined Arthroscopic and Open Surgical Treatment

In certain refractory cases, a posteromedial and/or posterolateral release may be necessary. These soft-tissue releases can be performed in conjunction with an arthroscopic procedure. The arthroscopic releases are performed first, followed by a limited open procedure if there is persistent stiffness caused by a tight posterior capsule. A limited posteromedial arthrotomy can be performed to release the posterior oblique ligament and posterior capsule (Figure 15-9).

The posterior edge of the superficial medial collateral ligament (MCL) is identified, and a small incision is made through the skin and subcutaneous tissue. The incision is deepened along the posterior MCL, and the capsule is entered. The posterior capsule is separated from its attachment to the femur. The release goes posterior, protecting the neurovascular structures. This interval is left open, and the knee is manipulated. Care must be taken to avoid injury to the medial meniscus as it is adjacent to the inferior limb of the capsular incision.

If extension lacks 5 degrees or less, the skin and subcutaneous tissues are closed. If extension lacks more than 5 degrees, the posteromedial incision is closed, and a posterolateral incision is made. This incision is made posterior to the fibular collateral ligament, and the capsule is elevated off the femur as it was on the medial side. Care must be taken to protect the peroneal nerve,

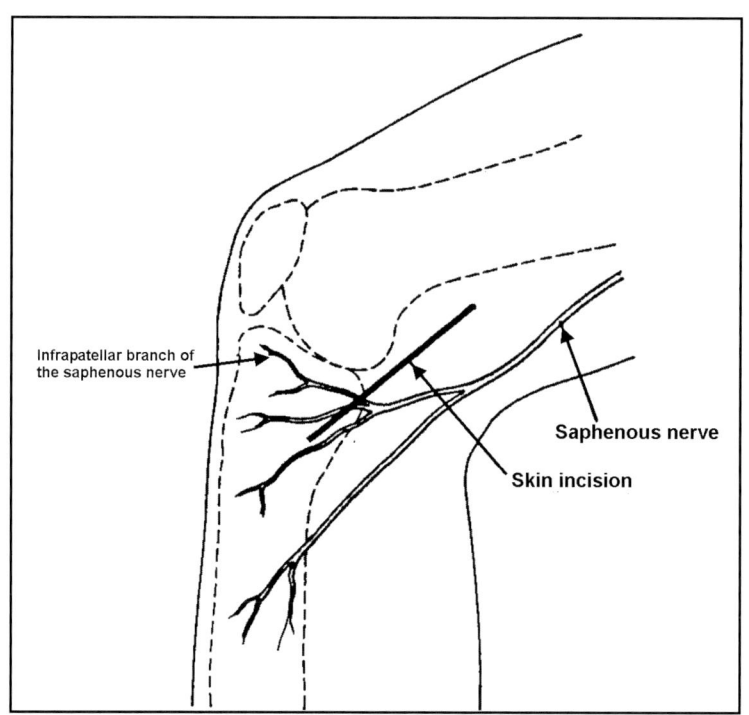

Figure 15-9. The incision line for a limited posteromedial arthrotomy.

popliteus tendon, posterior neurovascular structures, and lateral meniscus. This interval is also left open.

Osteophytes

Anterior osteophytes on the tibia sometimes block extension, particularly in degenerative joint arthrofibrosis (Figure 15-10). These osteophytes can be observed arthroscopically when the knee is extended. In the process of removing osteophytes, inflammatory elements from the bone marrow enter the joint. After osteophyte removal, the knee is extended as fully as possible. If there is any remaining impingement from bony osteophytes or even soft tissue, the offending structures are removed. An intra-articular drain is recommended during the initial postoperative period to aid removal of excessive blood or marrow elements released by the joint débridement. This drain is removed several hours later.

REHABILITATION

Rehabilitation is as important as the surgical procedure. Emphasis is placed on patellar mobility with manual mobilization (Figure 15-11) and regaining the lost motion with wall slides from a supine position, manual massage of the deep tissues, and devices such as the Elite Seat (Kneebourne Therapeutic, Noblesville, IN) and the JAS Splint (Joint Active System, Effingham, IL). Cryotherapy is used intermittently, and continuous passive motion (CPM) is employed until appropriate motion is obtained. The CPM machine is set at 0 to 50 degrees initially, increasing the range as the joint motion increases. The CPM machine is cycled once each minute. Use of the CPM machine may be necessary for several weeks. To minimize inflammation during the postoperative period, NSAIDs can be helpful. If this oral NSAID therapy is not successful, oral steroids and intra-articular steroids should be considered. Regardless, we believe that it is critical to

Figure 15-10. Anterior osteophyte blocking extension.

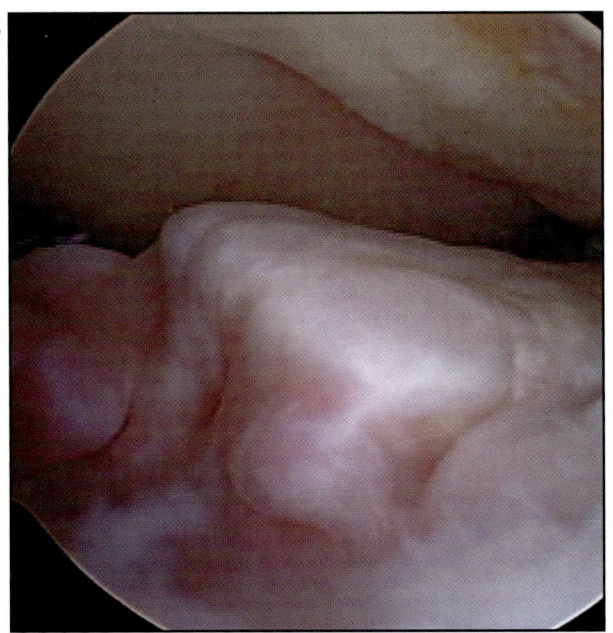

Figure 15-11. Patella mobility exercises consist of movement of the patella medial to lateral (A).

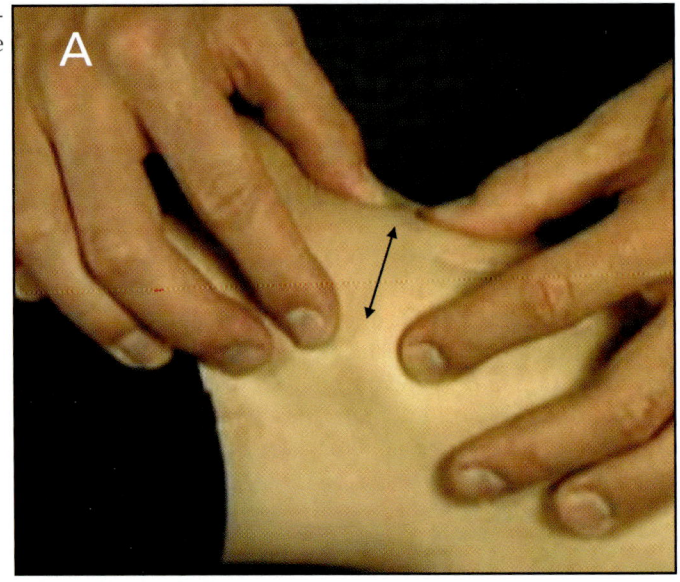

maintain the suprapatellar and infrapatellar spaces by using frequent manual patellar mobilization and emphasizing maximum tolerated flexion and extension with a goal of full range of motion.

In severe arthrofibrosis, repeat arthroscopic surgical procedures may be necessary as part of a staged approach to correct the problem. Each surgical intervention must be carefully considered and planned. We always counsel patients about this likelihood before the initial surgical procedure. If it appears that both full flexion and extension cannot be achieved after the first releases, then extension is emphasized.

Arthroscopic Treatment of Arthrofibrosis of the Knee 217

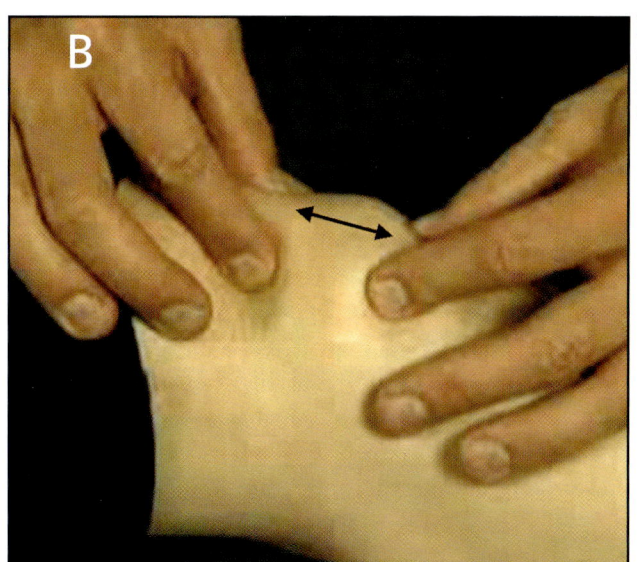

Figure 15-11. Patella mobility exercises consist of movement of the patella inferior to superior (B), medial to the patellar tendon (C), and quadriceps tendon (D).

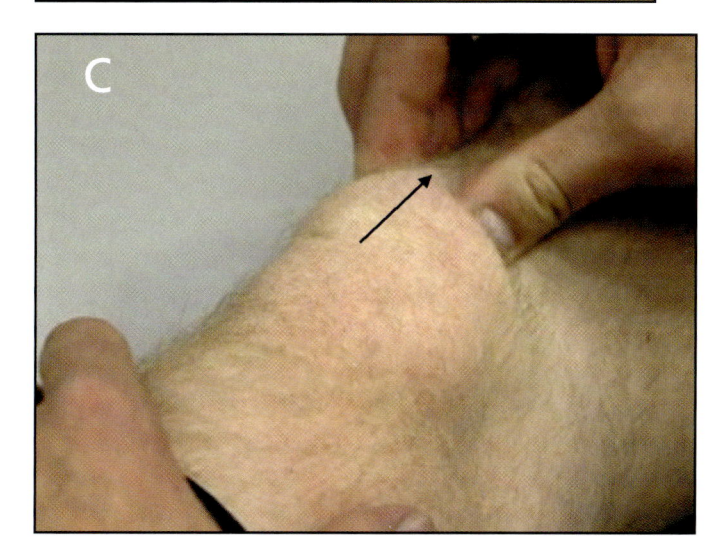

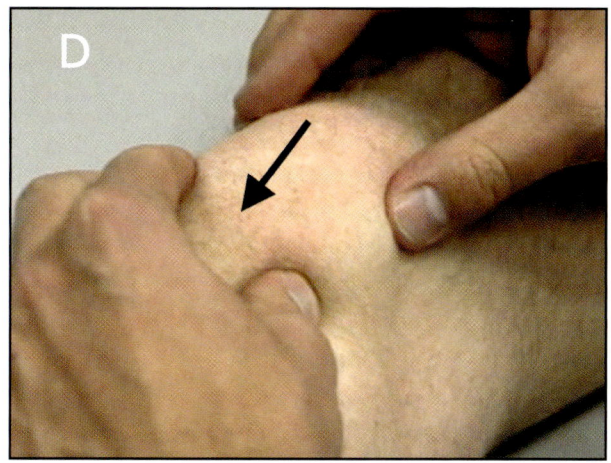

Tips and Pearls

✔ When insufflating the joint, it is important that the needle be fully in the joint, not in the subcutaneous tissue or the posterior capsule. Extreme caution should be taken to avoid the back wall of the capsule. If the joint is entered superolateral to the patella and the needle is angled down, it is more likely to enter the joint and avoid penetration of the back wall of the capsule. There should be an easy flow of solution into and out of the joint.

✔ The quadriceps muscle cannot relax properly when a flexion contracture is present because it prevents the knee from straightening and locking normally.

✔ Great care must be taken during anterior interval release to avoid cauterizing or causing thermal necrosis to the bone of the anterior tibia or to the patellar tendon. Meticulous hemostasis must be obtained in the anterior interval and infrapatellar fat pad to prevent postoperative bleeding or recurrent scarring.

✔ It may be possible to release less severe anterior interval contractures just posterior to the intermeniscal ligament, but care must be taken to avoid the anterior meniscal attachments.

✔ The suprapatellar plica can compartmentalize the suprapatellar pouch, thus decreasing joint volume. If compartmentalization is present, the quadriceps tendon cannot be visualized in the pouch. If the offending tissue is removed, increased joint volume results, and the quadriceps tendon can be visualized arthroscopically.

✔ It is important to realize that the CPM machine may not actually be able take the knee through the range of motion indicated on the machine settings. To overcome this shortcoming of the CPM machine, additional devices and manual techniques may be necessary to help the patient achieve full extension and flexion.

References

1. Dandy DJ, Edwards DJ. Problems in regaining full extension of the knee after anterior cruciate ligament reconstruction: does arthrofibrosis exist? *Knee Surg Sports Traumatol Arthrosc*. 1994;2:76-79.
2. Harner CD, Irrgang JJ, Paul J, et al. Loss of motion after anterior cruciate ligament reconstruction. *Am J Sports Med*. 1992;20:499-506.
3. Millett PJ, Wickiewicz TL, Warren RF. Motion loss after ligament injuries to the knee: part I: causes. *Am J Sports Med*. 2001;29:664-675.
4. Recht MP, Piraino DW, Cohen MA, et al. Localized anterior arthrofibrosis (cyclops lesion) after reconstruction of the anterior cruciate ligament: MR imaging findings. *Am J Roentgenol*. 1995;165:383-385.
5. Shelbourne KD, Wilckens JH, Mollabashy A, et al. Arthrofibrosis in acute anterior cruciate ligament reconstruction: the effect of timing of reconstruction and rehabilitation. *Am J Sports Med*. 1991;19:332-336.
6. Sprague NF III. Motion-limiting arthrofibrosis of the knee: the role of arthroscopic management. *Clin Sports Med*. 1987;6:537-549.
7. Sprague NF III, O'Connor RL, Fox JM. Arthroscopic treatment of postoperative knee fibroarthrosis. *Clin Orthop*. 1982;166:165-172.
8. Ahmad CS, Kwak SD, Ateshian GA, et al. Effects of patellar tendon adhesion to the anterior tibia on knee mechanics. *Am J Sports Med*. 1998;26:715-724.
9. Steadman JR, Dragoo JL, Hines SL, Briggs KK. Arthroscopic release for scarring of the anterior interval of the knee. *Am J Sports Med*. 2008;36:1763-1769.
10. Fisher SE, Shelbourne KD. Arthroscopic treatment of symptomatic extension block complicating anterior cruciate ligament reconstruction. *Am J Sports Med*. 1993;21:558-564.
11. Irrgang JJ, Harner CD. Loss of motion following knee ligament reconstruction. *Sports Med*. 1995;19:150-159.
12. Jackson DW, Schaefer RK. Cyclops syndrome: loss of extension following intra-articular anterior cruciate ligament reconstruction. *Arthroscopy*. 1990;6:171-178.

13. Marzo JM, Bowen MK, Warren RF, et al. Intra-articular fibrous nodule as a cause of loss of extension following anterior cruciate ligament reconstruction. *Arthroscopy*. 1992;8:10-18.
14. Petsche TS, Hutchinson MR. Loss of extension after reconstruction of the anterior cruciate ligament. *J Am Acad Orthop Surg*. 1999;7:119-127.
15. Steadman JR, Ramappa AJ, Maxwell RB, et al. An arthroscopic treatment regimen for osteoarthritis of the knee. *Arthroscopy*. 2007;23:948-955.

Index

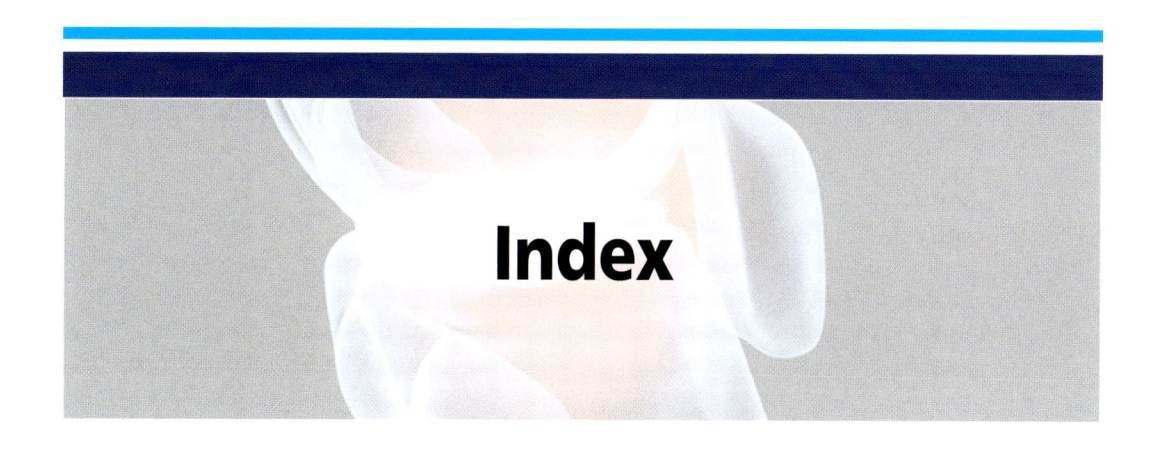

Achilles bone block, 175-176
  fixation of, 185
  in single-bundle tibial inlay PCL reconstruction, 181
all-inside repair
  advantages and indications for, 56
  limitations of, 56
  technique in, 56-58
  tips and pearls for, 60
allografts
  Achilles tendon
    harvesting of, 175-176
    in single-bundle PCL reconstruction, 147-150, 168-169
    in single-bundle tibial inlay PCL reconstruction, 172
  in single-bundle PCL reconstruction
    harvesting for, 175-176
    preparation of, 147-150
    tibial inlay, 172-176
  tibialis anterior
    in anatomic double-bundle ACL reconstruction, 123
    in transtibial double-bundle PCL reconstruction, 199
American Society of Anesthesiologists Classifications, 15
analgesia, epidural, 90
analgesia, in autologous chondrocyte implantation, 90
anatomic landmarks, 8
anesthesia. See also examination under anesthesia
  ambulatory versus inpatient, 15
  epidural, 18
  indwelling peripheral nerve catheters in, 23-24
  management of, 17-19
  preoperative issues in, 16
  regional, 19-23
anesthetics
  in general anesthesia, 18
  monitoring of, 17
  in neuroaxial anesthesia, 18
  in premedication, 17-18
  in regional anesthesia, 18-19
angle rasps, 49
anterior cruciate ligament (ACL)
  anatomic double-bundle reconstruction of, 123-133
  arthroscopic view of, 124
  damaged in tibial spine avulsion fractures, 139-141, 143
  examination of, 35-37
  single-bundle reconstruction of, 105-119
anterior interval, 210-211
  diagnostic examination of, 35
  widened, 213
anti-emetics, during anesthesia, 19
anxiolytics, 17
arthrofibrosis
  etiologies of, 209
  nonoperative treatment of, 210
  surgical treatment of, 210
    rehabilitation after, 216-217
    techniques in, 210-216
  tips and pearls for, 217-219
  types of, 209
arthroscopes
  with camera, 3
  camera orientation in, 40

introduction into joint, 3
types of, 27
arthroscopic tower, 4
arthroscopy
   in anatomic double-bundle ACL reconstruction, 124-125
   for arthrofibrosis, 210-219
   diagnostic
      10-point exam, 27-42
      for autologous chondrocyte implantation, 84
      pitfalls of, 42
      in single-bundle ACL reconstruction, 108
      in single-bundle PCL reconstruction, 150-151
      in single-bundle tibial inlay PCL reconstruction, 173-175
      surgical goals of, 27-40
      tips and pearls for, 40-41
      in transtibial double-bundle PCL reconstruction, 189, 190-191
   in tibial spine fracture reduction and internal fixation, 138-142
arthrotomy, 85-86
aspiration prophylaxis, 18
autografts
   for PCL single-bundle tibial inlay reconstruction, 172-173
   quadriceps tendon, in single-bundle tibial inlay PCL reconstruction, 172-173, 176-177
   in single-bundle tibial inlay PCL reconstruction
      harvesting of, 176-177
autologous chondrocyte implantation, 83
   operative technique in, 84-90
   pitfalls in, 91
   radiographic work-up for, 83-84
   rehabilitation after, 89-90
   surgical goals of, 84
   tips and pearls in, 90-91
   wound closure in, 89
awls, selection and placement of, 70

benzodiazepines, 17
bicitra, prophylactic, 18
bicycling exercise, postoperative, 186
BioScrew fixation, 169
bipolar defects, 63

blood pressure monitoring, in anesthesia, 17
BTB graft harvest, 106-107, 108
burrs, 5-6

cannulas, 4
   zone-specific, 54, 55
capnography, 17
capsular distention, 210
cartilage
   assessing quality of, 66
   biopsy for autologous chondrocyte implantation, 84-85
   calcified
      assessment of, 66
      debridement of, 65, 66, 67, 69
   lesions of
      autologous chondrocyte implantation for, 83-90
      avascular, 83
      debridement of, 86
      preparation of for autologous chondrocyte implantation, 86
catheters, indwelling peripheral nerve, 23-24
cautery devices, 6-7
chamfer reamer, 112, 115, 116
children, osteochondral injuries in, 93-102
chondral defects
   debridement of, 65, 66, 67
   depth of, 65
   duration of injury, 64
   location of, 64
   microfracture for, 63-70
   preparation of, 86
   size of, 64
chondral resurfacing, 100
compartmentalization, with suprapatellar plica, 213-215, 218
compressive loads, in meniscus tear rehabilitation, 60
computed tomographic scan, of tibial spine avulsion fractures, 135, 136
condylopatellar sulcus, 41
continuous passive motion (CPM)
   after autologous chondrocyte implantation, 89-90
   in arthrofibrosis rehabilitation, 216, 219
corticosteroids, 210
cruciate ligaments. *See also* anterior cruciate ligament (ACL); posterior cruciate ligament (PCL)

diagnostic examination of, 34-35
cryotherapy, 210
    rehabilitation after, 216
cyclops lesion, 36

débridement
    in single-bundle PCL reconstruction, 151, 153, 156
    in transarticular drilling, 102
deep tissue massage, for arthrofibrosis, 210
degenerative arthritis, 209
degenerative lesions, 64
dexamethasone, 19
Dial Test, 149
diazepam (Valium), 17

ECG monitoring, during anesthesia, 17
electrocautery, 6-7
empty wall sign, 35
EndButton drill, 127-128
EndoLoops, in transtibial double-bundle PCL reconstruction, 199, 203-204
examination under anesthesia, 1
    in single-bundle PCL reconstruction, 147
    for transtibial double-bundle PCL reconstruction, 189, 190, 192-193
eyelid sign, 48

fascia iliaca/femoral nerve block, 22
FasT-Fix technique, 56-58
femoral condyles, medial and lateral, 8
femoral nerve, anatomy of, 20
femoral nerve block, 19-20
    nerve stimulator for, 20-21
    ultrasound guidance in, 21-22
femoral notch, "clock face" orientation of, 114
femoral tunnel
    placement of
        in anatomic double-bundle ACL reconstruction, 127-129, 132, 133
        in single-bundle ACL reconstruction, 110-113, 115-116
    preparation of, 177-180
    reaming of, 115-116, 119
    in single-bundle PCL reconstruction, 159-164
fentanyl, premedication, 17
fibrin clot, 58-59
    augmentation, 61
fibrin glue sealing, 87-88

fixation. *See also* screws
    arthroscopically assisted internal, of tibial spine fractures, 135-143
    femoral
        in single-bundle ACL reconstruction, 118
        in single-bundle tibial inlay PCL reconstruction, 182-186
    in osteochondral dissecans lesions, 93
    of osteochondral fracture, 96-99
    in osteochondritis dissecans lesions, 96-99
    pitfalls in, 102
    in single-bundle PCL reconstruction, 166-168, 169
    in single-bundle tibial inlay PCL reconstruction, 182-186
    tibial
        in anatomic double-bundle ACL reconstruction, 130
        preparation for, 169
        in transtibial double-bundle PCL reconstruction, 203-204
    for traumatic osteochondral fractures, 93-94
fluid management, 7
fluid pressure, joint distention with, 41
fluid pump, 7
    complications related to, 7
fluoroscopic imaging, 204-205
fracture hematoma, tibial spine, 138, 143
fracture reduction, tibial spine, 138-142
fragment excision/reduction
    for osteochondritis dissecans lesions or osteochondral fracture, 100
    for traumatic osteochondral fractures, 93-94

grafts. *See also* allografts; autografts
    harvesting, in single-bundle tibial inlay PCL reconstruction, 175-177
    patellar tendon, in single-bundle ACL reconstruction, 105-119
    in PCL single-bundle tibial inlay reconstruction, 172-173
    posteromedial (PM) bundle, for transtibial double-bundle PCL reconstruction, 202
    in single-bundle PCL reconstruction, 164-166

guidepin fixation
  of tibial spine avulsion fractures, 139
  in transtibial double-bundle PCL reconstruction, 194-196, 197

haloperidol (Haldol), 19
heat/cold therapy, 210
high-tibial osteotomy, 90
hinged knee brace
  after patellar or trochlear groove lesion repair, 68
  in meniscus tear rehabilitation, 60
hip hyperextension, preventing, 1
Humphrey, ligament of, 36
hydromorphone (Dilaudid), 17

inferolateral portal, 9
inflammatory disorders, suprapatellar, 29
informed consent, with anesthesia, 16-17
inside-out repair
  advantages and indications for, 52
  limitations to, 53
  techniques in
    lateral meniscus, 55-56
    medial meniscus, 53-55
  tips and pearls for, 60
intercondylar notch, diagnostic examination of, 33
intra-articular pressure, in fluid management, 7
iontophoresis, 210

JAS Splint, 216
joint insufflation, 217-218

kinetic chain exercises, postoperative, 186
Kirschner wire
  in osteochondritis dissecans lesion repair, 94-95
  in transarticular drilling, 100
"kissing" lesions, 63
knee alignment, contraindicating microfracture technique, 65

laboratory studies, preoperative, 16
Lachman examination, 35
lateral compartment
  diagnostic examination of, 35-38
  postoperative protocols for lesions of, 69-70

lateral gutter, diagnostic examination of, 30-32
lateral post, in patient positioning, 1-2
"laundromat" effect, 27
leg holder, 2-3
ligamentous insufficiency, 84
ligamentum mucosum, 34
loose bodies, access for removal of, 39-40
lorazepam (Ativan), 17

magnetic resonance imaging (MRI)
  of articular cartilage defects, 84
  of tibial spine avulsion fractures, 135
malaligned knee, 65
malalignment, 84
medial compartment
  diagnostic examination of, 32-33
  postoperative protocols for lesions of, 69-70
medial femoral condyle, 34
medial gutter, diagnostic examination of, 32
medial synovial plica, 31
meniscal flounce, 41
meniscal repair
  rehabilitation after, 60
  techniques of, 48
    all-inside, 56-58
    fibrin clot in, 58-59
    inside-out, 52-56
    outside-in, 49-52
    patient positioning for, 46-47
    patient selection for, 45-46
    tear preparation in, 48-49
    tips and pearls for, 60-61
meniscal tears
  complete radial, 47
  partial-thickness, 46
  preparation of for repair, 48-49
  prognostic criteria for, 45-46
  rim width of, 45
  variable patterns of, 47
meniscus
  examination of, 32
  lateral, 37-38
  medial, 33
meperidine (Demerol), 17
metoclopramide (Reglan), prophylactic, 18
microfracture
  contraindications to, 64-65
  goal of, 64
  indications for, 63

operative technique in, 65
pitfalls in, 67
postoperative protocol for
    in medial or lateral compartment lesions, 69-70
    in patellar or trochlear groove lesions, 68-69
tips and pearls for, 65-67
midazolam, 17
monitors, during anesthesia, 17
monopolar radiofrequency devices, 6
morphine, premedication, 17
mosaicplasty, 73
"Mulberry" knot technique, 51-52
muscle stimulation, 210

naloxone, 18
narcotics, premedication, 17-18
nerve blocks
    complications of, 22-23
    contraindications to, 23
nerve stimulator, 20-21
nitinol wires, 166-168
nonsteroidal anti-inflammatory drugs (NSAIDs), 210
    rehabilitation after, 216
notchplasty, 108-109

ondansetron (Zofran), 19
open lateral release, 96, 101
operating room set-up, 5
opioids, 17-18
osteochondral autograft (OAT) plugs, 73
    size of, 74
osteochondral defect, Grade IV, 77
osteochondral fracture
    fixation of, 96-99
    fragment excision and chondral resurfacing of, 100
    pediatric, 93-102
        treatment of, 93-94
osteochondral grafting
    allograft technique, 77-80
        tips and pearls for, 81
    autograft technique, 74-77
        tips and pearls for, 80
    contraindications to, 73
    graft sinkage, 81
    harvester for, 75
    indications for, 73
    pitfalls for, 81
    recipient site preparation for, 75
    surgical goals of, 73-74
    tips and pearls for, 80-81
osteochondral injuries, pediatric, 93-94
    operative technique for, 94-100
    pitfalls for, 102
    surgical goals for, 94
    tips and pearls for, 100-102
osteochondral plug
    allograft
        before implantation, 79
        in recipient socket, 80
    full-thickness, 79
osteochondritis dissecans lesions
    fixation of, 96-99
    fragment excision and chondral resurfacing of, 100
    pediatric, 93-102
    surgical treatment of, 93
    transarticular drilling of, 94-96
osteophytes, 216
    along femoral condyle, 30
outflow cannula, 28
    incorrect positioning of, 29
outside-in repair
    advantages and indications for, 49
    fibrin clot augmentation in, 58
    limitations to, 49
    principles of, 50
    technique in, 49-52
    tips and pearls for, 60
oxygen analyzer, 17

padding, in patient positioning, 1
patella, 8
    articular surface of, 30
    lesions, postoperative protocols for, 68-69
    loss of mobility of, 209
    maltracking and instability of, 84
patella mobility exercises, 216-217
patellar tendon, 8
patellofemoral joint, diagnostic examination of, 29-30
patellofemoral ligament, lateral, 31
patient positioning, 1-3
    in anatomic double-bundle ACL reconstruction, 125
    in meniscal repair, 46-47

in single-bundle ACL reconstruction, 106-107
in single-bundle PCL reconstruction, 147, 148
in single-bundle tibial inlay PCL reconstruction, 173
patient selection, for meniscal repair, 45-46
periosteal patch
   fixation and testing of, 87-88
   harvesting, 86-87, 90, 91
physical therapy, for arthrofibrosis, 210
pivot shift exam, 106, 107
popliteal hiatus, 37
popliteus tendon, 31
portals, 9-10
   accessory anteromedial (AAM), 124-125, 132
   anterolateral (AL), 124-125, 132
   anteromedial (AM), 124-125, 132
   in arthrofibrosis treatment, 211
   inferolateral, 9
   outflow, in intra-synovial location, 40
   parapatellar, in transtibial double-bundle PCL reconstruction, 203
   posteromedial (PM), 9-11
      in single-bundle PCL reconstruction, 151-152
      in transtibial double-bundle PCL reconstruction, 203
   superolateral, 9
   superomedial, 9
posterior compartments, diagnostic examination of, 38-40
posterior cruciate ligament (PCL)
   debridement of, 151, 153, 156, 169
   examination of, 38-40
   injuries to, 171, 189
      classification of, 189-190
   single-bundle reconstruction of, 147-169
   single-bundle tibial inlay reconstruction of
      graft selection for, 172-173
      indications for, 171-172
      operative technique in, 173-186
      options for, 171-172
      pitfalls in, 186-187
      surgical goals for, 173
      tips and pearls for, 186
   transtibial double-bundle reconstruction of, 189-205
posteromedial arthrotomy, 215

postoperative pain, 19
postoperative protocol
   for medial or lateral compartment lesions, 69-70
   for patellar or trochlear groove lesions, 68-69
premedication, 17-18
preoperative consultation, 16
propofol, 18
pulse oximetry, 17
push-in technique, 113-118

quadriceps exercises
   after PCL injuries, 189
   after single-bundle tibial inlay PCL reconstruction, 186

radiofrequency probe, 6
radiographic examination
   of articular cartilage defects, 83-84
   of tibial spine avulsion fractures, 135-136
range of motion
   after arthrofibrosis treatment, 216-217, 219
   in meniscus tear rehabilitation, 60
ranitidine (Zantac), prophylactic, 18
reconstruction
   anatomic double-bundle ACL
      indications for, 123
      operative steps in, 124-131
      pitfalls in, 132-133
      surgical goals for, 123-124
      tips and pearls for, 132
   single-bundle ACL
      indications for, 105
      pitfalls in, 119
      surgical goals of, 105-106
      technique in, 106-118
      tips and pearls for, 118
   single-bundle PCL arthroscopic transtibial technique, 147-169
   single-bundle tibial inlay PCL technique, 171-187
      graft selection for, 173
      indications for, 171-172
      operative technique in, 173-186
      pitfalls in, 186-187
      tips and pearls for, 186
   transtibial double-bundle PCL
      pitfalls in, 205
      portals and incisions in, 203-204

surgical goals of, 189-190
    technique in, 190-203
    tips and pearls for, 204-205
rehabilitation
    after autologous chondrocyte implantation, 89-90
    after meniscus repair, 60
    after PCL injuries, 189
    after single-bundle tibial inlay PCL reconstruction, 186
    for arthrofibrosis, 216-217
    for tibial spine avulsion fractures, 135
"roller coaster" effect, 27

scopolamine, 19
screws
    bioabsorbable
        in anatomic double-bundle ACL reconstruction, 131
        in osteochondritis dissecans lesions and osteochondral fractures, 97, 99
        in single-bundle PCL reconstruction, 166
    biocompression, 97
    cannulated, in arthroscopic fixation of tibial spine fractures, 138-142
    Herbert, for osteochondritis dissecans lesions and osteochondral fractures, 96-97, 98
semimembranosus bursa, aperture of, 39
set-up
    pitfalls of, 11-12
    portals and, 9-10
shavers, 3-5
slide board, 186
SmartNail fixation, 99
soft-tissue masses, suprapatellar, 29
spinal anesthesia, 18
spinal needle, orientation for outside-in repair, 51
sulcus terminalis, 41
suprapatellar plica, 29
suprapatellar pouch
    adhesions in, 212-215
    diagnostic examination of, 28-29
    fluid in, 211
    plica in, 213-215, 218
    scarred, 214
surgical approach, in single-bundle tibial inlay PCL reconstruction, 181-182

surgical site "time-out," 3
sutures
    in arthroscopic reduction and fixation of tibial spine fractures, 141-142
    horizontal mattress, 52
    OrthoCord, in single-bundle PCL reconstruction, 149-150
    in single-bundle PCL reconstruction, 149-150, 164-166
    in tibial spine fracture repair, 143
    for transtibial double-bundle PCL reconstruction, 199-201
    vertical mattress, 52, 55, 59
synovial hypertrophy, suprapatellar, 29

thermal ablation
    for arthrofibrosis, 211-212
    for suprapatellar pouch adhesions, 212-215
thermal necrosis, 218
tibial guidepin
    in single-bundle ACL reconstruction, 109-110, 111
    in single-bundle PCL reconstruction, 152-157
tibial implantations, osteochondral autograft, 80
tibial joint line, proximal, 8
tibial spine fractures
    avulsion
        arthroscopically assisted internal fixation of, 135-143
        suture fixation of, 141-142
    classification of, 135, 136-137
    fixation of
        cannulated screws in, 138-142
        indications for, 135-137
        postoperative management of, 142
        surgical goals for, 137
        tips and pitfalls in, 143
tibial tunnel
    in anatomic double-bundle ACL reconstruction, 132
    fixation of
        pin depth in, 169
        in single-bundle PCL reconstruction, 167
    placement of
        in anatomic double-bundle ACL reconstruction, 128
        pitfalls in, 119

in single-bundle PCL reconstruction, 157-159
tourniquet
  in autologous chondrocyte implantation, 91
  in patient positioning, 1
  in transarticular drilling, 102
transarticular drilling, 93, 100-101
  goal of, 94
  operative technique in, 94-96
  pitfalls in, 102
transtibial tunnel reconstruction, PCL, 171-172
traumatic osteochondral fractures, pediatric, 93-102
trochlear groove, lesions of, postoperative protocols for, 68-69

ultrasound
  for arthrofibrosis, 210
  in femoral nerve block placement, 21-22
unipolar defects, 63

vertical strut sign, 35

weightbearing
  after medial or lateral compartment repair, 69
  after osteochondral grafting, 81
  after patellar or trochlear groove lesion repair, 68
  after single-bundle tibial inlay PCL reconstruction, 186
  in meniscus tear rehabilitation, 60
wound closure, after autologous chondrocyte implantation, 89

WAIT
...There's More!

SLACK Incorporated's Health Care Books and Journals offers a wide selection of products in the field of Orthopedics. We are dedicated to providing important works that educate, inform and improve the knowledge of our customers. Don't miss out on our other informative titles that will enhance your collection.

As minimally invasive surgeries for commonly scoped joints increase, the *Visual Arthroscopy Series* led by Dr. James R. Andrews and Dr. Tal S. David will answer the call for all in orthopedic surgery seeking succinct and highly visual books that will provide step-by step-instructions on arthroscopic techniques for the shoulder, knee, and hip. Each book serves as a quick reference, easy-to-use manual that succinctly highlights the relevant details a resident, fellow, or orthopedic surgeon must know prior to performing an arthroscopic procedure.

Arthroscopic Techniques of the Shoulder: A Visual Guide
Tal David MD; James Andrews MD
200 pp., Soft Cover, 2009, ISBN 13 978-1-55642-838-8, Order #18388, **$99.95**

Some chapter topics include:
* Diagnostic Arthroscopy
* Subacromial Decompression
* Rotator Cuff Repairs—supraspinatus, subscapularis and massive tears

Arthroscopic Techniques of the Knee: A Visual Guide
Thomas J. Gill MD
200 pp., Soft Cover, 2009, ISBN 13 978-1-55642-858-6, Order #18586, **$99.95**

Some chapter topics include:
* Articular Cartilage Resurfacing—microfracture; osteochondral transplantation; autologous chondrocyte implantation
* Pediatric Osteochondral Injuries—special issues and techniques
* ACL—current topics in both single and double bundle reconstruction

Arthroscopic Techniques of the Hip: A Visual Guide
Bryan T. Kelly MD; Marc J. Philippon MD
200 pp., Soft Cover, 2009, ISBN 13 978-1-55642-886-9, Order #18869, **$99.95**

Some chapter topics include:
* Diagnostic Arthroscopy
* Removal of Loose Bodies/Excision of PVNS/Synovial Chondromatosis
* Femoroacetabular Impingement

Please visit
www.slackbooks.com
to order any of these titles!
24 Hours a Day…7 Days a Week!

Attention Industry Partners!
Whether you are interested in buying multiple copies of a book, chapter reprints, or looking for something new and different—we are able to accommodate your needs.

Multiple Copies
At attractive discounts starting for purchases as low as 25 copies for a single title, SLACK Incorporated will be able to meet all of your needs.

Chapter Reprints
SLACK Incorporated is able to offer the chapters you want in a format that will lead to success. Bound with an attractive cover, use the chapters that are a fit specifically for your company. Available for quantities of 100 or more.

Customize
SLACK Incorporated is able to create a specialized custom version of any of our products specifically for your company.

Please contact the Marketing Communications Director of Health Care Books and Journals for further details on multiple copy purchases, chapter reprints or custom printing at 1-800-257-8290 or 1-856-848-1000.

*Please note all conditions are subject to change.

CODE: 328

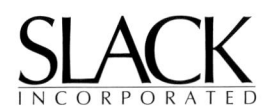

SLACK
INCORPORATED

SLACK Incorporated • Health Care Books and Journals
6900 Grove Road • Thorofare, NJ 08086
1-800-257-8290 or 1-856-848-1000
Fax: 1-856-848-6091 • E-mail: orders@slackinc.com • Visit: www.slackbooks.com